Surgery in Thyroid Eye Disease

Suryasnata Rath • Milind N. Naik
Editors

Surgery in Thyroid Eye Disease

A Conceptual Approach

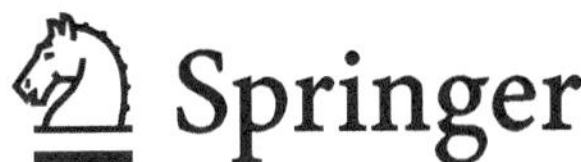

Editors
Suryasnata Rath
Ophthalmic Plastic Surgery Service
LV Prasad Eye Institute
Bhubaneswar
India

Milind N. Naik
Ophthalmic Plastic Surgery Service
LV Prasad Eye Institute
Hyderabad
India

ISBN 978-981-32-9222-2 ISBN 978-981-32-9220-8 (eBook)
https://doi.org/10.1007/978-981-32-9220-8

This Springer imprint is published by the registered company Springer Nature Singapore Pte Ltd.
The registered company address is: 152 Beach Road, #21-01/04 Gateway East, Singapore 189721, Singapore

Foreword

Thyroid eye disease (TED) is the most common orbital disorder worldwide and can result in distressing changes in appearance, periocular discomfort, or visual disturbance. These complications often disrupt quality of life, ability to perform daily activities, and both social and work lives.

Recent discoveries concerning the pathogenesis of this autoimmune condition have identified more targeted medical therapies, raising hope that someday the more severe manifestations of TED may be avoided. Until then, however, surgery remains a vital component of management, either during the progressive active phase to prevent vision loss from optic nerve compression or corneal exposure, or during the quiescent stable phase to reduce proptosis, straighten eyes, and normalize eyelid position and appearance.

This surgical atlas is an invaluable asset for oculoplastic surgeons, comprehensive ophthalmologists, and their students, who wish to learn the most current surgical techniques to manage complications of TED. While there exist chapters on TED-related surgery in oculoplastic atlases, and there are textbooks devoted to Graves' disease and/or orbitopathy, this manual represents the first surgical atlas solely devoted to surgery for TED.

The book is organized within a conceptual framework that recognizes the natural course of the disease (active versus inactive), the periocular structures that are affected, and the order in which the surgeries are usually performed. High-quality intraoperative photographs and illustrations document key steps for each procedure, while succinct text highlights important tips, preoperative considerations, indications, and possible complications. Newer approaches such as endoscopic orbital decompressions, and smaller incisions for orbital and eyelid surgeries, and avoidance of late slippage in strabismus surgery are reviewed. Contributors include well recognized international experts in ophthalmic anatomy and surgery.

The text is authored and edited by two experienced and dedicated oculoplastic and orbital surgeons at the LV Prasad Eye Institute (LVPEI) in India, Dr. Suryasnata Rath and Dr. Milind N Naik. Both share similar educational backgrounds, a strong interest in managing TED and a passion for teaching nationally and internationally.

Suryasnata completed ophthalmology residency followed by fellowship at LVPEI and subsequently joined as faculty in 2006. From 2011 to 2012, he took leave to pursue further fellowship training with me and my colleagues at The University of British Columbia, Canada, where he developed a keen interest in TED. I remember Surya fondly for his jovial personality that endeared him to patients and colleagues, his enthusiasm and skill as a clinician, surgeon and teacher, and his love of the outdoors, wildlife, and gardening. I also noticed his considerable leadership skills, so was not surprised that following his return to India, he was soon promoted to head the Mithu Tulsi Chanrai Campus in Bhubaneswar as well as director of the division of oculoplastics and orbit at that campus.

Milind completed his ophthalmology training at Christian Medical College, Vellore and joined the faculty of LVPEI in 2001. He took leave for a fellowship in oculoplastics and orbital surgery with Bob Goldberg and colleagues in 2006. I first met Milind at a conference on TED at Jules Stein Campus, a seminal meeting that subsequently led to the formation of the International Thyroid Eye Disease Society. Milind impressed me with his polite manner, quiet sense of humor, and highly analytic mind. His talents as a surgeon, teacher, and writer have led to his highly respected position in the field of ophthalmic plastic surgery in India and globally. Milind has delivered numerous lectures nationally and internationally, and I always feel lucky to attend these, as they are consistently lucid, carefully crafted, entertaining, and highly informative.

This textbook on surgical management of TED reflects the dedication and experience of the two co-editors and of all the contributing authors. The rich dividend of this combined effort will be better surgeons and enhanced quality of life for their patients suffering from TED.

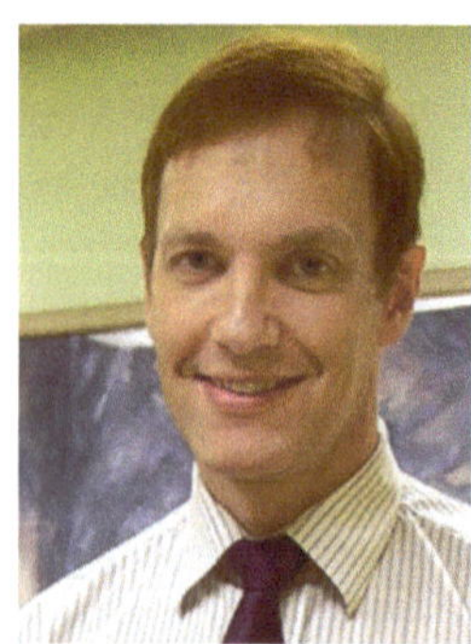

Peter J. Dolman
Eye Care Centre, Vancouver General Hospital,
The University of British Columbia,
Vancouver, BC, Canada

Foreword

Thyroid eye disease (TED) can make patients miserable. On the horizon, perhaps, are medical treatments that will treat the underlying medical disease: hopefully, future doctors will look back at our surgical treatment of an autoimmune disease as barbaric. In the meantime, we have to go to the operating room to deal with the sequelae of TED. Fortunately, surgery has evolved substantially so that we can truly help our patients with their disfigurement, vision, and comfort. Drs. Rath and Naik, highly regarded international experts in TED, have assembled an outstanding compendium of cutting-edge surgical techniques, clearly described and illustrated, that will allow physicians to improve and refine their ability to help their patients.

It is worth noting that the authors are Ophthalmologists. An anecdote regarding Henry Baylis, the Founding Chief of Orbital and Ophthalmic Plastic Surgery at UCLA and one of the pioneers of our specialty, might provide an informative perspective on the history of orbital decompression. Dr. Baylis had a vision of a robust discipline of Ophthalmic Plastic Surgery, and was a leader in expanding the field beyond treatment of eyelid disorders. In the 1970s, when orbital decompression was performed almost exclusively by otolaryngologists, Hank took the initiative to learn and refine techniques of transantral orbital decompression. He used to enjoy telling the story that when he first presented this work at the AAO meeting in San Francisco, Crowell Beard, one of his mentors, commented that it was malpractice for an ophthalmologist to do orbital decompression. Henry was dismayed but not deterred. To today's trainees, it seems obvious that orbital decompression is a core Oculofacial procedure, but it was not always that way.

That anecdote reflects a fairly recent history. Now, oculofacial surgeons are at the leading edge of developing new surgical treatments for TED, and surgical rehabilitation has continued to improve. We now have minimally invasive techniques for orbital decompression that can be individualized and graded, and are associated with decreased morbidity. Eye muscle surgery continues to evolve conceptually and technically. Taking advantage of developments in aesthetic surgery, we now approach eyelid repositioning and soft tissue rehabilitation with customized, small incision approaches that allow us to more closely recreate our patients' premorbid comfort and appearance. In the chapters that follow, the fruits of these years of hard work and innovation are on display.

We are preceded by giants. Their passion and generosity in teaching, their dedication to their patients, and their unwavering commitment to advancing the discipline, is their legacy. Drs. Rath and Naik pay homage to this legacy by creating this textbook. I am sure they will be very gratified when their efforts result in better surgeons who improve the quality of life of the patients they treat.

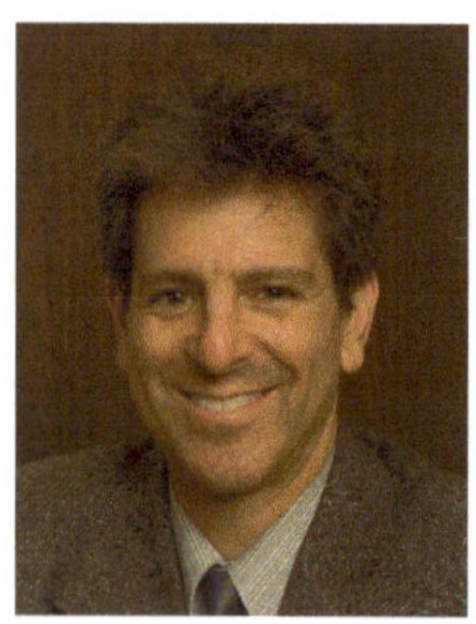

Robert Alan Goldberg, Md, FACS
Professor and Division Head,
Orbital and Ophthalmic Plastic Surgery,
Stein Eye Institute,
UCLA, Los Angeles. USA

Preface

The Making of "Surgery in Thyroid Eye Disease: A Conceptual Approach"

Thyroid eye disease (TED) is a debilitating disease that affects the orbit and adnexal structures. While severe TED can affect visual function, even mild to moderate disease can disrupt the work, family, and social life of individuals. Management of TED usually takes months to years. Surgical interventions in TED are spread over a wide spectrum, and choosing the right surgical option can be daunting.

Several excellent comprehensive textbooks and treatises exist that deal with the pathogenesis and management of TED. However, most are descriptive in nature. An oculoplastic surgeon managing TED is often intimidated by the surgical challenges that lie ahead. These challenges are different in the active phase, as against the quiescent phase.

Some of these challenges include the choice of anesthesia, single-stage vs. multi-stage intervention, surgical approach, and finally, the optimum outcome that is just right for the patient. This surgical manual intends to fill this void by focusing on surgery through pictures, schematics, flowcharts, and complementing text to share nuances and pearls to guide the oculoplastic surgeon in this path and improve their outcome.

Dr Rath's interest with TED grew after managing a young lady more than a decade ago. She presented with bilateral severe proptosis with exposure changes. Her disfigurement was the sequel of burnt-out TED, and she had covered her face when she arrived. She had been blind for several years. Disowned by her parents, she was brought to the institute by a local non-governmental charity.

As a young oculoplastic surgeon, Dr Rath was overwhelmed by achieving euthyroid status (which took months), followed by sequential staged orbital decompression, and eyelid surgeries to correct the exposure and improve her appearance. Finally, vision salvage was attempted with penetrating keratoplasty in the right eye after lengthy discussions and considerable counseling. She improved to 20/50 in the right eye. When she walked into the clinic several months later along with a smile and her parents, her appearance said it all (Fig. 12.11a-b). The journey took six long years, but Dr Rath had managed to restore useful vision and rehabilitate her in society. Lessons learned were for life—TED can devastate an individual physically and emotionally. Nevertheless, a planned, systematic approach comprising a team of specialists can restore normalcy.

For Dr Naik, his trigger patient was a middle-aged lady presenting in 2002 with inactive TED who was depressed because her grandchildren were scared to come close to her. Dr Naik realized how despite vision being normal, TED could change a person's appearance leading to psychosocial disharmony. She was asked by her ophthalmologist to "hide" her eyes behind dark glasses, as orbital decompressions were not being performed in India back then.

There was much learning that happened over a decade and a half for both Dr Rath and Dr Naik while managing patients with TED. For Dr Rath, an international fellowship with Prof. Peter Dolman at the University of British Columbia, Vancouver, Canada, helped vertical learning. The exposure goaded him to delve into understanding the pathogenesis of TED and the role of disease-modifying agents to flatten the curve. For Dr Naik, his International Fellowship in Orbitofacial Plastic Surgery at UCLA, Los Angeles, with Prof. Robert Goldberg paved the way for a deep liking towards TED and minimally invasive surgical approaches for the same.

As Dr Rath and Dr Naik metamorphosed from novice surgeons to experts in the surgical management of TED, on several occasions, both felt the need for a surgical manual that could guide fellow surgeons in this journey.

The process of building the chapter outline, its flow, and highlighting the nuances of surgery was based on this need and turned out to be a fantastic experience for both. As this was a surgical atlas, there was a perpetual obsession to get the best clinical photographs. On several occasions, the precise surgical photograph in their mind took months before it depicted the intended surgical pearl. Their contributing authors across the globe made their job easier by giving their best of talent and photographs!

Finally, both editors had the difficult task of meeting deadlines and sending reminders. The turning point, however, was a marathon session when both of them disappeared from the surface of the earth for 3 days: dug in a secret cove and focused only on the completion of the book! The rest is history.

While new medical therapies keep emerging, there would be a day when surgeries would not be required for new patients of TED, and we could medically avoid the progression of proptosis, strabismus, and lid retraction. Until then, and for the benefit of those patients who are in quiescent phase already, surgical intervention, would remain relevant for rehabilitation. This manual will prove to be a useful, engaging, and ready-reference guide for the oculoplastic surgeons managing TED, both in the clinic and the operating room.

Bhubaneswar, India — Suryasnata Rath
Hyderabad, India — Milind N. Naik

Acknowledgements

This book has been a collaborative project from the start. Being a surgical book, the role of our photographers and artists were pivotal. We thank our lead medical photographers, SBN Chary, Naresh Gattu, Pradeep Moharana, and Nishanth B. Their zeal for perfection in clinical and intraoperative photographs has contributed immensely to the making of this book. We also thank Dr. Virangi Doshi, our Ophthalmology resident and Dr. Varshitha H. Vasanthapuram, clinical fellow for their medical illustrations of the highest quality.

We gratefully acknowledge the thoughtful comments and advice of the many clinical fellows in Ophthalmic plastic surgery, visiting scholars, mentors, and well-wishers, both national and international, who supported us through the making of *Surgery in Thyroid Eye Disease: A Conceptual Approach*.

Thanks to our publisher, Springer, for the valuable assistance of their staff, including Kumar Athiappan and Mariesha Justin.

Thanks to Drs. Jonathan Dutton, Jacqueline Mupas-Uy, Hirohiko Kakizaki, Mahasweta Mishra, Varshitha Vasanthapuram, Peter Dolman, Javed Ali, Robert Goldberg, Michael Burnstine, Mica Bergman, Ramesh Kekunnaya, Mithila Negalur, and Gangadhar Sundar for their outstanding chapter contributions.

For submitting contributions and corrections on the proofs, many thanks to Akhila Mallu, Oshin Bansal, Ashi Morawala, Virangi Doshi, Varshitha H. Vasanthapuram, Priyanka Walvekar, and Gautam Dendukuri.

Contents

About the Editors

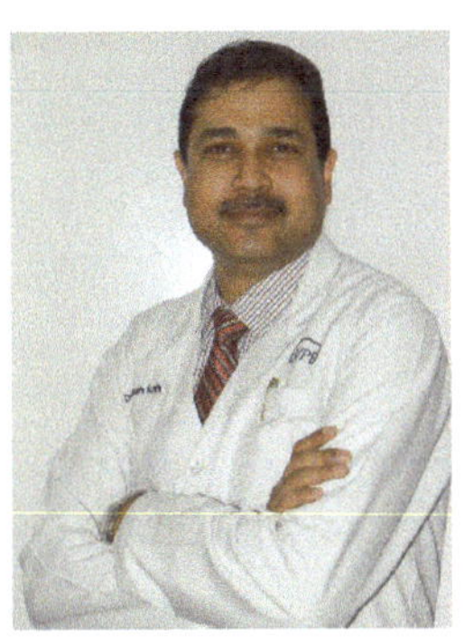

Suryasnata Rath, FRCS Dr. Suryasnata Rath is currently Head of the Mithu Tulsi Chanrai (MTC) campus of LV Prasad Eye Institute, Bhubaneswar, India and of the Ophthalmic Plastics, Orbit and Ocular Oncology Services at MTC. Following his basic medical training in Odisha, he completed long-term fellowships (2001–2003 and 2005–2006) at the LV Prasad Eye Institute, Hyderabad, India before joining as faculty in July 2006.

He became a fellow of the Royal College of Physicians and Surgeons (FRCS), Glasgow, in 2004. Since his training in Oculoplastics with Dr. Peter Dolman at the University of British Columbia, Canada, in 2011–2012, he has developed a keen interest in thyroid eye disease and endonasal lacrimal surgery. Suryasnata is the principal investigator of several ongoing projects, including a multicenter randomized trial on orbital radiotherapy in thyroid eye disease and a Department of Biotechnology (DBT)-funded project to explore the role of infection in ocular adnexal lymphoma. Suryasnata recently stepped into the realm of innovation as a recipient of the Biotechnology Industry Research Assistance Council–Biotechnology ignition grant (BIRAC-BIG) to develop a device for the minimally invasive treatment of chronic dacryocystitis. He has written 47 peer-reviewed, indexed publications, and several chapters on non-endoscopic endonasal dacryocystorhinostomy.

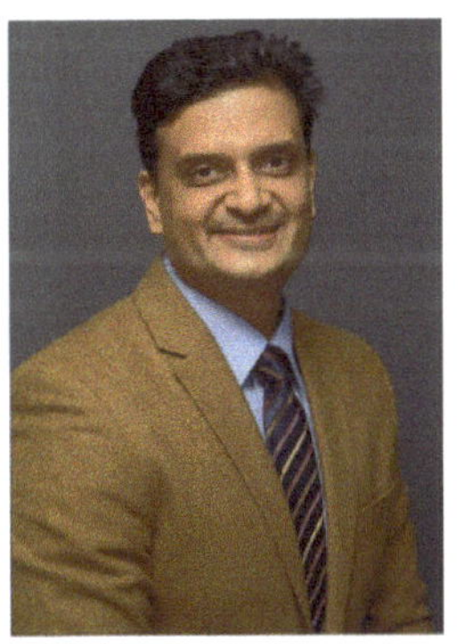

Milind N. Naik, MD Dr Milind N. Naik completed his postgraduate training in Ophthalmology at the Christian Medical College, Vellore, India. In 2001, he then completed a fellowship in Ophthalmic plastic surgery at LV Prasad Eye Institute, Hyderabad, India. He completed his Orbitofacial plastic surgery fellowship at the Stein Eye Institute, University of California, Los Angeles, in 2006–2007. His areas of interest include thyroid eye disease, aesthetic orbitofacial surgery, and minimally invasive ophthalmic plastic surgery.

He received the American Academy of Ophthalmology's Senior Achievement Award in 2015 and is a member of the

American Society of Ophthalmic Plastic and Reconstructive Surgery (ASOPRS). He served as the Vice President of the Asia Pacific Society of Ophthalmic Plastic and Reconstructive Surgery (APSOPRS) from 2010 to 2012.

Dr Naik has published over 200 peer-reviewed articles in international journals and lectures extensively around the globe in the field of Ophthalmic plastic surgery and facial aesthetics. Dr Naik is a senior Consultant, Ophthalmic Plastic Surgery Services at LV Prasad Eye Institute, Hyderabad, India. He also serves as Associate Professor, Department of Ophthalmology and Visual Sciences, University of Rochester, New York, USA.

Part I

Anatomy and Pre-operative Planning

1 Anatomy of the Eyelids Pertaining to Thyroid Eye Disease

Jonathan J. Dutton

1.1 Introduction

The major clinical eyelid findings associated with thyroid eye disease (TED) are varied, but most often involve upper and lower eyelid retraction, contour abnormalities, eyelid edema, prolapsed orbital fat, conjunctival injection and chemosis, and meibomian gland dysfunction. The exact causes of these changes remain a matter of controversy, but numerous hypotheses have been proposed, most with limited experimental support.

Eyelid retraction is probably the most significant manifestation of TED. Not only because of it's obvious aesthetic implications for the patient, but because of its relation to corneal exposure and it's potential for vision loss. Three theories related to the etiology of eyelid retraction have been mentioned in the literature and repeated in numerous publications on TED. The first is a mechanical factor related to globe proptosis. Rajabi et al. [1] evaluated 166 TED eyes and found no correlation between lower lid position and inferior fornix depth as a measure of retractor fibrosis, but they did find a significant correlation between proptosis and degree of lid retraction. The authors concluded that the mechanical draping of the lid over a proptotic globe was the main cause of lower lid retraction. This is partially supported by the observation that retraction usually improves following orbital decompression.

Upper eyelid retraction appears to be more complicated. Although proptosis might play some role, it is considered to be a rather minor factor [2]. A more widely quoted mechanism is Müller sympathetic muscle overaction, ever since it was proposed by Pochin in 1939 [3]. One basis for this is that many of the clinical symptoms in hyperthyroidism, such as palpitations, tachycardia, tremor, sweating, and heat intolerance are related to beta-adrenergic activity [4, 5]. Also, beta-adrenergic blockade is well-known to modify these symptoms in Graves patients [6–8]. Morton et al. [9] demonstrated a lateral extension of Müller smooth muscle fibers accompanying the lateral horn of the levator aponeurosis between the lobes of the lacrimal gland. They proposed that overaction of this portion could contribute to the lateral flare frequently seen with eyelid retraction in TED patients. Although Noh et al. [10] found sympathetic overactivity in intraocular smooth muscles of hyperthyroid patients, there was no difference in this activity in patients with or without eyelid retraction. They concluded that eyelid retraction was not caused by sympathetic overactivity alone, but by other factors in addition.

J. J. Dutton (✉)
Department of Ophthalmology, University of North Carolina, Chapel Hill, NC, USA
e-mail: jonathan_dutton@med.unc.edu

S. Rath, M. N. Naik (eds.), *Surgery in Thyroid Eye Disease*,
https://doi.org/10.1007/978-981-32-9220-8_1

Other factors that likely contribute to upper lid retraction are inflammation and fibrosis of Müller muscle, but the histologic data are inconsistent. Lowinger et al. [11] found no significant histologic difference in Müller muscle specimens from inactive TED patients compared with normal controls. However, Cokerham et al. [12] and Shih et al. [13] found increased inflammation, fibrosis, and fat infiltration in the Müller muscles of inactive euthyroid TED patients.

Another mechanism proposed to contribute to upper lid retraction is overaction of the levator palpebrae superioris (LPS) muscle. Small [14] showed CT evidence of enlargement of the levator muscle proximal to Whitnall ligament in TED patients compared with controls, and suggested hypertrophy as the likely cause of eyelid retraction. Wesley et al. [15] also demonstrated LPS enlargement and proposed that inferior rectus muscle restriction caused overaction of the superior rectus and levator muscles from Hering law.

Some degree of levator connective tissue system fibrosis and of the suspensory ligaments of the superior conjunctival fornix may be at least partially responsible for upper lid retraction. It is not uncommon to find persistent retraction during surgery even when the levator aponeurosis and Müller muscle are completely detached up to the level of Whitnall ligament. This view is supported further by the observation of diminished levator excursion associated with increasing levels of lid lag and lagophthalmos in TED patients with lid retraction [16].

One final mechanism for eyelid retraction was suggested by Harrison et al. [16] who noted a significant reduction of myofibers in the preseptal orbicularis muscle of hyperthyroid rabbits compared with controls. The weakened tone in the orbicularis muscle could allow overaction of the less opposed levator muscle.

Eyelid edema is a common manifestation of thyroid eye disease that may be unilateral or bilateral. Histologic evidence has shown dilated lymphatic vessels and perivascular cellular infiltrate, mostly lymphocytic, in the dermis of eyelid skin in hyperthyroid patients, but with no deposition of mucopolysaccharides [17]. The mechanism is not clear, but has been suggested to possibly be from reduced lymphatic drainage associated with decreased eyelid motility associated with lid retraction and globe proptosis, or from periorbital venous stasis related to orbital fat prolapse, proptosis, and inflammation [18].

TED patients typically show ocular surface changes with an unstable tear film and severe symptoms of dry eyes [19]. The etiology is not completely understood, and there are some conflicting studies. Gürdal et al. [20] and Ozkan et al. [21] demonstrated increased squamous metaplasia associated with decreased Schirmer tear test and increased tear breakup time in Graves patients compared with controls. However, Kikkawa [22] reported only a trend toward higher conjunctival inflammation that was not significant when compared with normal controls.

With these clinical manifestations of eyelid features in TED patients in mind, we will review eyelid anatomy.

1.2 Anatomy of the Eyelids

In young adults, the interpalpebral fissure measures 10–11 mm vertically, but with advancing age this decreases to only about 8–10 mm. The horizontal length of the fissure is 30–31 mm, and the upper and lower eyelids meet at an angle of approximately 60° medially and laterally (Fig. 1.1) [2]. In primary position, the upper eyelid margin normally lies at the superior corneal limbus in children and 1.5–2 mm below it in adults. The lower eyelid margin rests at the inferior corneal limbus. A well-defined eyelid crease and supra-crease fold in the upper lid mark the approximate zone of attachment of levator aponeurosis fibers to the orbicularis muscle and skin. The lacrimal puncta are situated medially, 6–8 mm from the canthal angle. In thyroid eye disease, the upper and lower eyelids are often retracted so that white sclera is visible between the cornea and the eyelid margins.

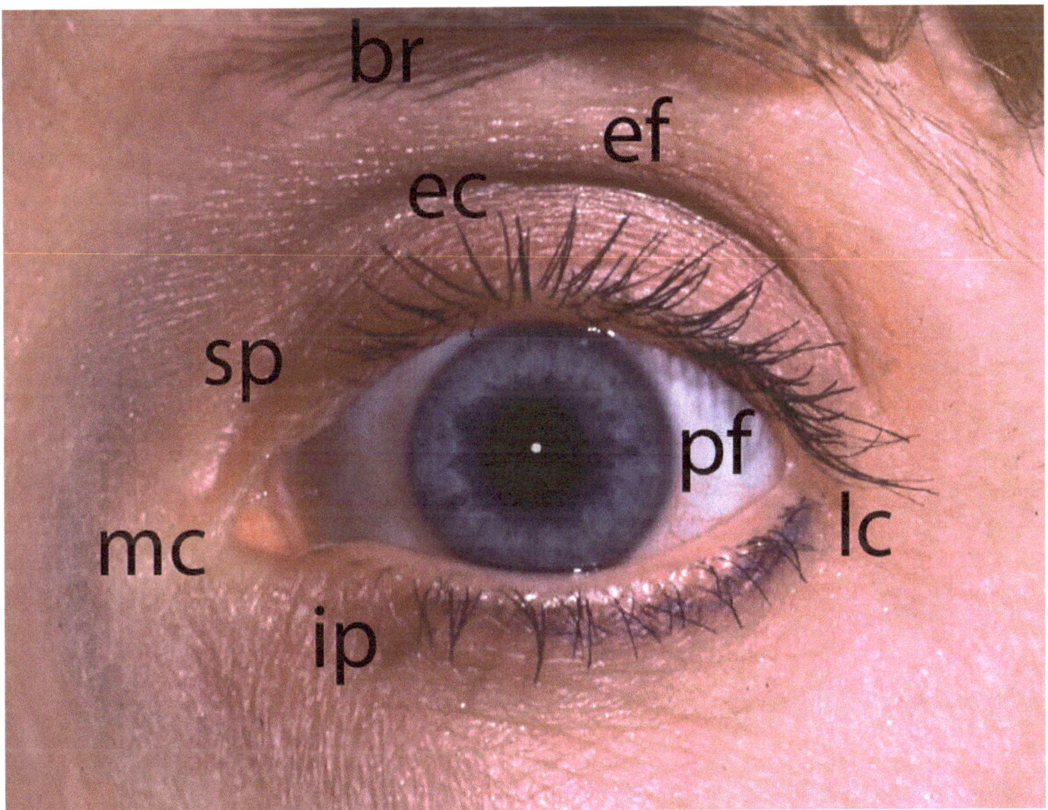

Fig. 1.1 Anatomy of the normal eyelids. This frontal photograph shows the brow (br), the eyelid crease (ec), eyelid fold (ef), inferior punctum (ip), lateral canthus (lc), medial canthus (mc), palpebral fissure (pf), and superior punctum (sp)

1.3 Eyelid Margin

The eyelid margin is about 2-mm thick (Fig. 1.2). It is covered posteriorly by conjunctival epithelium interrupted by the meibomian gland orifices, about 25 in the upper eyelid and 20 in the lower. Anteriorly, the margin is covered with skin from which emerge several rows of eyelashes. Separating these posterior and anterior lamellae, is a faint gray line that represents the marginal projection of specialized horizontal fibers of Riolan muscle that may in part function in meibomian secretion [23]. Tissue lamellae are seen in sagittal section through the lateral upper eyelid in Fig. 1.3.

During eyelid recession procedures for lid retraction, an interpositional graft is usually placed on the posterior lamella to lengthen the capsulopalpebral fascia. A three-dimensional layered dissection through the upper and lower eyelids is demonstrated in Figs. 1.4 and 1.5.

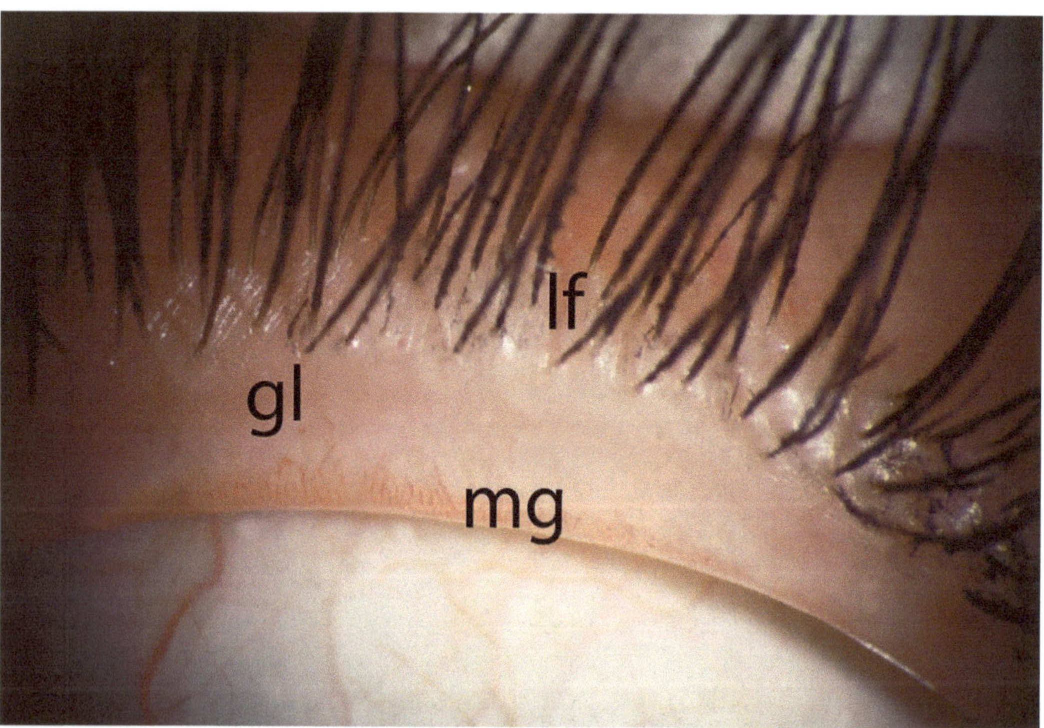

Fig. 1.2 Eyelid margin, showing the meibomial glands (mg), grey line (gl), and lash follicles (lf) arranged posterior to anterior

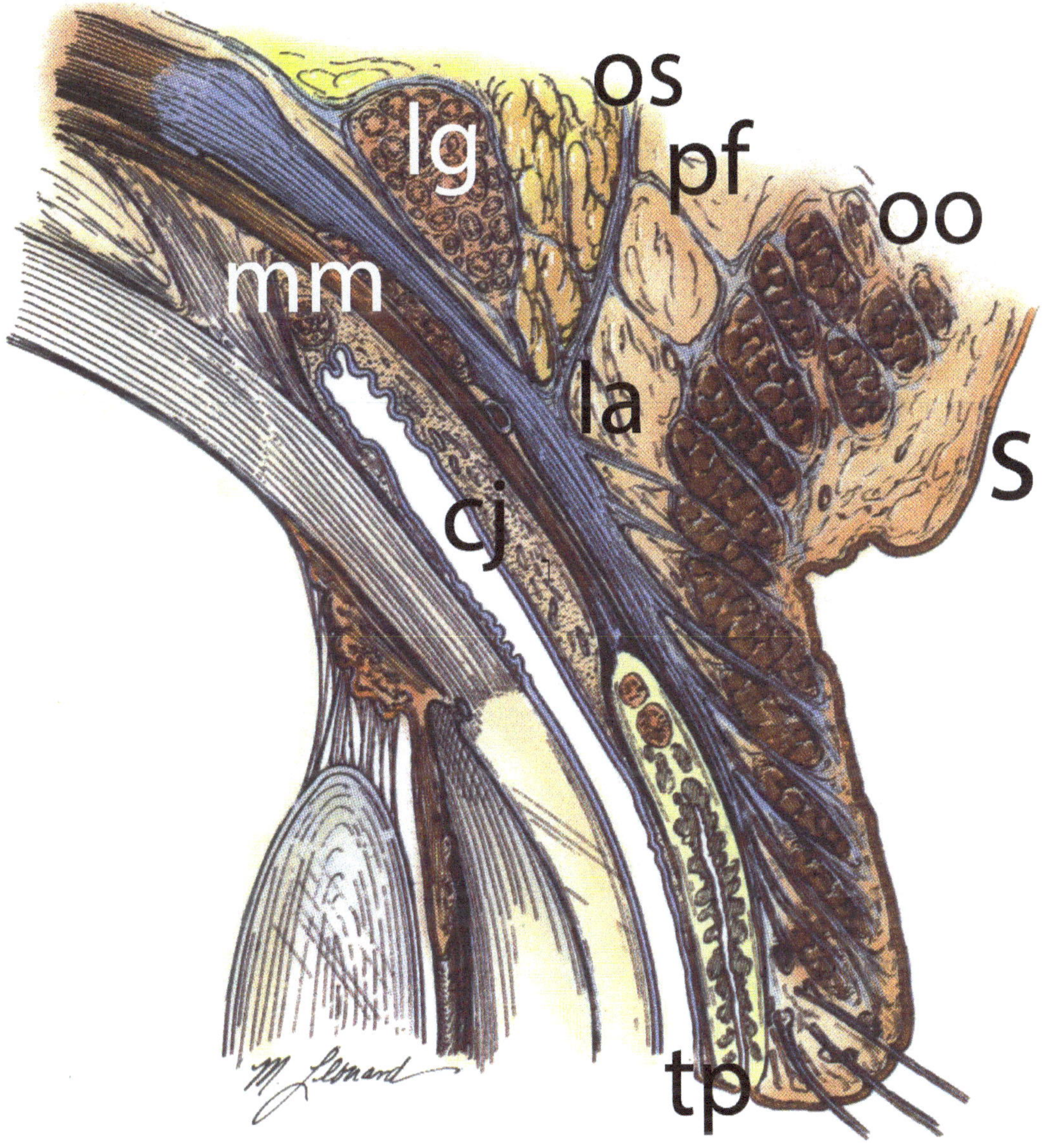

Fig. 1.3 Sagittal section of the upper eyelid showing skin (s), orbicularis oculi muscle (oo), post-orbicular fascial plane (pf), orbital septum (os), levator aponeurosis (la), Muller muscle (mm), lacrimal gland (lg), conjunctiva (cj), and tarsal plate (tp)

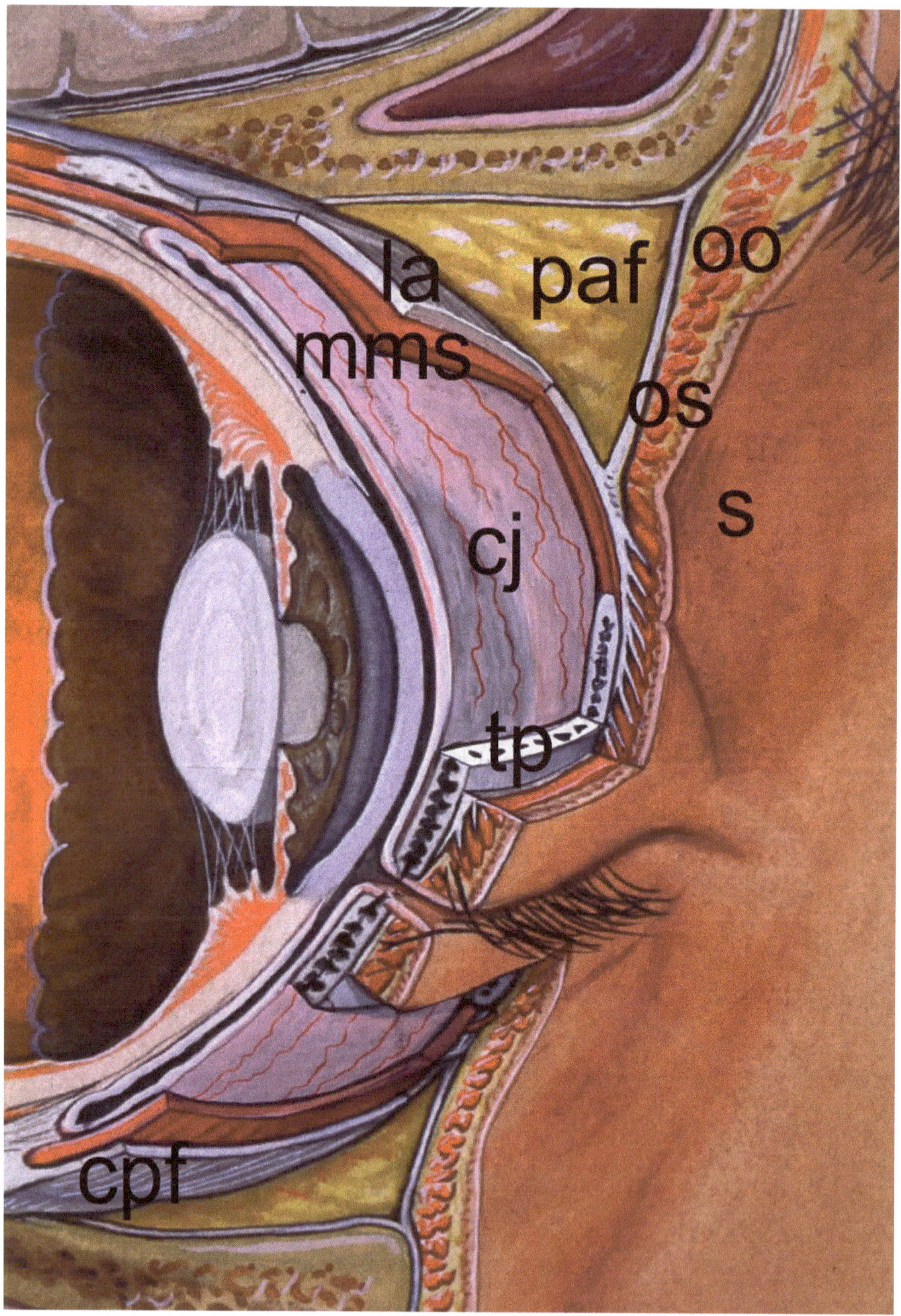

Fig. 1.4 A three-dimensional layered dissection through the upper and lower eyelids showing the skin(s), orbicularis oculi muscle(oo), tarsal plate (tp), conjunctiva (cj), orbital septum (os), preaponeurotic fat (paf); levator aponeurosis (la), superior Muller muscle (mms), and capsuloplalpebral fascia (cpf)

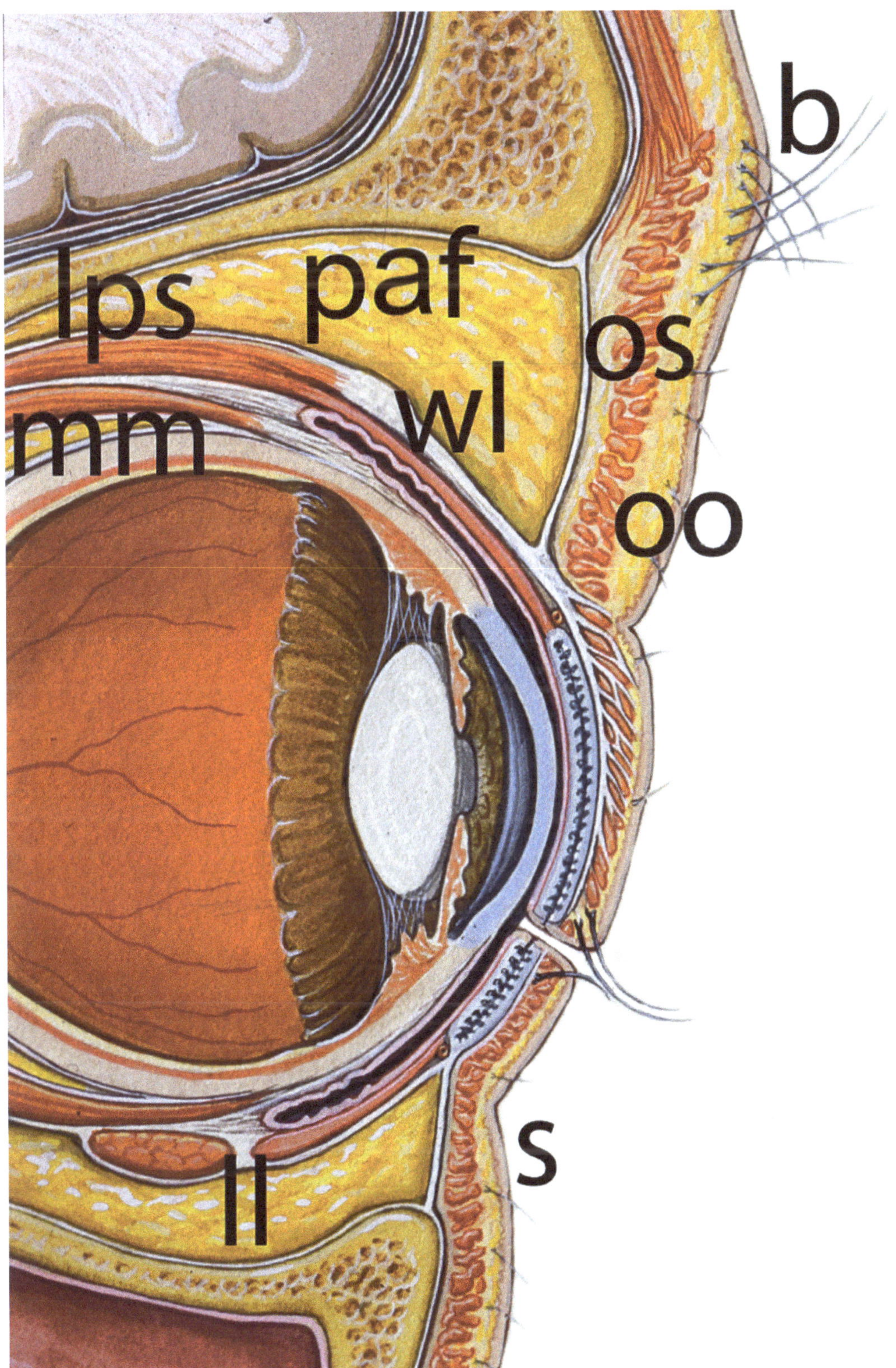

Fig. 1.5 Sagittal section through the globe, upper and lower eyelids showing the brow (b), orbital septum (os), orbicularis oculi muscle (oo), skin (s), Whitnall ligament (wl), Lockwood ligament (ll), levator palpebrae superioris (lps), Muller muscle (mm), and preapnoneurotic fat (paf)

1.4 Orbicularis Oculi

The orbicularis oculi is a complex striated muscle that lies just below the skin (Fig. 1.6). It is divided anatomically into three contiguous parts: orbital, preseptal, and pretarsal [24, 25]. The orbital portion overlies the bony orbital rims. Its fibers pass around the orbital rim to form a continuous ellipse. The palpebral portion overlies the mobile eyelid from the orbital rims to the eyelid margins. It is divided topographically into the preseptal and pretarsal portions (Fig. 1.6). The preseptal portion overlies the orbital septum in both upper and lower eyelids and the pretarsal portion overlies the tarsal plates. Medially, the deep heads of the pretarsal fibers fuse to form Horner muscle that runs behind the posterior limb of the canthal tendon to insert onto the posterior lacrimal crest. Horner muscle helps maintain the posterior position of the canthal angle and may aid in the lacrimal pump mechanism [26].

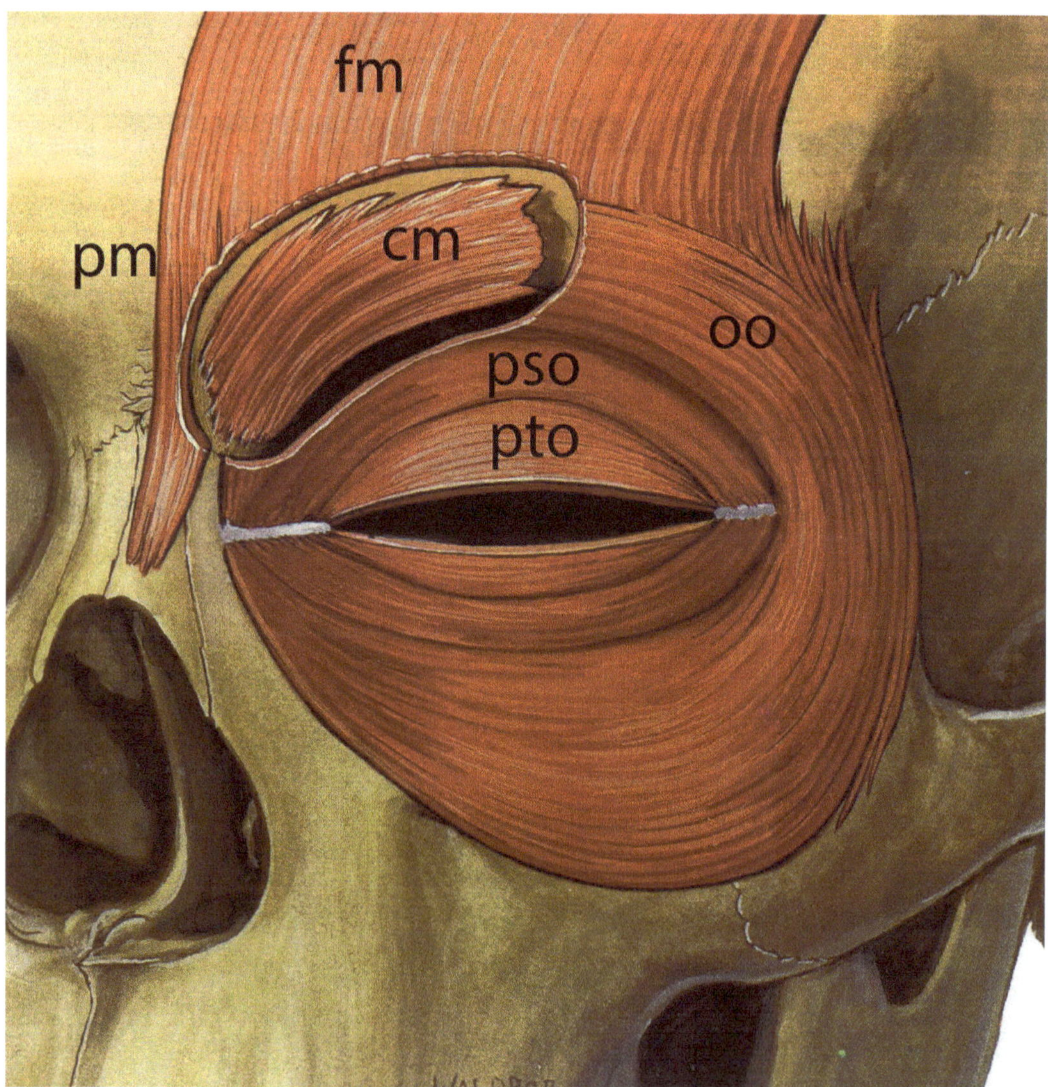

Fig. 1.6 Periorbital musculature. Procerus muscle (pm), frontalis muscle (fm), orbicularis oculi muscle(oo), pre-septal orbicularis (pso), pre-tarsal orbicularis (pto), and corrugator muscle (cm)

The preseptal orbicularis muscles are attached to the medial canthal tendon via deep and superficial heads (Fig. 1.7). The superficial heads partially surround the lacrimal canaliculi and contraction during the eyelid blink cycle helps fold these structures to prevent reflux of tears. Along the eyelid margins, Riolan muscle is a specialized portion of the orbicularis with short horizontal fibers that surround the orifices of the Meibomian glands and may help with secretion. The deep heads pass posterior to the canthal tendon where they merge with Riolan muscles to form Horner muscle just posterior to the lacrimal sac.

The muscles of Riolan are distinct bundles of fibers along the eyelid margins (Fig. 1.8). The main portion of the muscle inserts around the lacrimal puncta and ampullae. Deep fibers form short bundles that run in various directions along the lid margin and between tarsus and conjunctiva. Fine bundles surround the eyelash follicles and excretory ducts of the Meibomian glands.

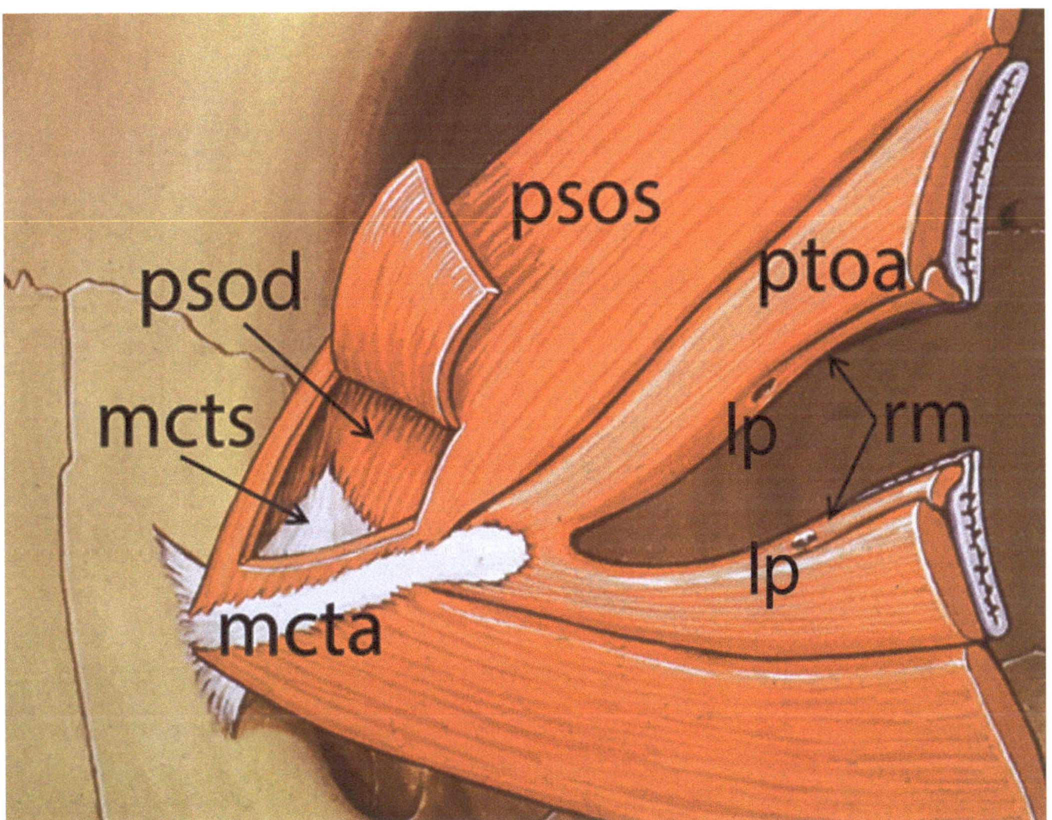

Fig. 1.7 Medial canthal soft tissue anatomy, showing the medial canthal tendon, anterior arm (mcta), medial canthal tendon, superior arm (mcts); Riolan muscle (rm), pre-septal orbicularis superficial head (psos), pre-septal orbicularis, deep head (psod), pretarsal orbicularis, anterior (ptoa), and lacrimal puncta (lp)

The *medial canthus* supports structures that maintain alignment and orientation of the medial eyelids [27]. Medially, the tarsal plates pass into fibrous bands that form the crura of the medial canthal tendon. The superior and inferior crura fuse to form a stout common tendon that inserts via three arms (Fig. 1.9). The *anterior arm* inserts onto the orbital process of the maxillary bone in front of and above the anterior lacrimal crest. The *posterior arm* arises from the common tendon and passes between the canaliculi to insert onto the posterior lacrimal crest in front of Horner muscle. The *superior arm* arises as a broad arc of fibers from both the anterior and the posterior limbs. It passes upward to insert onto the orbital process of the frontal bone. It provides vertical support to the canthal angle and appears to play a role in the lacrimal pump mechanism [28].

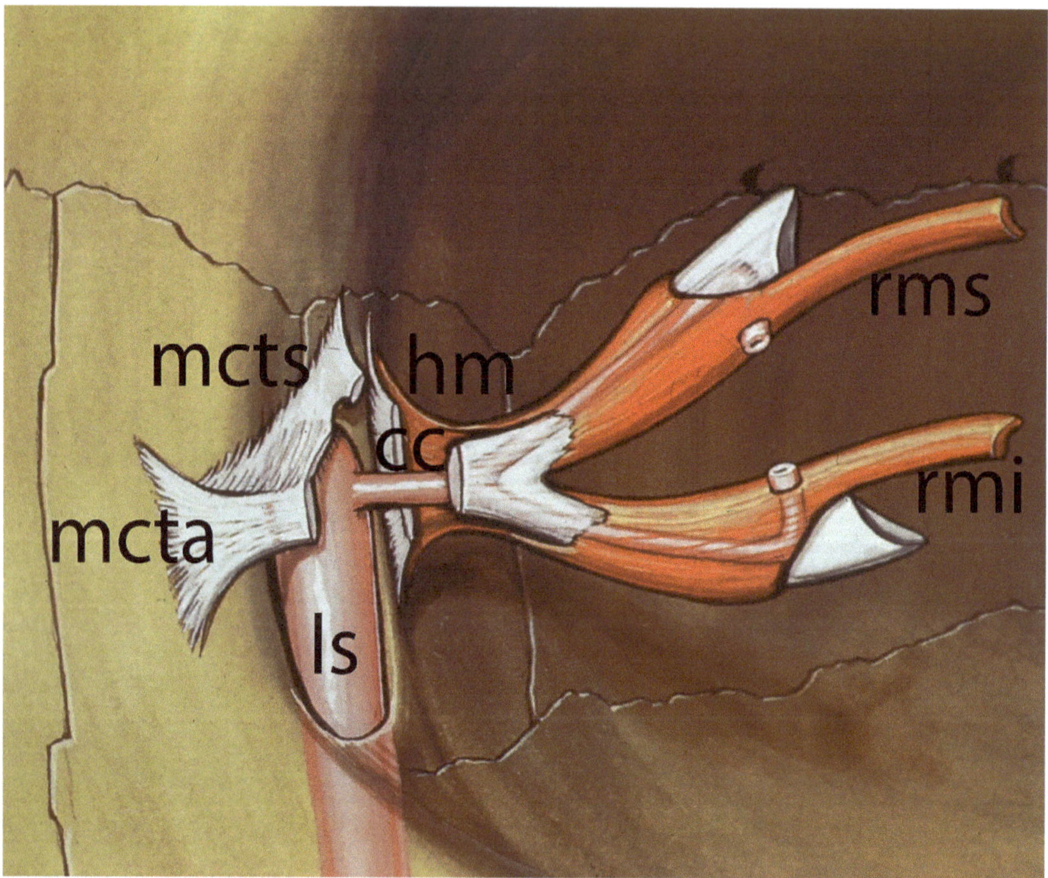

Fig. 1.8 Medial canthal anatomy describing the muscle of Riolan. Lacrimal sac (ls), medial canthal tendon, anterior arm (mcta), medial canthal tendon, superior arm (mcts), superior Riolan muscle (rms), inferior Riolan muscle (rmi), Horner muscle (hm), and common canaliculus (cc)

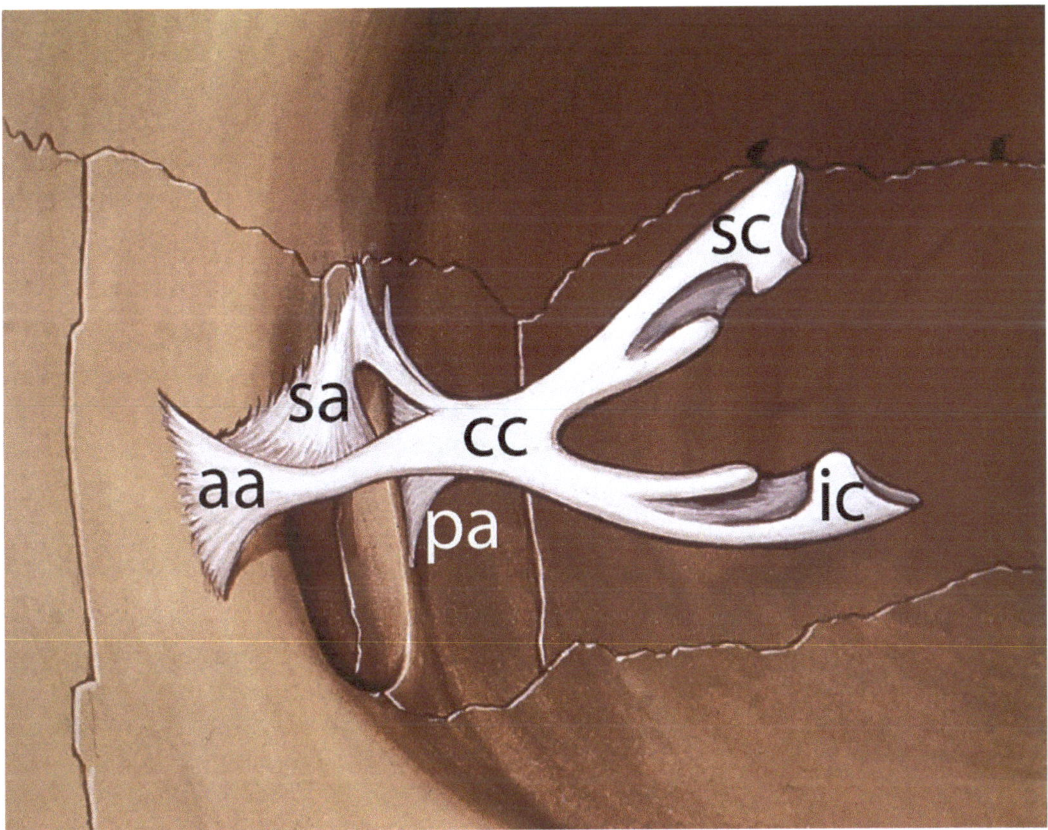

Fig. 1.9 Anatomy of the medial canthal tendon. Medial canthal tendon, anterior arm (aa), medial canthal tendon, superior arm (sa), medial canthal tendon, posterior arm (pa), common canaliculus (cc), superior crus (sc), and inferior crus (ic)

1.5 Orbital Septum

The *orbital septum* is a thin, fibrous, multilayered membrane that begins anatomically at the arcus marginalis along the orbital rims (Fig. 1.10). Distally in the upper eyelid fibers merge into the anterior surface of the levator aponeurosis [29]. The point of insertion usually is about 3–5 mm above the tarsal plate, but it may be as much as 10–15 mm above it [30]. In the lower eyelid, the septum fuses with the capsulopalpebral fascia several millimeters below the tarsus, and the common fascial sheet inserts onto the inferior tarsal edge [31, 32].

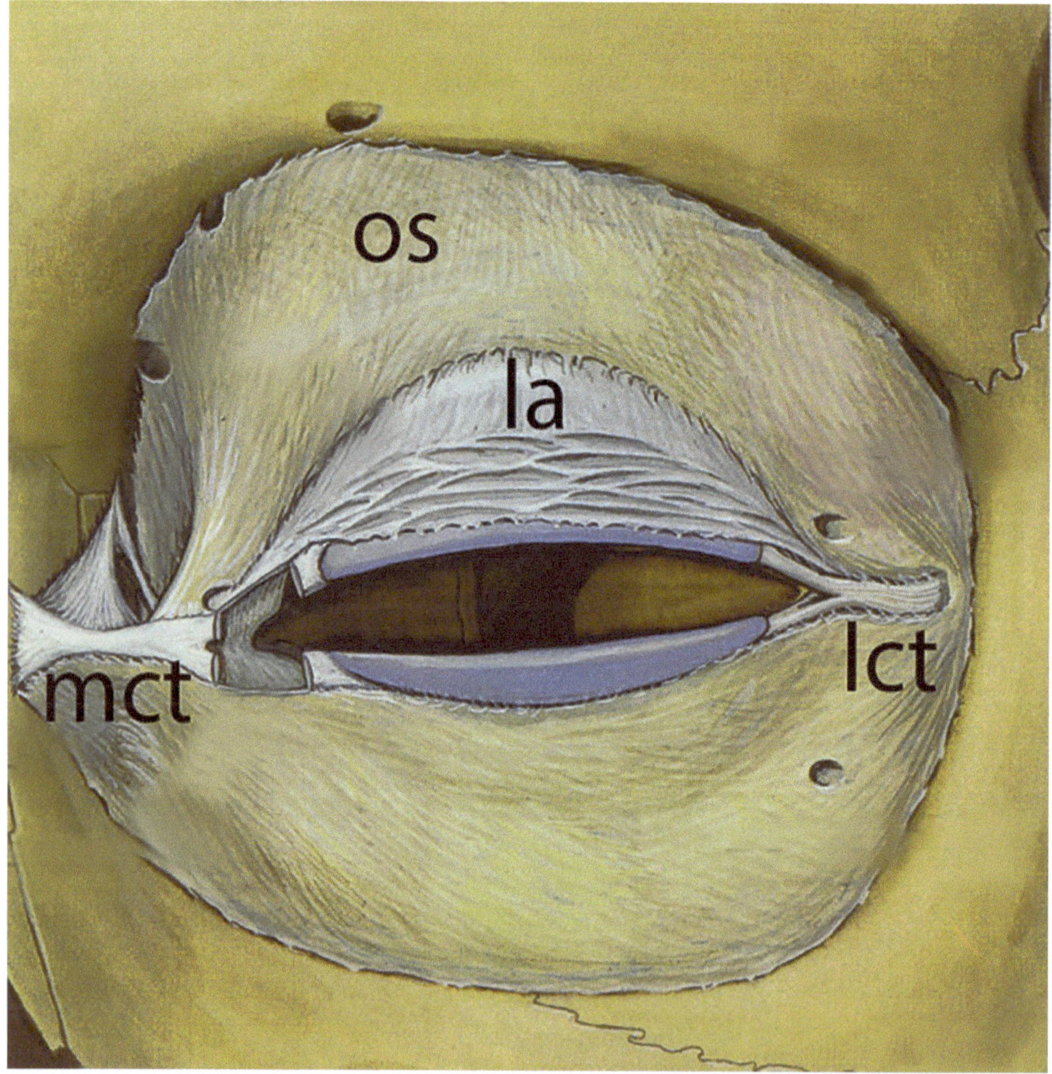

Fig. 1.10 Anatomy of the orbital septum. Medial canthal tendon (mct), lateral canthal tendon (lct), orbital septum (os), and aponeurosis of levator muscle (la)

The preaponeurotic fat pockets in the upper eyelid and the precapsulopalpebral fat pockets in the lower eyelid are anterior extensions of extraconal orbital fat (Fig. 1.11). These are surgically important landmarks and help identify a plane immediately behind the orbital septum and anterior to the major eyelid retractors (levator aponeurosis in the upper lid and capsulopalpebral fascia in the lower lid). In the upper eyelid, two fat pockets are noted: a medial pocket and a central one [33]. Laterally, the lacrimal gland is present but it may be surrounded by a thin layer of fat. In the lower eyelid three fat pockets are noted: medial, central, and lateral [34]. Prolapse of these fat pockets is seen as an aging phenomenon, but also in thyroid eye disease secondary to adipogenesis and proptosis.

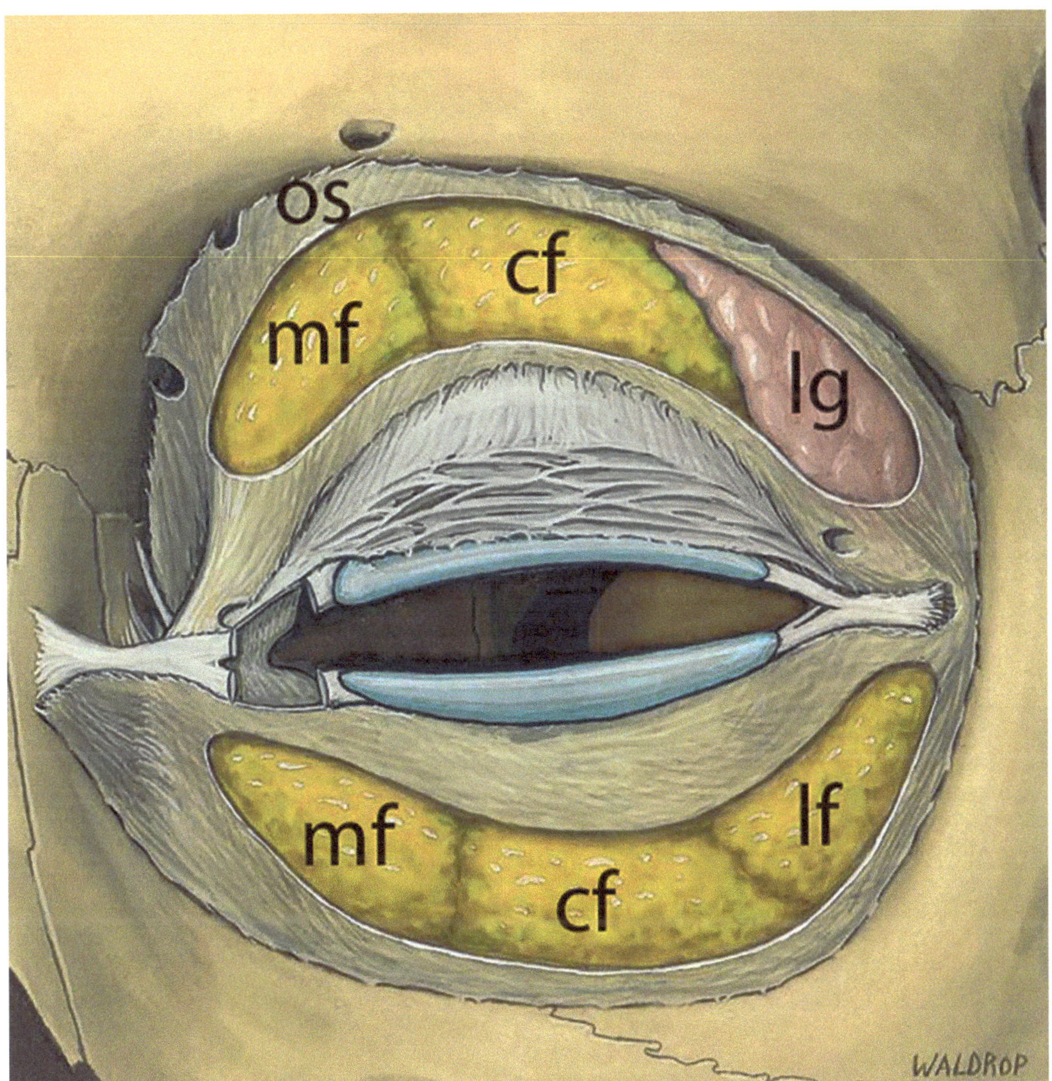

Fig. 1.11 Fat pockets of the upper and lower eyelids. Orbital septum (os), medial fat pocket (mf), central fat pocket (cf); lateral fat pocket (lf), and the lacrimal gland (lg)

1.6 Eyelid Retractors

The retractors of the upper eyelid consist of the levator palpebrae superioris and Müller muscle [35, 36]. The levator palpebrae superioris arises from the lesser sphenoid wing in the orbital apex and runs forward just above the superior rectus muscle. Near the superior orbital rim, a condensation along the muscle sheath attaches medially and laterally to the orbital walls. This is the superior transverse orbital suspensory ligament of Whitnall (Fig. 1.12). The muscle passes into its aponeurosis and continues downward 14–20 mm to its insertion near the marginal tarsal border, about 3–4 mm above the eyelid margin [36, 37]. It also sends delicate slips forward and downward to insert onto the interfasicular septa of the pretarsal orbicularis muscle. These slips maintain the close approximation of the skin, muscle, aponeurosis, and tarsal lamellae, and defines the upper eyelid crease. During eyelid recession procedures, these retractors are recessed upward, usually without a graft. In the lower eyelid, the capsulopalpebral fascia (Fig. 1.12) is a fibrous sheet that arises from Lockwood's ligament and the sheaths around the inferior rectus and inferior oblique muscles [38]. It passes upward and generally fuses with the orbital septum about 4–5 mm below the tarsal plate. From this junction, a common fascial sheet continues upward and inserts onto the lower border of the tarsus.

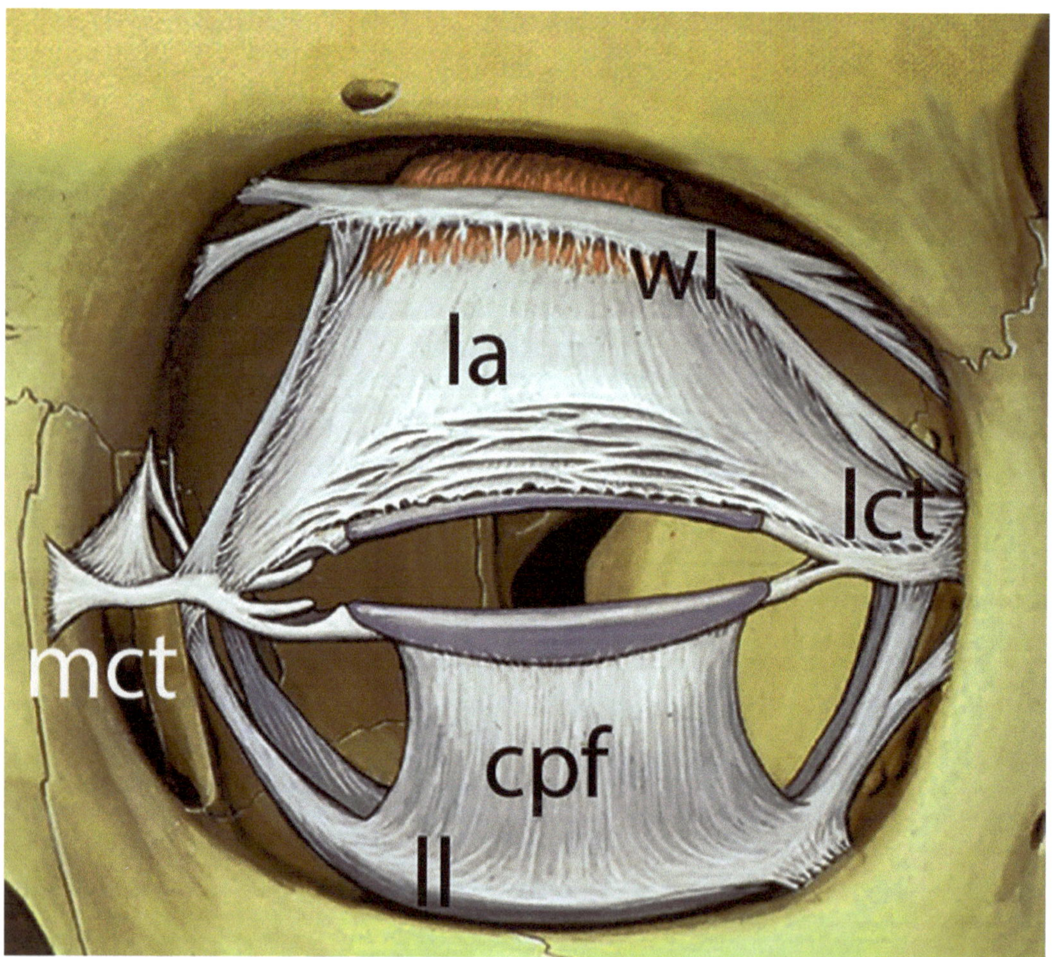

Fig. 1.12 Medial canthal tendon (mct), lateral canthal tendon (lct), levator aponeurosis (la), capsulopalpebral fascia (cpf), Whitnall ligament (wl), and Lockwood ligament (ll)

The eyelids are supported by a complex suspensory system (Fig. 1.13) that supports the canthal angles and redirect vector forces from horizontal in the orbit to vertical in the eyelids [24]. The superior suspensory ligament of Whitnall is a condensation of the levator sheath. It inserts medially and laterally onto the periosteum of the orbital walls. Fine fibers extend from Whitnall ligament to suspend the superior conjunctival fornix. Fibrosis is partially responsible for the eyelid retraction seen in thyroid eye disease. In the lower eyelid, Lockwood ligament forms a fascial condensation involving Tenon capsule, and the conjoined sheaths of the inferior oblique and inferior rectus muscles. The capsulopalpebral fascia extends from this ligament to the inferior tarsus and facilitates retraction of the lower lid in downgaze. In correction of lower lid retraction in thyroid eye disease, this structure is often disinserted or lengthened with an interpositional graft.

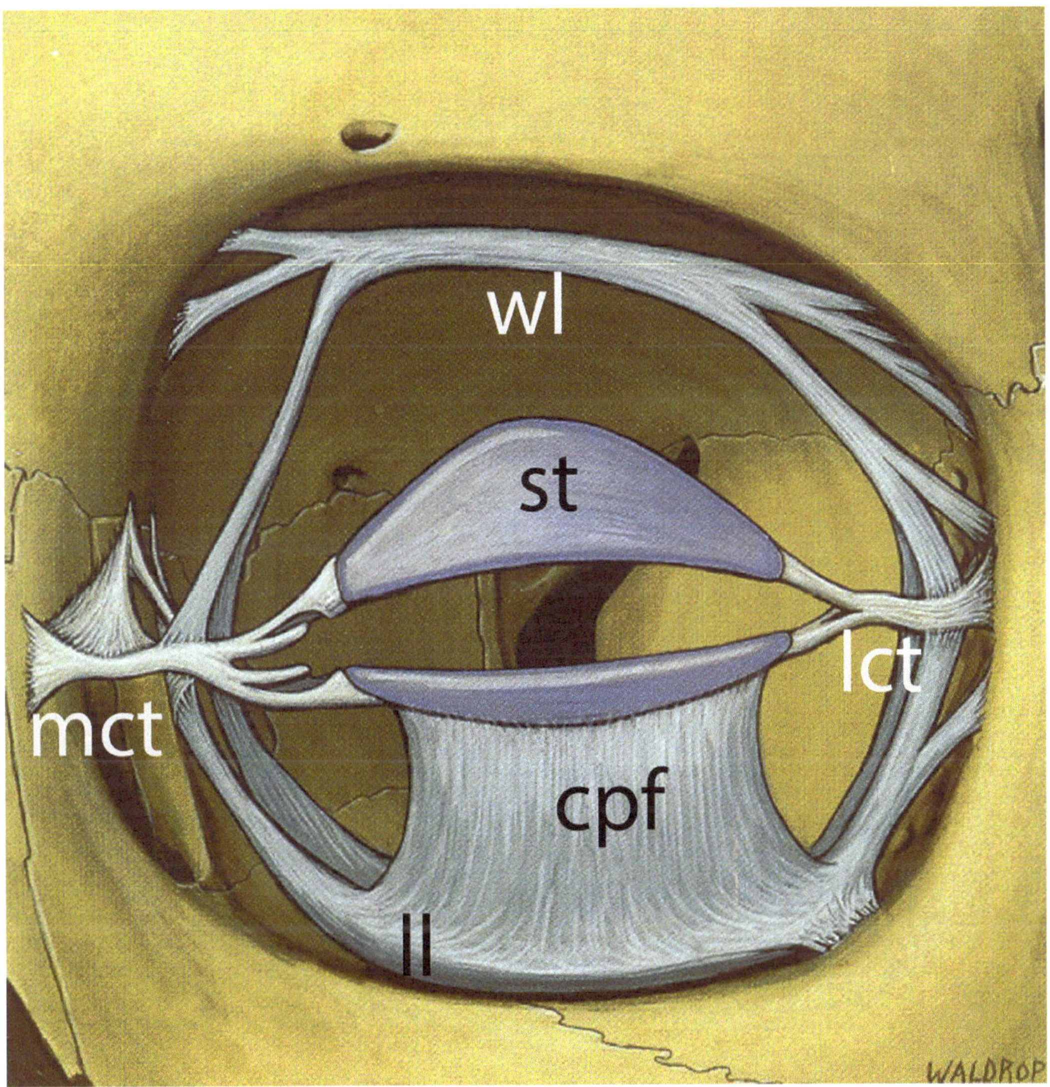

Fig. 1.13 Suspensory system of the eyelids. Whitnall ligament (wl); Lockwood ligament (ll), superior tarsus (st), capsulopalpebral fascia (cpf), medial canthal tendon (mct), and lateral canthal tendon (lct)

1.7 Nerve Supply of the Eyelids

The facial nerve (CN VII) provides motor innervation to the muscles of facial expression. Branches to the periorbital muscles originate in the temporal and zygomatic branches (Fig. 1.14). The temporal branch primarily innervates the frontalis muscle and the upper half of the orbicularis muscle. The zygomatic branch crosses the zygomatic arch and innervates the lower half of the orbicularis muscle. The buccal, mandibular, and cervical branches innervate muscles of the lower face and neck [39].

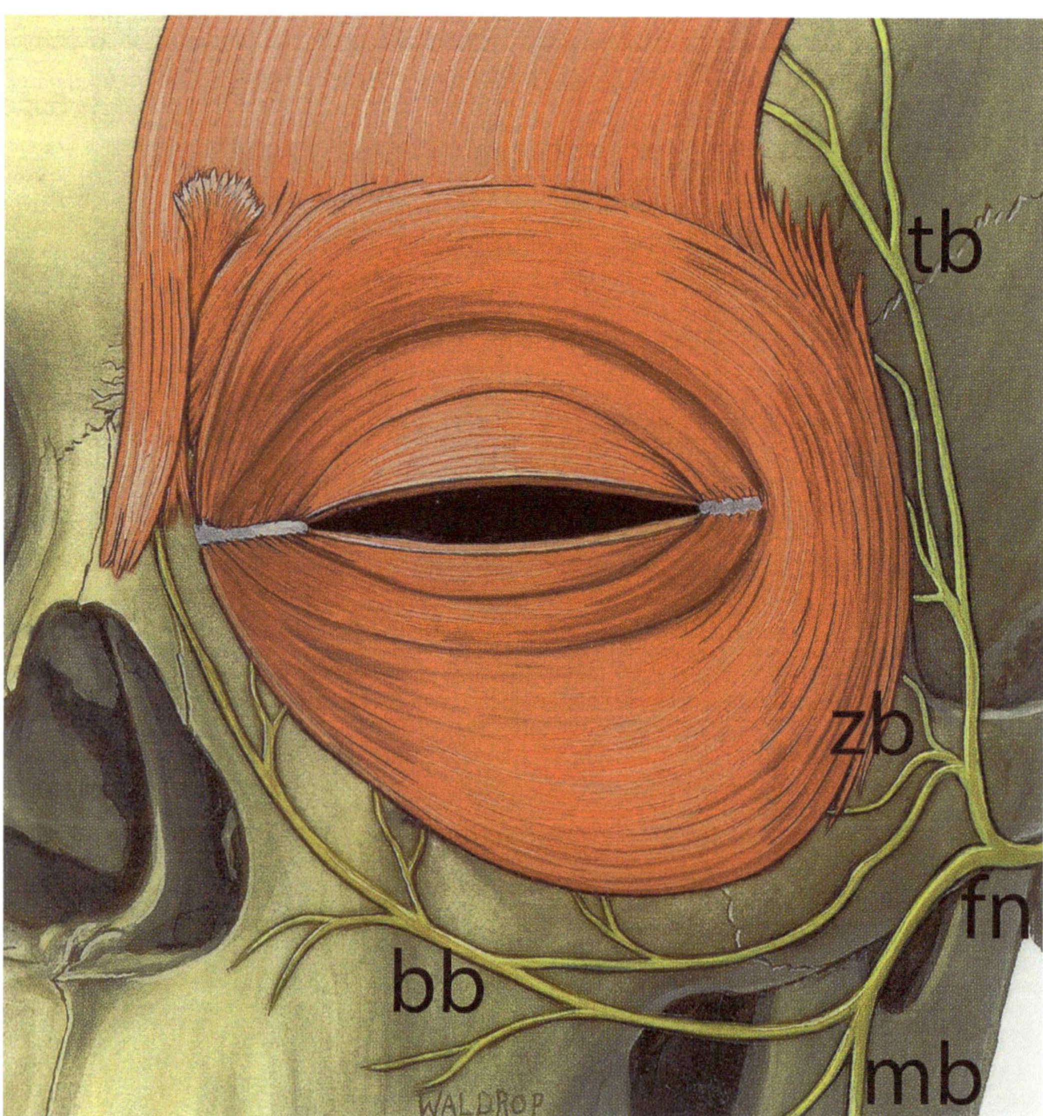

Fig. 1.14 Branches of the Facial nerve. Temporal branch (tb), zygomatic branch (zb), buccal branch (bb), mandibular branch (mb), and facial nerve (fn)

Sensory nerves from the eyelids (Fig. 1.15) derive from the ophthalmic and infraorbital branches of the trigeminal nerve (CN V). These branches pass backward along the orbital walls to the middle cranial fossa. The infraorbital nerve lies within a canal in the orbital floor and is particularly vulnerable to injury during decompression for thyroid eye disease. The zygomaticofacial and zygomaticotemporal nerves pass through the orbital rim and lateral wall where they can be damaged during surgery to advance the rim or decompress the lateral wall.

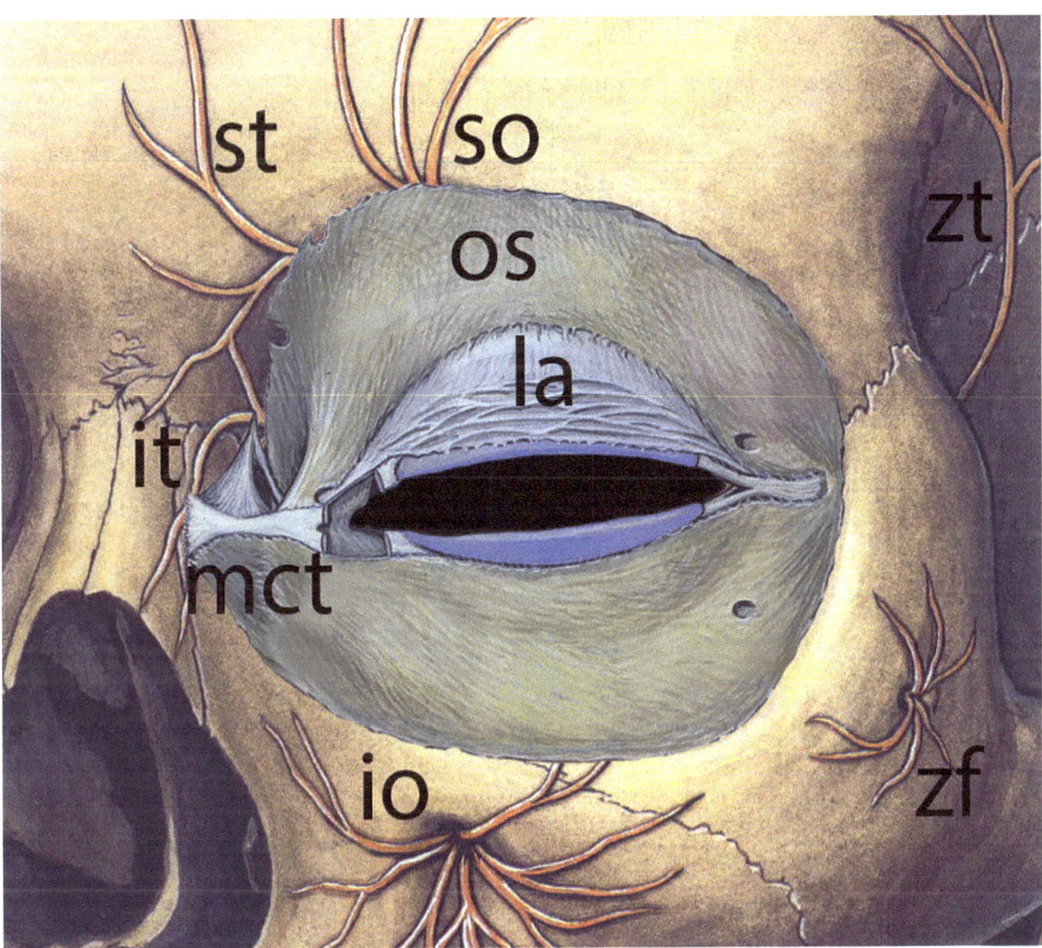

Fig. 1.15 Sensory nerves of the eyelids. Orbital septum (os), supratrochlear nerve (st); *so,* supraorbital nerve (so), levator aponeurosis (la), zygomaticofacial nerve (zf), zygomaticotemporal nerve (zt), infraorbital nerve (io), infratrochlear nerve (it), and medial canthal tendon (mct)

1.8 Vascular Supply of the Eyelids

The posterior eyelid lamellae receive arterial blood through the vascular arcades (Fig. 1.16). In the upper eyelid, a marginal arcade runs about 2 mm from the eyelid margin, and a peripheral arcade extends along the upper border of the tarsus between the levator aponeurosis and Müller muscle. These arcades are supplied medially by the superior medial palpebral vessel from the terminal ophthalmic artery, and laterally by the superior lateral palpebral vessel from the lacrimal artery. They anastomose extensively with the facial arterial system. The lower eyelid arcade receives blood from the medial and lateral inferior palpebral vessels.

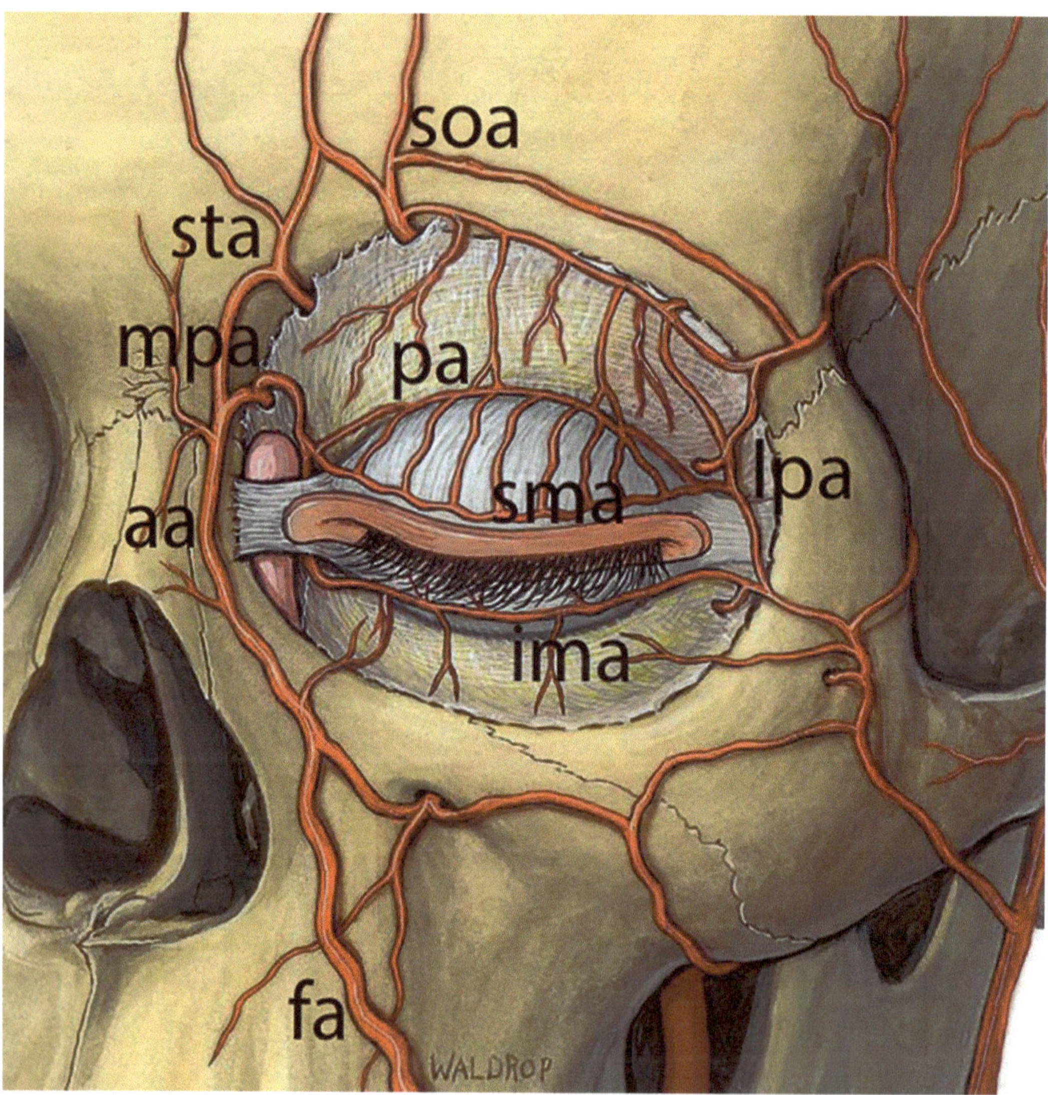

Fig. 1.16 Arterial supply of the Eyelids. Angular artery (aa), medial palpebral artery (mpa), lateral palpebral artery (lpa), supratrochlear artery (sta), supraorbital artery (soa), transverse facial artery (fa), peripheral arcade (pa), superior marginal arcade (sma), and inferior marginal arcade (ima)

The venous drainage system is not as well defined as the arterial system. Drainage is mainly into several large vessels of the facial system and drains both anteriorly into the facial veins, and posteriorly to the cavernous sinus (Fig. 1.17).

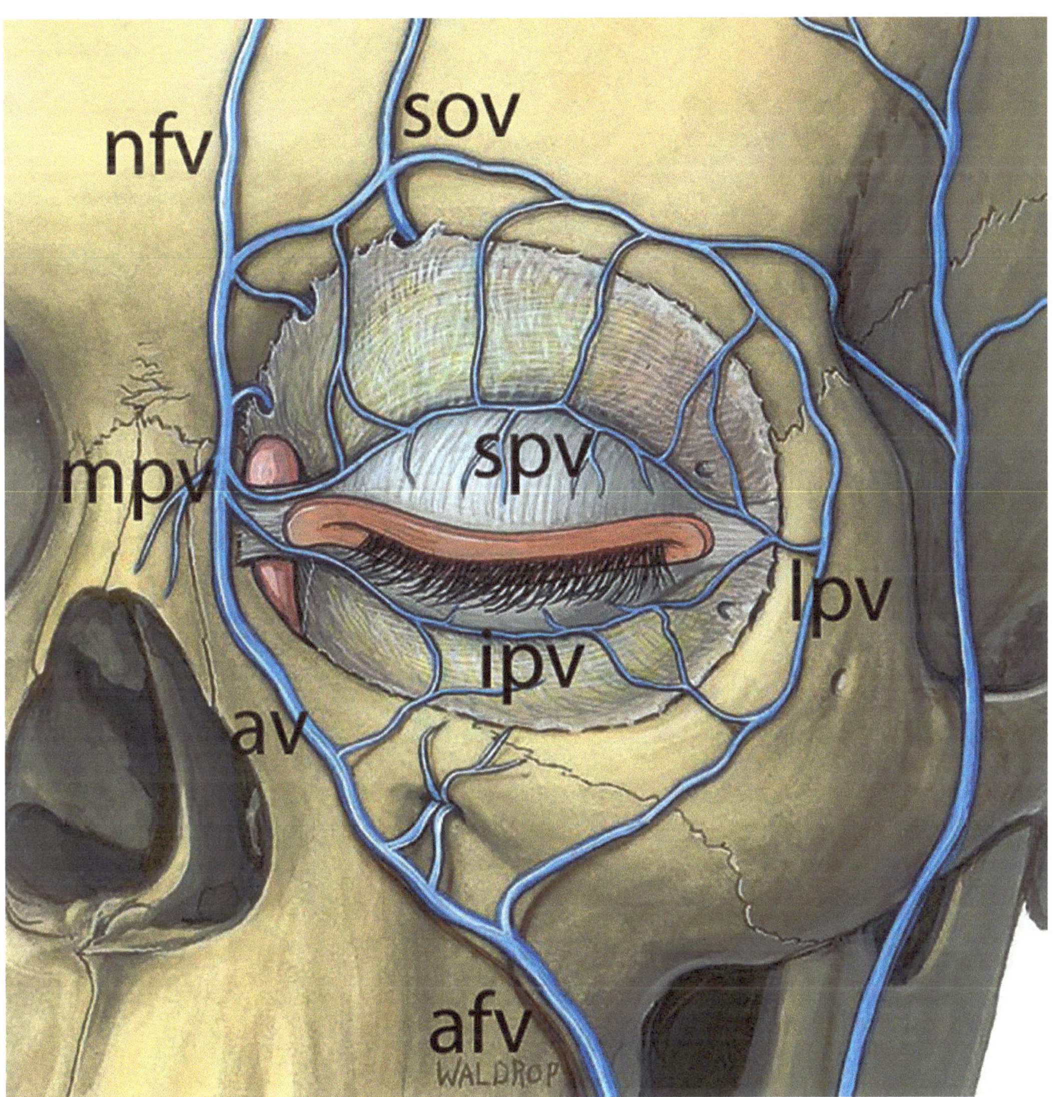

Fig. 1.17 Venous drainage of the Eyelids. Medial palpebral vein (mpv), lateral palpebral vein (lpv), superior palpebral vein (spv), inferior palpebral vein (ipv), nasofrontal vein (nfv), supraorbital vein (sov), angular vein (av), and anterior facial vein (afv)

1.9 Lymphatic Drainage of the Eyelids

The lymphatic drainage from the eyelids is restricted to the region anterior to the orbital septum. Traditional teaching is that lymphatic flow from the lateral two-thirds of the upper eyelid and the lateral one-third of the lower eyelid drain laterally into the deep and superficial parotid nodes, and flow from the medial one-third of the upper eyelid and the medial two-thirds of the lower eyelid drains inferiorly into the submandibular and anterior cervical nodes (Fig. 1.18). However, recent studies have shown a more diffuse drainage from all areas of the eyelids into the parotid nodes [40].

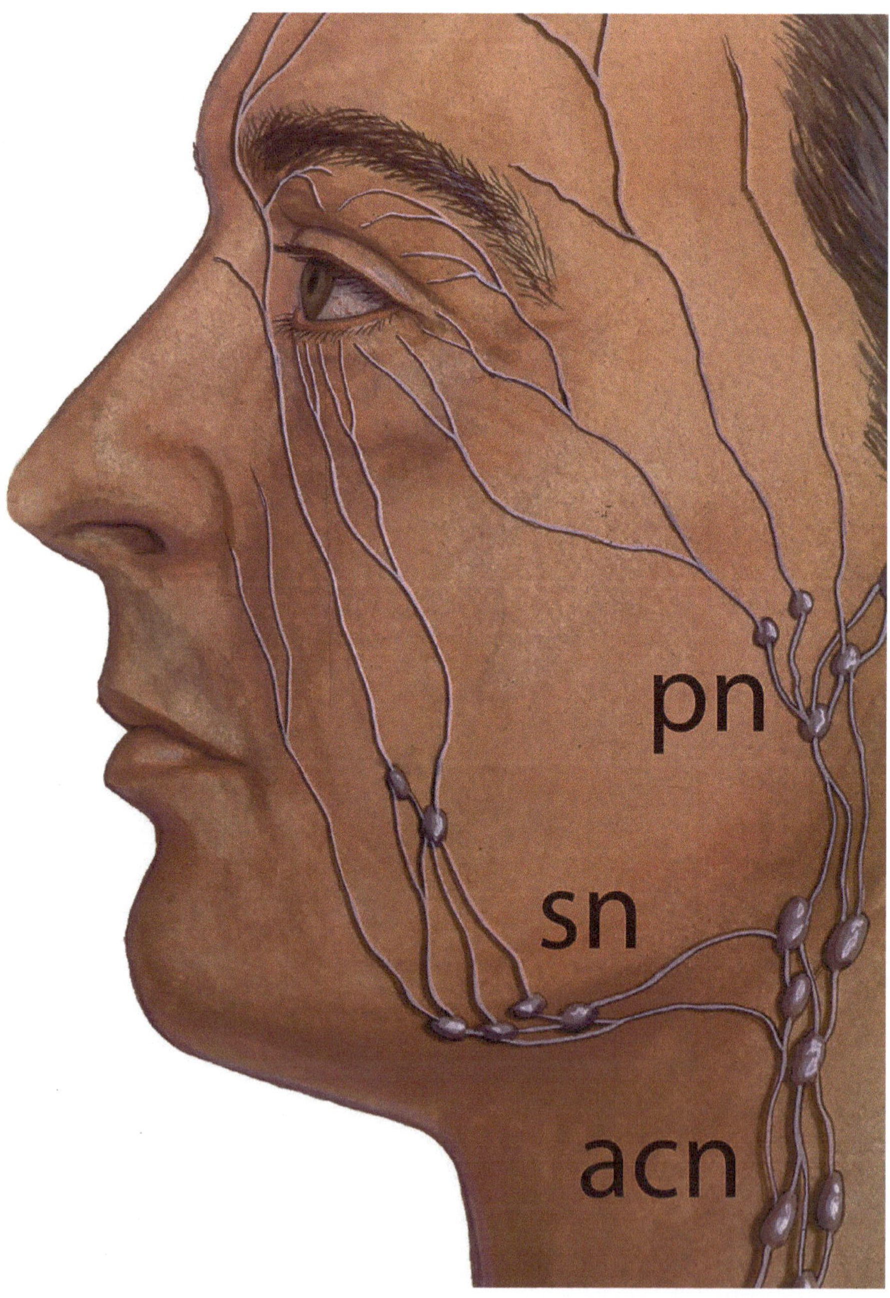

Fig. 1.18 Lymphatic drainage of the Eyelids. Parotid nodes (pn), submandibular nodes (sn), and anterior cervical nodes (acn)

References

1. Rajabi MT, Jafari H, Mazloumi M, et al. Lower lid retraction in thyroid orbitopathy: lamellar shortening or proptosis? Int Ophthalmol. 2014;34:801–4.
2. Cruz AA, Ribeiro SF, Garcia DM, et al. Graves upper eyelid retraction. Surv Ophthalmol. 2013;58:63–76.
3. Pochin EE. The mechanism of lid retraction. Clin Sci. 1939;4:91–101.
4. Levey GS, Klein I. Catecholamine-thyroid hormone interactions and the cardiovascular manifestations of hyperthyroidism. Am J Med. 1990;88:642–6.
5. Silva JE, Bianco SD. Thyroid-adrenergic interactions: physiological and clinical implications. Thyroid. 2008;18:157–65.
6. Turner P. Beta-adrenergic receptor blocking drugs in hyperthyroidism. Drugs. 1974;7:48–54.
7. Utiger RD. Beta-adrenergic-antagonist therapy for hyperthyroid greaves' disease. N Engl J Med. 1984;31:1597–8.
8. Geffner DL, Hershman JM. Beta-adrenergic blockade for treatment of hyperthyroidism. Am J Med. 1992;93:61–8.
9. Morton AD, Elner VM, Lemke BN, White VA. Lateral extensions of the Müller muscle. Arch Ophthalmol. 1996;114:1486–8.
10. Noh JY, Makamura Y, Ito K, et al. Sympathetic overactivity of intraocular muscles evaluated by accommodation in patients with hyperthyroidism. Thyroid. 1996;6:289–93.
11. Lowinger A, Gill HS, Phan I, et al. Histology of Müller's muscle observed in quiescent graves' orbitopathy. Can J Ophthalmol. 2013;48:468–70.
12. Cockerham KP, Hidayat AA, Brown HG, et al. Clinicopathologic evaluation of the Müller muscle in thyroid-associated orbitopathy. Ophthalmic Plast Reconstr Surg. 2002;18:11–7.
13. Shih MJ, Liao SL, Kuo KT, et al. Molecular pathology of Müller's muscle in Grave's ophthalmopathy. J Clin Endocrinol Metab. 2006;91:1159–67.
14. Small RG. Enlargement of levator palpebrae superioris muscle fibers in Grave's ophthalmopathy. Ophthalmology. 1989;96:424–30.
15. Wesley RE, Bond JB. Upper eyelid retraction from inferior rectus restriction in dysthyroid orbit disease. Ann Ophthalmol. 1987;19:34–6.
16. Harrison AR, McLoon LK. Effect of hyperthyroidism on the orbicularis oculi muscle in rabbits. Ophthalmic Plast Reconstr Surg. 2002;18:289–94.
17. Higadi T, Satoh T, Yokozeki H, et al. Palpebral edema as a cutaneous manifestation of hyperthyroidism. J Am Acad Dermatol. 2003;48:617–0.
18. Imazumi M. Recurrent upper eyelid edema as first sign of graves' disease. Thyroid. 2006;16:95–6.
19. Kim YS, Kwak AY, Lee SY, et al. Meibomian gland dysfunction in graves' orbitopathy. Can J Ophthalmol. 2015;50:278–82.
20. Gurdal C, Sarac O, Genc I, et al. Ocular surface and dry eye in graves' disease. Curr Eye Res. 2011;36:8–13.
21. Ozkan SB, Söylev MF, Vahapoglu H, et al. Evaluation of conjunctival morphology in thyroid associated eye disease by use of impression cytology. Acta Ophthalmol Scand. 1997;75:145–7.
22. Kikkawa DO. Histologic analysis of palpebral conjunctiva in thyroid-related orbitopathy (an American ophthalmological society thesis). Trans Am Ophthalmol Soc. 2010;108:46–61.
23. Lipham WJ, Tawfik HA, Dutton JJ. A histologic analysis and three-dimensional reconstruction of the muscle of Riolan. Ophthalmic Plast Reconstr Surg. 2002;18:93–8.
24. Dutton JJ. Atlas of clinical and surgical orbital anatomy. 2nd ed. London: Elsevier Saunders; 2011. p. 129–64.
25. Ridgway JM, Larrabee WE. Anatomy for blepharoplasty and brow-lift. Facial Plast Surg. 2010;26:177–85.
26. Kakizaki H, Zako M, Miyaishi O, et al. The lacrimal canaliculi and sac bordered by the Horner's muscle form a functional lacrimal drainage system. Ophthalmology. 2005;112:710–6.
27. Kang H, Takahshi Y, Ichinosae A, et al. Lateral canthal anatomy: a review. Orbit. 2012;31:279–85.
28. Poh F, Kakizaki H, Selva D, et al. The anatomy of the medial canthal tendon in Caucasians. Clin Exp Ophthalmol. 2012;40:170–3.
29. Kakizaki H, Selva D, Asamoto K, et al. Orbital septum attachment sites on the levator aponeurosis in Asians and whites. Ophthalmic Plast Reconstr Surg. 2010;26:265–8.
30. Lim HW, Paik DJ, Lee YJ. A cadaveric anatomical study of the levator aponeurosis and Whitnall's ligament. Korean J Ophthalmol. 2009;23:183–7.
31. Kakizaki H, Jinsong Z, Zako M, et al. Microscopic anatomy of Asian lower eyelids. Ophthalmic Plast Reconstr Surg. 2006;22:430–3.
32. Meyer DR, Linberg JV, Wobig JL, et al. Anatomy of the orbital septum and associated eyelid connective tissue. Ophthalmic Plast Reconstr Surg. 1991;7:104–13.
33. Persichetti P, Di Lella F, Delfino S, et al. Adipose compartments of the upper eyelid: anatomy applied to blepharoplasty. Plast Reconstr Surg. 2004;113:373–8.
34. Oh CS, Chung IH, Kim YS, et al. Anatomic variations of the infraorbital fat compartments. J Plast Reconstr Aesthet Surg. 2006;59:376–9.
35. Kakizaki H, Malhotra R, Selva D. Upper eyelid anatomy: an update. Ann Plast Surg. 2009;63:336–43.
36. Anderson RL, Beard C. The levator aponeurosis. Attachments and their clinical significance. Arch Ophthalmol. 1977;95:1437–41.
37. Collin JRO, Beard C, Wood I. Experimental and clinical data on the insertion of the levator palpebrae superioris muscle. Am J Ophthalmol. 1987;85:792–801.
38. Kakizaki H, Malhotra R, Madge SN, et al. Lower eyelid anatomy: an update. Ann Plast Surg. 2009;63:344–51.
39. Saylam C, Ucerler H, Orham M, et al. Anatomic guides to precisely localize the zygomatic branches of the facial nerve. J Craniofac Surg. 2006;17:50–3.
40. Nijhawan N, Marriott C, Harvey JT. Lymphatic drainage patterns of the human eyelid: assessed by lymphoscintigraphy. Ophthalmic Plast Reconstr Surg. 2010;26:281–5.

2 Anatomy of the Orbit Pertaining to Thyroid Eye Disease

Jacqueline Mupas-Uy and Hirohiko Kakizaki

2.1 Introduction

Patients with thyroid eye disease often require orbital decompression surgery to expand the orbital space. This is performed by widening the bony orbit and removal of excessive orbital fat. This decreases the venous congestion and mechanical pressure on the optic nerve, and also reduces proptosis. Theoretically, there are four bony orbital walls available for decompression: medial, inferior, lateral and superior wall. A thorough knowledge of the pertinent orbital anatomy is very essential for safe and successful orbital surgery. This chapter will focus on the orbital anatomy with regard to thyroid eye disease and its management.

J. Mupas-Uy · H. Kakizaki (✉)
Department of Oculoplastic, Orbital & Lacrimal Surgery, Aichi Medical University Hospital, Aichi, Nagakute, Japan
e-mail: cosme@d1.dion.ne.jp

S. Rath, M. N. Naik (eds.), *Surgery in Thyroid Eye Disease*,
https://doi.org/10.1007/978-981-32-9220-8_2

2.2 Lateral Orbital Wall

The lateral orbital wall is composed of the sphenoid bone, frontal bone, zygomatic bone, and maxillary bone (Fig. 2.1). When thinking of orbital decompression, however, it is useful to think in terms of "conceptual" bony anatomy rather than strictly "anatomical" bones that form the orbit. The lateral wall is therefore divided into 3 thick "conceptual" areas that are amenable for removal in deep lateral orbital decompression surgery. The areas are called lacrimal keyhole, sphenoid door jamb, and basin of the inferior orbital fissure (Fig. 2.2) [6].

The *lacrimal keyhole* consists of the frontal bone, part of the lesser wing of the sphenoid, and a small portion of the greater wing of sphenoid. It extends into the entire fossa of the lacrimal gland. It is limited medially by the point at which the orbital roof thins as the thin frontal bone, and posteriorly by the anterior cranial fossa and the posterior thick border of the lesser wing of the sphenoid [6]. Inferiorly, it blends into the sphenoid door jamb.

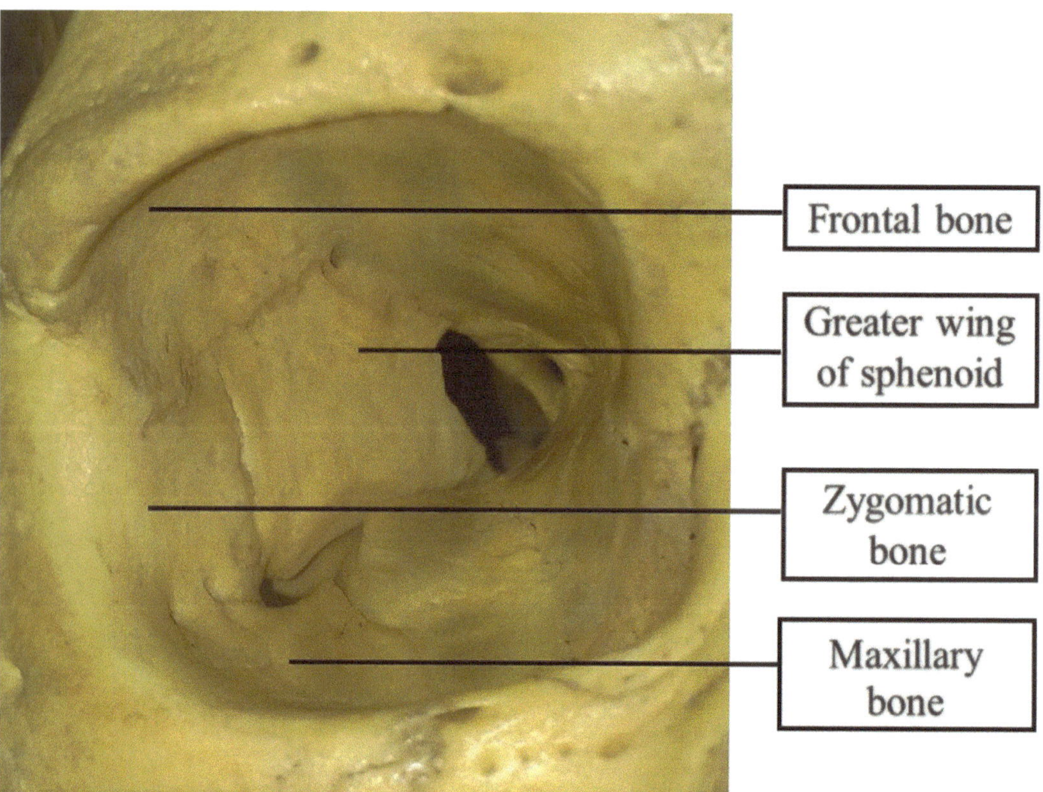

Fig. 2.1 The "anatomic" description of the right lateral orbital wall

The *sphenoid door jamb* consists of the greater wing of the sphenoid (Fig. 2.3). It is called the "trigone" of the greater wing and is filled with a large amount of bone marrow. Its lateral border forms the inferotemporal fossa in which temporalis muscle exists. The *basin of the inferior orbital fissure* is formed by the zygomatic bone and part of the lateral maxilla. It comprises the anterior and lateral parts of the inferior orbital fissure.

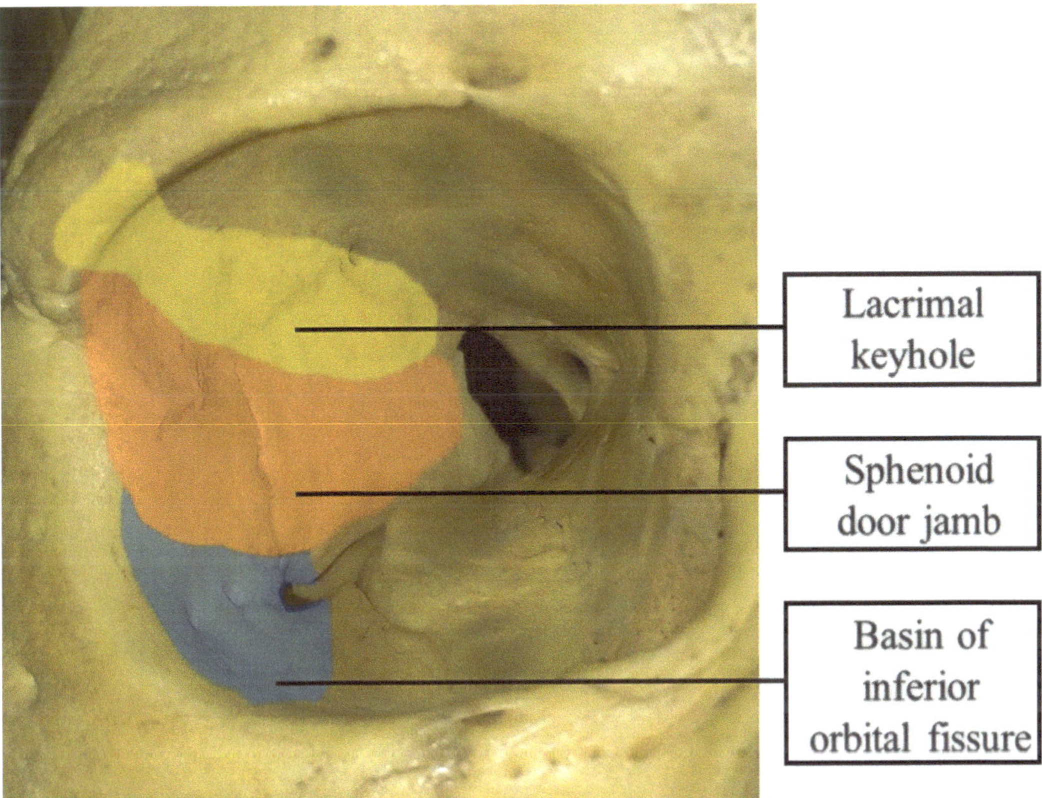

Fig. 2.2 The "conceptual" description of the right lateral orbital wall showing 3 areas of thick bone: lacrimal keyhole (yellow), sphenoid door jamb (orange) and basin of the inferior orbital fissure (blue)

The superior border of the lateral orbital wall is a thin cortical bone that underlies the anterior cranial fossa [7]. Anteriorly, it lies in parallel with the orbital roof, which serves as a guide for grinding (Fig. 2.4). Posteriorly, the orbital roof curves inferiorly and becomes perpendicular to the superior border of the lateral orbital wall [7].

The posterior border of the lateral orbital wall is also a thin cortical bone that is adjacent to the middle cranial fossa [8]. It is 12–24 mm wide and is located 26–33 mm posterior to the lateral orbital rim [8]. As the shape of the deep lateral orbital wall is a trigone and its posterior border is anteriorly curved, the posterior border is better observed when the surgeon stands contralateral to the operated orbit (Fig. 2.5) [6, 9].

In the junction between the superior and posterior border of the lateral orbital wall, a thick bone marrow exists (Fig. 2.6) [7]. However, this area corresponds to the junction of anterior and middle cranial fossa in the intracranial cavity (Fig. 2.7) [7]. Hence, the surgeons are advised to grind this junction smoothly. The superior orbital fissure, which is located medial to this junction, is used as a landmark to identify this area [7].

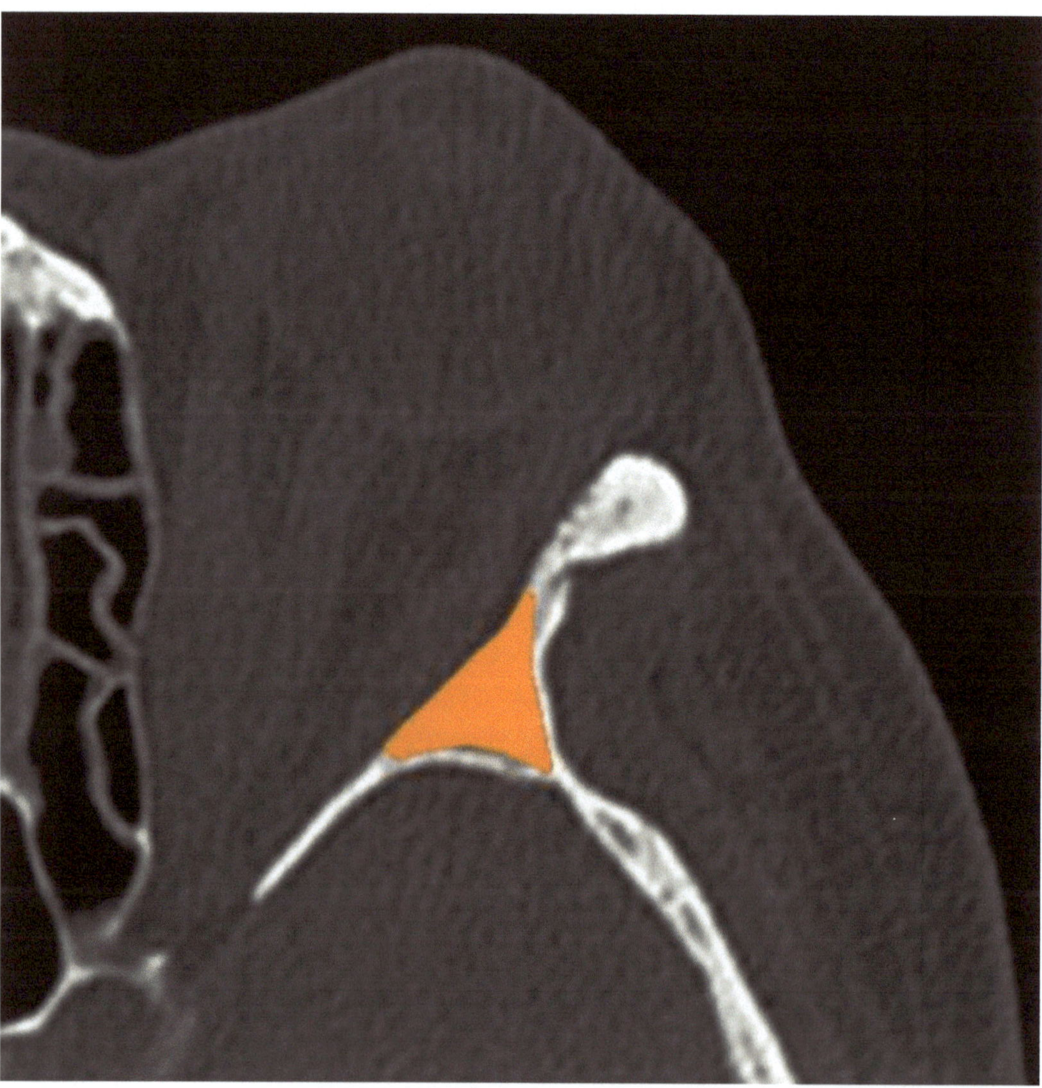

Fig. 2.3 Left axial computed tomographic image showing the orbital door jamb (orange)

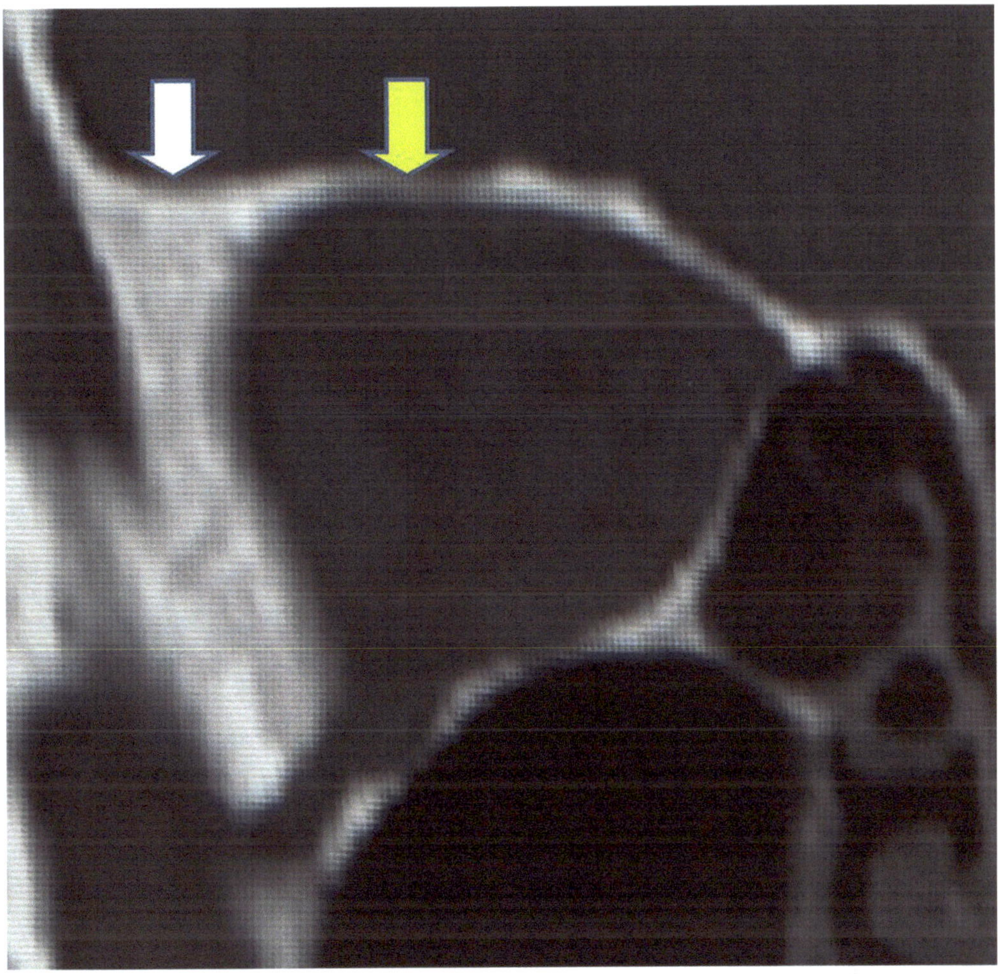

Fig. 2.4 Right coronal computed tomographic image shows superior border of door jamb. Anterior part of the superior border of door jamb (white arrow) lies parallel with the orbital roof (yellow arrow)

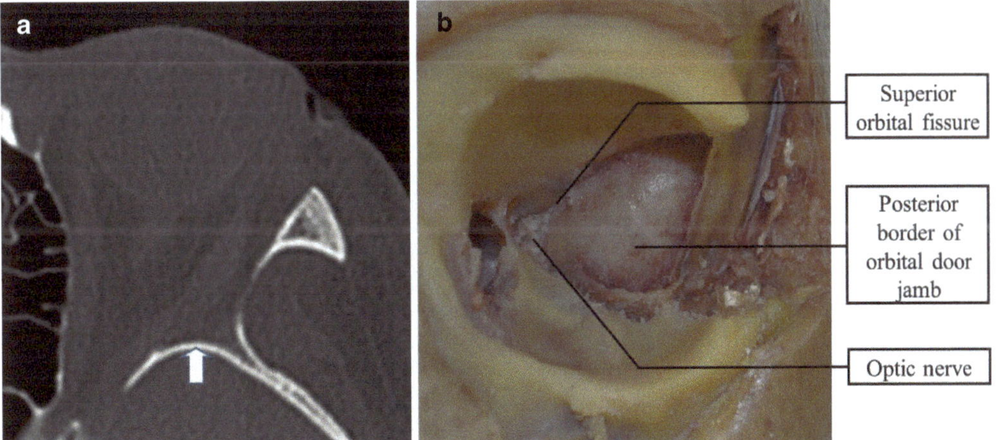

Fig. 2.5 Left axial computed tomographic image after deep lateral decompression shows the posterior border of door jamb (white arrow) is anteriorly curved (**a**). The same posterior border of orbital door jamb shown on the cadaver skull after bone removal from the left orbit (**b**)

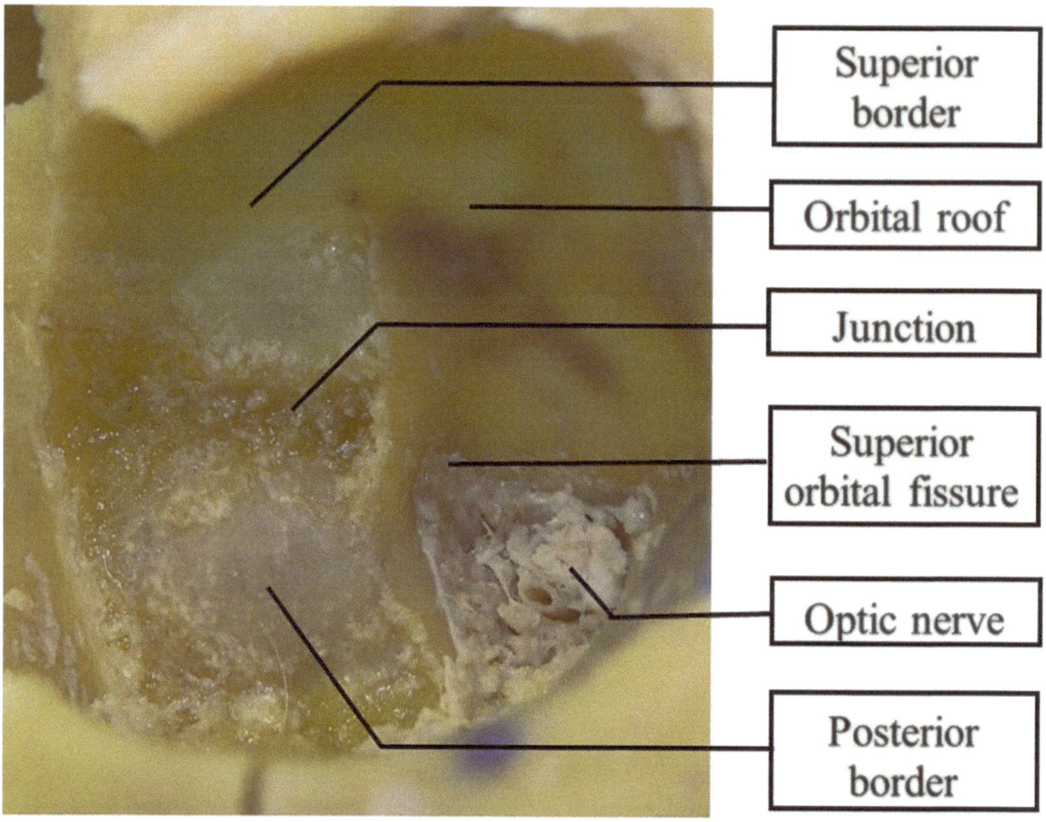

Superior border

Orbital roof

Junction

Superior orbital fissure

Optic nerve

Posterior border

Fig. 2.6 Right lateral orbital wall, depicting the thick junction between the superior and posterior borders of door jamb, lying just lateral to the superior orbital fissure

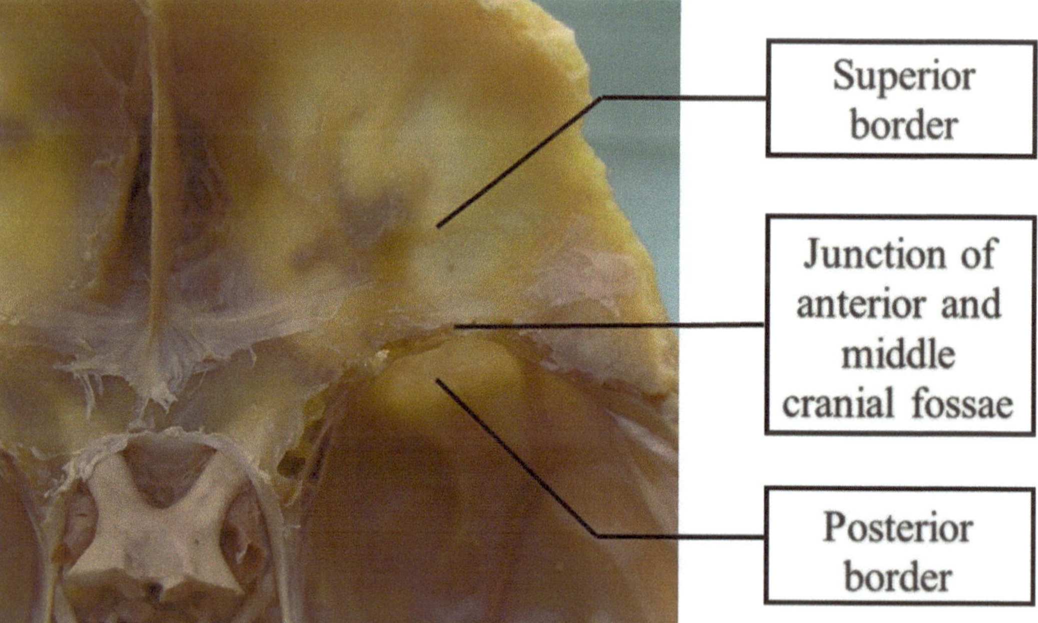

Fig. 2.7 Intracranial view showing the junction of superior and posterior borders of the door jamb that corresponds to the junction between the anterior and middle cranial fossae

2.3 Medial Orbital Wall

The medial orbital wall is composed of the lesser wing of the sphenoid, ethmoid bone, lacrimal bone, and frontal process of maxilla (Fig. 2.8). At its anterior aspect, it contains the lacrimal sac fossa that is bounded by the anterior (frontal process of maxilla) and posterior lacrimal crests (lacrimal bone). The lamina papyracea of the ethmoid, which forms the large part of the medial wall, is a paper-thin bone that is adjacent to the middle and posterior ethmoid cells. At the posterior aspect of medial wall, thick part of the sphenoid bone adjoins the optic canal. The inferior limit of medial wall removal is the thick inferomedial orbital strut [1], which is usually left intact anteriorly to support the globe [10]. This is marked by the maxilla-ethmoid suture [10].

The anterior limit of medial wall removal is the origin of Horner's muscle. It is located 2-4 mm posterior to the posterior lacrimal crest. The posterior limit of medial wall removal is posterior ethmoidal foramen, where the posterior ethmoidal nerves and vessels leave the orbit [11]. Bone removal beyond this level may cause optic nerve injury [11]. It is located 32–36 mm posterior to the anterior lacrimal crest [12–18].

Accessory ethmoidal foramina, namely middle and deep middle ethmoidal foramen, are occasionally present between the anterior and posterior foramina [12, 15, 16, 18]. These foramina are located 29.8 mm and 32.0 mm posterior to the anterior lacrimal crest, respectively [18]. Misidentification of these foramina as posterior ethmoidal foramen may result in insufficient bone removal [18].

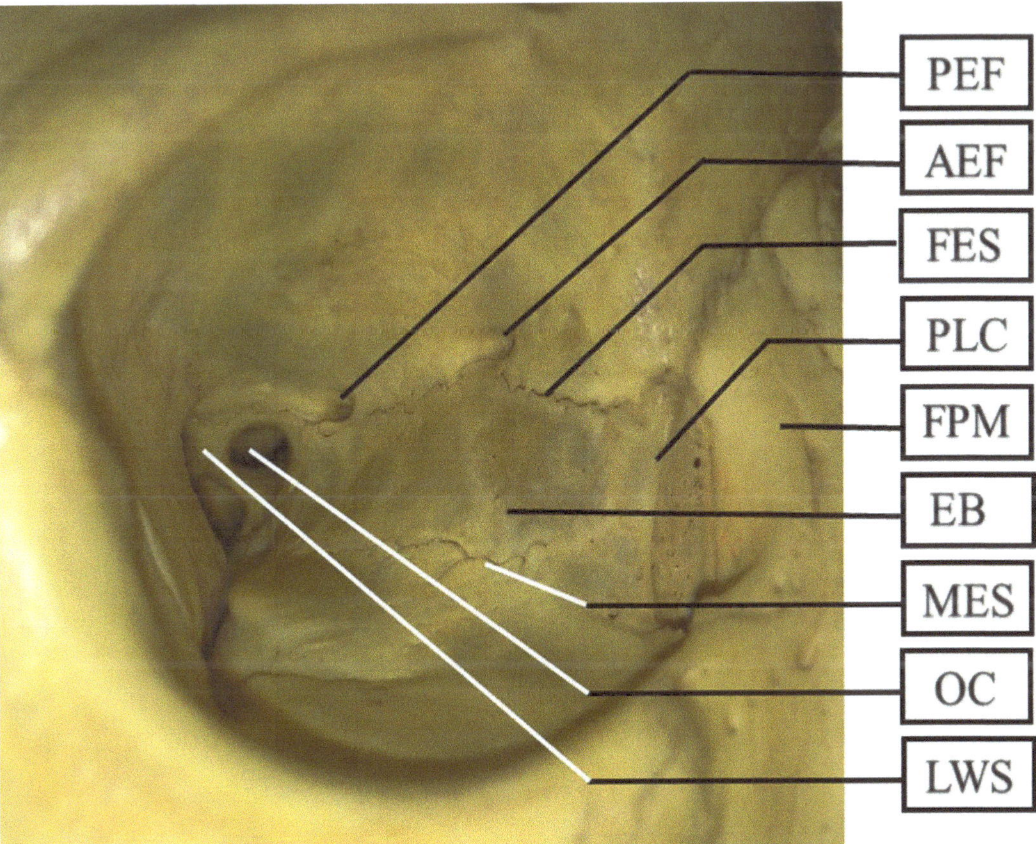

Fig. 2.8 Right medial orbital wall, slightly temporal coronal view. *PEF* posterior ethmoidal foramen, *AEF* anterior ethmoidal foramen, *FES* frontoethmoidal suture, *PLC* posterior lacrimal crest, *FPM* frontal process of maxilla, *EB* ethmoid bone, *MES* maxilla–ethmoid suture, *OC* optic canal, *LWS* lesser wing of sphenoid

The superior limit of medial wall removal is the frontoethmoidal suture [19]. Anteriorly at the level of this suture, the frontal sinus occupies between medial wall and ethmoidal roof. Posteriorly, the medial wall is directly attached to the ethmoidal roof (Fig. 2.9) [19]. Therefore, bone removal above the frontoethmoidal suture in the posterior orbit may cause CSF leakage [19].

Ethmoidal foramina serve as a landmark in patients with an obscure frontoethmoidal suture [20]. Anterior ethmoidal foramen is located approximately 9-mm above the superior border of the medial canthal tendon and 20-mm posterior to the anterior lacrimal crest [18, 2]. Ethmoidal foramina are commonly located on the frontoethmoidal suture. However, they are occasionally situated 0.5–4.0 mm above the suture [3, 12, 16, 20, 21, 22]. Extrasutural foramina are most frequently seen in anterior ethmoidal foramina, followed by accessory and posterior foramina, respectively [20].

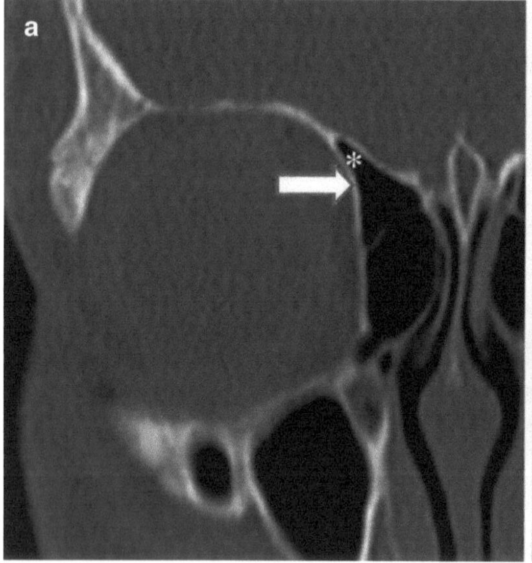

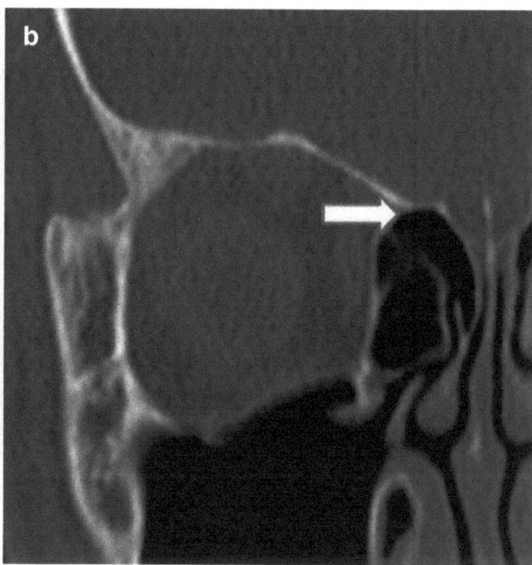

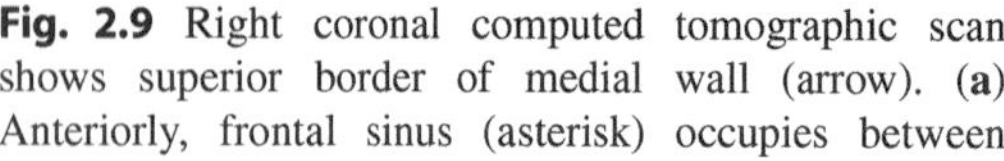

Fig. 2.9 Right coronal computed tomographic scan shows superior border of medial wall (arrow). (**a**) Anteriorly, frontal sinus (asterisk) occupies between medial wall superior border and skull base. (**b**) Posteriorly, the medial wall directly attaches to the skull base

2.4 Inferior Orbital Wall

The inferior orbital wall is composed of the zygomatic bone, palatine bone, and orbital process of the maxillary bone (Fig. 2.10). The inferior orbital wall is the roof of the maxillary sinus as well.

Anterior end of the inferior orbital fissure is located approximately 2 cm posterior to the inferolateral orbital rim [23]. It connects the pterygopalatine fossa with the inferior orbit and it also separates the inferior orbital wall from the lateral wall. On the posterior part of the fissure, the maxillary division of trigeminal nerve (V_2) enters the orbit after traversing the pterygopalatine fossa from the foramen rotundum. The nerve lies exposed in a sulcus in the anterior part of the inferior orbital wall where it is prone to surgical injury [10]. The infraorbital branch of the maxillary artery, inferior ophthalmic vein, and autonomic branches of pterygopalatine ganglion also cross the posterior part of the inferior orbital fissure.

The lateral limit of conservative inferior orbital wall removal is the infraorbital groove, which transmits the infraorbital artery and infraorbital nerve (Figs. 2.10 and 2.11). These continue anteriorly in the infraorbital canal through the inferior orbital wall and exit at the infraorbital foramen. The infraorbital foramen is located on the anterior side of maxilla at approximately 6.4 mm inferior to the inferior orbital rim and approximately 4.9 mm lateral to lateral margin of ala nasi [24, 4]. Medial to the infraorbital groove, the inferior orbital wall is anatomically weak [5, 25–28]. Inferior orbital wall decompression is usually commenced in this area. The bone lateral to this groove is occasionally fractured in case the bone is thinner than the medial [29].

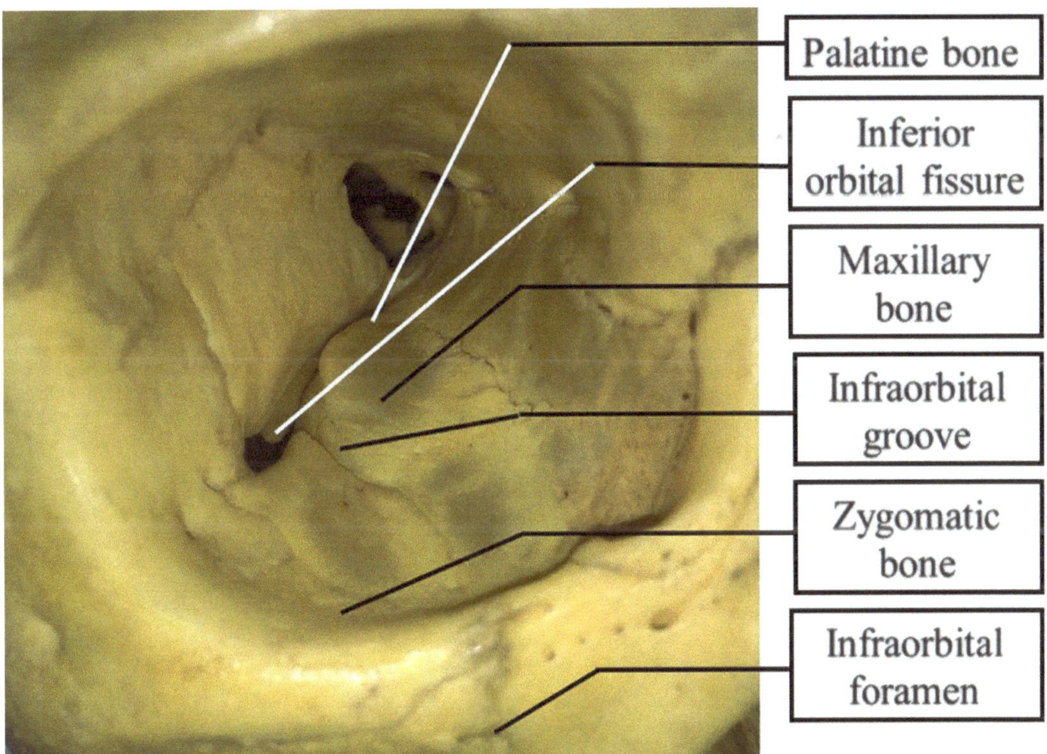

Fig. 2.10 Right inferior orbital wall, slightly top coronal view

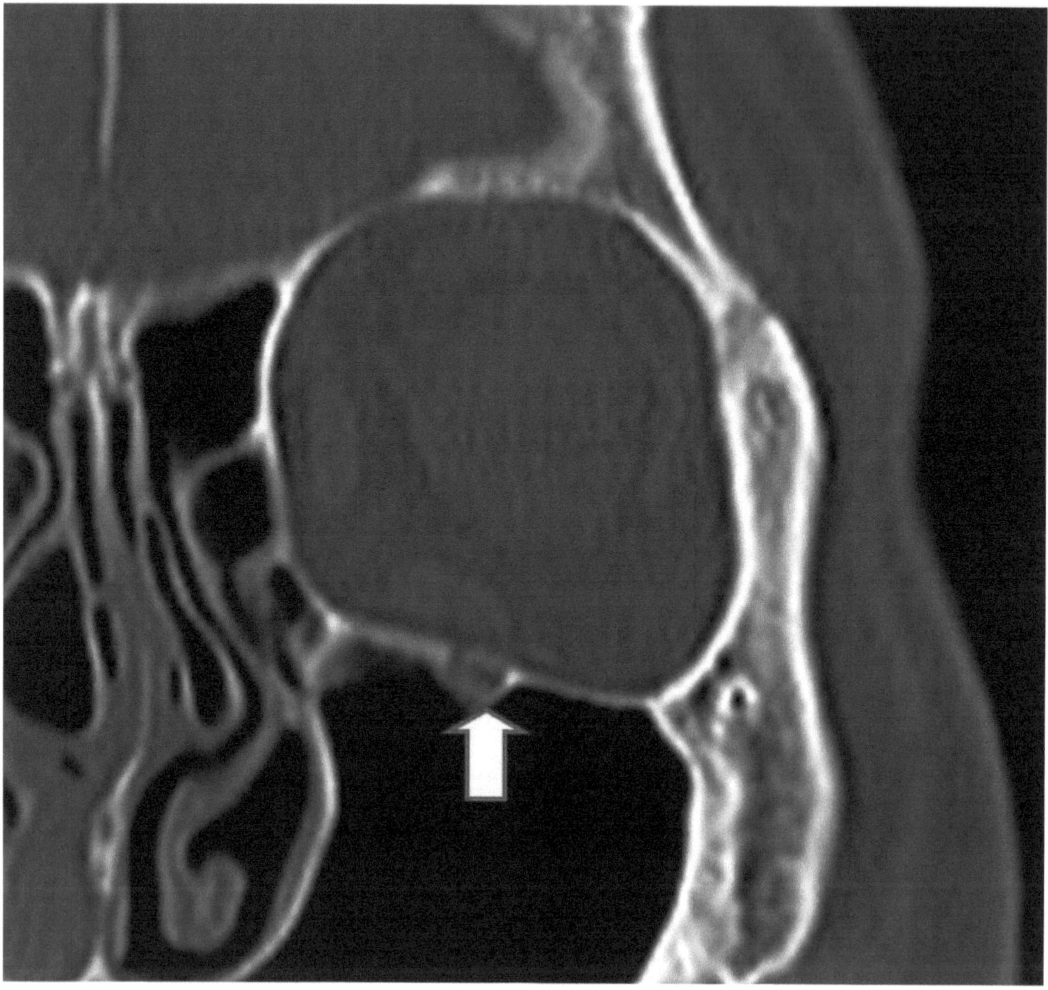

Fig. 2.11 Coronal computed tomographic image showing the left infraorbital nerve (arrow)

Acknowledgment All cadavers were Japanese and were registered with Aichi Medical University. Proper consent and approval were obtained prior to their use. The methods used to secure the tissues were humane and complied with the tenets of the Declaration of Helsinki.

References

1. Mahoney N, Grant MP, Susarla SM, Merbs S. Computer-assisted three-dimensional planning for orbital decompression. Craniomaxillofac Trauma Reconstr. 2015;8:211–7.
2. Takahashi Y, Kinoshita H, Nakano T, Asamoto K, Ichinose A, Kakizaki H. Anatomy of anterior ethmoidal foramen, medial canthal tendon, and lacrimal fossa for transcutaneous anterior Ethmoidal nerve block in Japanaese individuals. Ophthalmic Plast Reconstr Surg. 2014;30:431–3.
3. Berry AC, Berry RJ. Epigenetic variation in the human cranium. J Anat. 1967;101:361–79.
4. Takahashi Y, Kakizaki H, Nakano T. Infraorbital Foramen. Horizontal location in relation to ala nasi Ophthalmic Plast Reconstr Surg. 2011;27:295–7.
5. Takahashi Y, Nakano T, Miyazaki H, Kakizaki H. An anatomical study of the orbital floor in relation to the orbital groove: implications of predisposition to orbital floor fracture site. Graefes Arch Clin Exp Ophthalmol. 2016;254:2049–55.
6. Goldberg RA, Kim AJ, Kerivan KM. The lacrimal keyhole, orbital door jamb, and basin of the inferior orbital fissure. Three areas of deep bone in the lateral orbit. Arch Ophthalmol. 1998;116(12):1618–24.
7. Kakizaki H, Takahashi Y, Asamoto K, et al. Anatomy of the superior border of the lateral orbital wall: surgical implications in deep lateral orbital wall decompression surgery. Ophthalmic Plast Reconstr Surg. 2011;27:60–3.
8. Kakizaki H, Nakano T, Asamoto K, Iwaki M. Posterior border of the deep lateral orbital wall-appearance, width, and distance from the orbital rim. Ophthalmic Plast Reconstr Surg. 2008;24:262–5.
9. Kakizaki H. Advantageous surgeon's position in deep lateral orbital wall decompression. Orbit. 2011;30:131.
10. Rene C. Update on orbital anatomy. Eye. 2006;20:1119–29.
11. Choe CH, Cho RI, Elner VM. Comparison of lateral and medial orbital decompression for the treatment of compressive optic neuropathy in thyroid eye disease. Ophthalmic Plast Reconstr Surg. 2011;27:4–11.
12. Rontal E, Rontal M, Guilford FT. Surgical anatomy of the orbit. Ann Otol Rhinol Laryngol. 1979;88:382–6.
13. McQueen CT, DiRuggiero DC, Campbell JP, Shockley WW. Orbital osteology: a study of the surgical landmarks. Laryngoscope. 1995;105:783–8.
14. Hwang K, Baik SH. Surgical anatomy of Korean adults. J Craniofac Surg. 1999;10:129–34.
15. Karakas P, Bozkir MG, Oguz O. Morphometric measurements from various reference points in the orbit of male Caucasians. Surg Radiol Anat. 2003;24:358–62.
16. Cheng AC, Lucas PW, Yuen HK, et al. Surgical anatomy of the Chinese orbit. Ophthalmic Plast Reconstr Surg. 2008;24:136–41.
17. Nitek S, Wysocki J, Reymond J, Plasecki K. Correlations between selected parameters of the human skull and orbit. Med Sci Monit. 2009;15:370–7.
18. Takahashi Y, Kakizaki H, Nakano T. Accessory ethmoidal foramina: an anatomical study. Ophthalmic Plast Reconstr Surg. 2011;27:125–7.
19. Takahashi Y, Kakizaki H, Nakano T, et al. The ethmoidal sinus roof: anatomical relationships with the intracranial cavity. Ophthalmic Plast Reconstr Surg. 2010;26:372–4.
20. Takahashi Y, Kakizaki H, Nakano T, et al. An anatomical study of the positional relationship between the ethmoidal foramina and the frontoethmoidal suture. Ophthalmic Plast Reconstr Surg. 2011;27:457–9.
21. Kirschner JA, Yanagisawa E, Crelin ES. Surgical anatomy of the ethmoidal arteries: a laboratory study of 150 orbits. Arch Otolaryngol. 1961;74:382–6.
22. Isaacson G, Monge JM. Arterial ligation for pediatric epistaxis: developmental anatomy. Am J Rhinol. 2003;17:75–81.
23. Turvey T, Golden B. Orbital anatomy for the surgeon. Oral Maxillofac Surg Clin North Am. 2012;24(4):525–36.
24. Cutright B, Quillopa N, Schubert W. An anthropometric analysis of the key foramina for maxillafacial surgery. J Oral Maxillofac Surg. 2003;61(3):354–7.
25. Kang H, Takahashi Y, Kakizaki H. Isolated orbital floor fracture lateral to the infraorbital nerve: report of two pediatric patients. Can J Ophthalmol. 2015;50:121–2.
26. Strong EB, Tollefson TT. Sinonasal trauma. In: Kennedy DW, Hwang PH, editors. Rhinology: diseases of the nose, sinuses, and skull base. New York: Thieme Medical Publishers; 2012.
27. Jones DE, Evans JN. Blow-out fractures of the orbit: an investigation into their anatomical basis. J Laryngol Otol. 1967;81:1109–20.
28. Park JS, Lew H, Lee SY. Role of inferior orbital wall morphologic properties in isolated orbital blow-out fracture. Ophthalmic Res. 2012;47:1–6.
29. Ishida Y, Takahashi Y, Kitaguchi Y, Kakizaki H. Orbital floor thickness in adult patients with isolated orbital floor fracture lateral to the infraorbital nerve. J Craniofac Surg. 2016;27(7):e638–40.

3 Orbital Imaging for Orbital Decompression

Milind N. Naik

3.1 Introduction

Graves' disease is an autoimmune disorder characterized by thyroid gland hyperplasia and excessive production of thyroid hormones [1]. Involvement of the eye, also known as Graves' Ophthalmopathy or Thyroid Eye Disease (TED) is the most common extrathyroidal manifestation of Graves' disease [2]. TED results from infiltration of the orbital soft tissues with autoreactive T lymphocytes, proliferation of orbital fibroblasts, and increased adipocytes [3]. Clinically recognizable TED has been reported to occur in 25–50% of GD patients, and sight-threatening disease in 3–5% cases in the Western literature [4]. The diagnosis of TED is usually based on obvious clinical findings such as lid retraction and unilateral or bilateral proptosis in a person with systemic thyroid dysfunction [5]. Orbital imaging aids in ruling out the differential diagnosis, to assess disease activity (MRI), and surgical planning prior to orbital decompression [5]. It has been shown that orbital imaging reveals abnormalities in 90% of patients with Graves' disease [6].

3.2 Indications for Imaging in TED

Neuroimaging is important in the differential diagnosis and management of patients with TED. The indications for neuroimaging in TED are summarized in Table 3.1.

Table 3.1 Indications and advantages of orbital imaging in the management of TED

Phase of TED	Indication/Advantage
Acute phase or initial presentation	1. To rule out non-thyroid differential diagnosis in unilateral/atypical cases 2. Patient with TED and reduced vision, to rule out compressive optic neuropathy 3. Serial imaging to assess clinical activity (MRI) 4. Serves as early marker of TED in Euthyroid patients
Quiescent phase	5. Surgical planning for orbital decompression (CT scan)

M. N. Naik (✉)
Ophthalmic Plastic Surgery Service,
LV Prasad Eye Institute, Hyderabad, India

University of Rochester, Rochester, New York, USA
e-mail: milind@drmilindnaik.com

S. Rath, M. N. Naik (eds.), *Surgery in Thyroid Eye Disease*,
https://doi.org/10.1007/978-981-32-9220-8_3

3.3 Imaging Modalities

Despite adequate literature, there is no consensus on the imaging protocol for patients with TED. A European study showed variability among experts in the use of CT scan, MRI, ultrasound, and octreoscan for TED [7, 8]. The imaging modalities available are Computed Tomography (CT) scan, Magnetic Resonance Imaging (MRI), Orbital Ultrasound, and Octreotide scanning.

3.3.1 Computed Tomography Scan

Computed tomography uses X-rays to distinguish tissues by measuring their densities. The fat within the orbit forms an excellent natural intrinsic contrast within the orbital tissue, against which other soft tissues can be assessed with high anatomic accuracy [9]. The recent spiral (helical) technique and the multi-slice spiral (helical) techniques (MS-spiral-CT) allow quick data acquisition and increased axial resolution devoid of artifacts [10]. Radiation exposure is an important disadvantage of CT. The intraocular lens is the most sensitive organ, and a dose between 0.5 and 2 Gray can cause detectable opacities within the lens.

3.3.2 Magnetic Resonance Imaging

MRI does not use ionizing radiation, but generates cross-sectional images of the tissues using the physical phenomena of nuclear magnetic resonance. Atomic nuclei with an odd number of protons have a magnetic dipole moment (spin). Hydrogen (H+) is the most abundant ion in human tissue. In the presence of a magnetic field, the normally randomly arranged small magnetic dipoles tend to align in the direction of the magnetic field, and tumble around the direction of the external static magnetic field. Each nucleus has a specific precession frequency (Larmor frequency). These nuclei are then subjected to an external radio frequency pulse. The change in the spin and its return to normal emits electromagnetic waves that are specific to tissues. The energy of these waves is measured, and reconstructed to form an MR image [11].

MRI protocol for TED patients is T1-weighted images, and T2-weighted fat suppression or short tau inversion recovery (STIR) images in axial, coronal, and sagittal planes with 3-mm slice thickness. In addition, the calculation of T2 relaxation time of the enlarged rectus muscles enables one to define an objective degree of the inflammation [12]. The increased amount of polysaccharides in the inflamed extraocular muscles results in high amount of protons, thereby causing the lengthening of the T2-time. In this sequence, the echo time (TE from 20 to 400 ms) is measured in a long repetition time (TR > 3000 ms), resulting in a definite T2-time. It is measured over the affected rectus muscle, and compared to the unaffected temporalis muscle. The individual T2 time of both is compared, and the difference of both can be defined as the edema. (Fig. 3.1).

3.3.3 Orbital Ultrasound

Orbital ultrasound is easily accessible in an eye hospital, is low on cost and quick, and avoids radiation [13]. Low precision in tissue assessment, and inability to characterize disease activity are the drawbacks. Visualization of contiguous orbital structures is not as precise as CT scan, and it is not effective in assessing the orbital apex or bony walls. The muscle measurements are investigator dependent and not as accurate as MRI [14]. Therefore, orbital ultrasound though possible, is not the imaging modality of choice.

3.3.4 Octreotide Scan

Scanning with the labelled octreotide (octreoscan) has a high sensitivity in the evaluation of patients with TED. A positive orbital octreoscan indicates clinically active disease in which immunosuppressive treatment might be of therapeutic benefit [15]. It is helpful in the initial stages as well as during treatment. However, it is an expensive method, has radiation exposure, and a high interobserver variability [16]. It is not specific, and does not offer detailed morphological orbital imaging provided by CT scan or MRI.

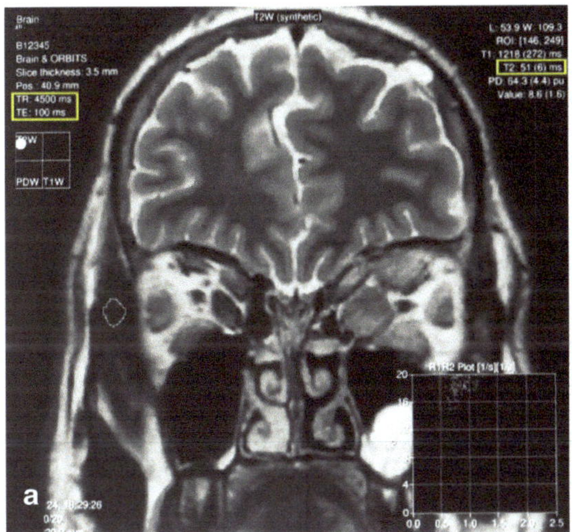

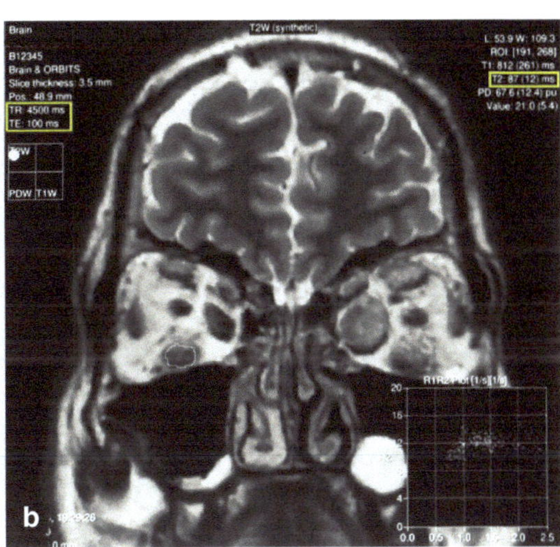

Fig. 3.1 Utility of magnetic resonance imaging in detecting thyroid eye disease activity. Coronal view showing measurement of the T2 time. Measurement of noninvolved right temporalis muscle with Echo Time (TE) 100 and a long repetition time (TR) of 4500 showing a short T2 time of 56 ms (**a**). Corresponding measurement of right inferior rectus with same TE and TR parameters, showing a prolonged T2 time of 87 ms indicating a "wet" or "inflammed" muscle (**b**)

3.4 Role of Imaging in Active Phase of the Disease

In the active phase or at the initial presentation, imaging is useful in 3 ways (Table 3.2). Firstly, to rule in the clinically suspected TED, or rule out other differential diagnoses. Secondly, to assess disease activity (amount of inflammatory component), and thirdly assessment of suspected compressive optic neuropathy.

Table 3.2 Role of imaging in active TED

Indication	Useful radiological signs
To *rule-in* the diagnosis of TED	1. Classic muscle enlargement 2. Optic nerve straightening/ stretching 3. Radiologic measurement of proptosis (Hilal and Trokel method)
To *rule-out* the differential diagnosis of TED	1. Muscle tendon not spared 2. Orbital mass mimicking TED
To assess disease activity	1. Increased T2 relaxation time in the extraocular muscles on MRI 2. High signal intensity in T2 images on MRI 3. Dynamic contrast enhanced MRI
To assess suspected Compressive Optic neuropathy	1. Barrett's muscle index 2. Nugent grading scale

3.4.1 *Rule in* the Diagnosis of TED

TED is the most frequent cause of unilateral or bilateral proptosis in adults [17]. In most cases, diagnosis of TED is clinically obvious: lid retraction with unilateral or bilateral proptosis. The classic radiological finding in TED is spindle-shaped enlargement of one or more extraocular muscles (>4 mm) without the involvement of the corresponding tendon, seen best on axial views of CT or MRI (Fig. 3.2) [18].

Preferential muscle involvement, in order of frequency includes inferior rectus, followed by the medial, the superior and finally the lateral rectus muscle seen best on coronal views (Fig. 3.3).

Another radiologic finding in TED is the increase in orbital fat space, leading to proptosis and straightening or stretching of the optic nerves (Fig. 3.4).

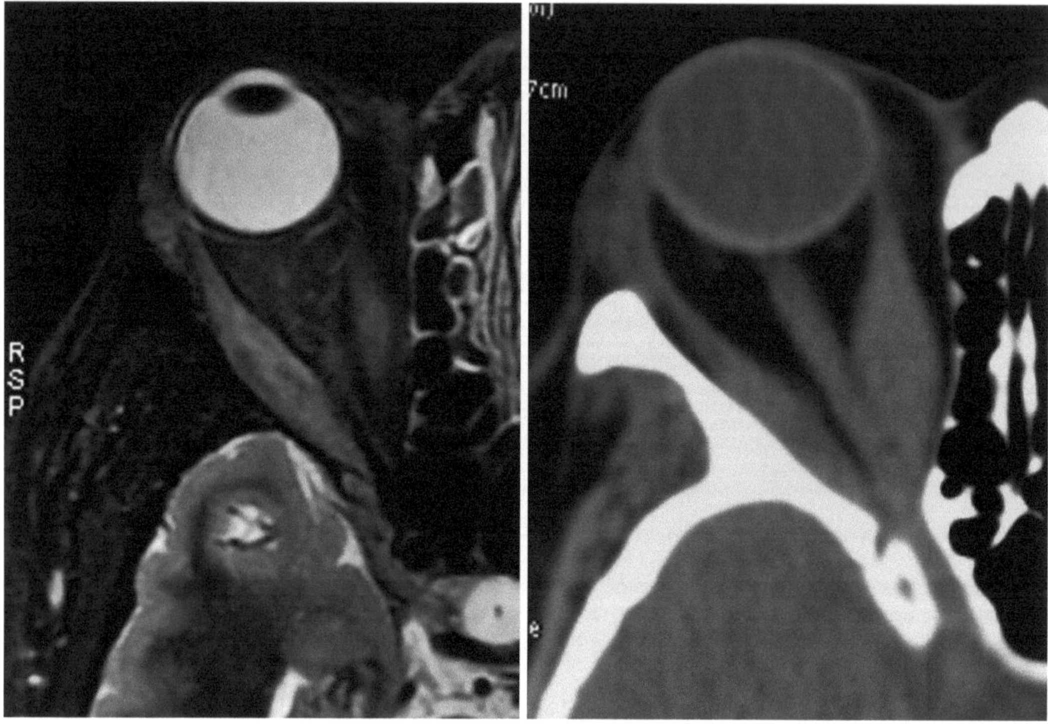

Fig. 3.2 Axial magnetic resonance imaging (left) and computed tomography (right) scan images showing the classic spindle-shaped enlargement of extraocular muscles in thyroid eye disease. Note the sparing of the tendons closer to the globe

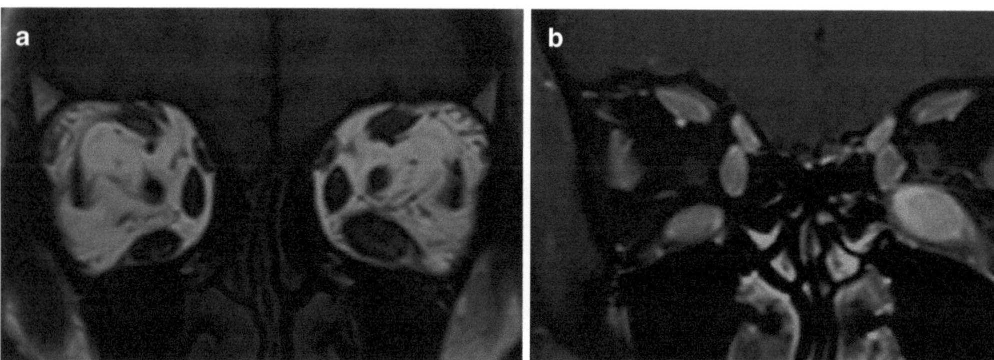

Fig. 3.3 Axial MRI scans with T2 image (**a**) and with fat suppression (**b**) showing the classic enlargement of extraocular muscles in thyroid eye disease. The inferior rectus is the commonest muscle affected, followed by medial rectus, superior rectus, and the lateral rectus

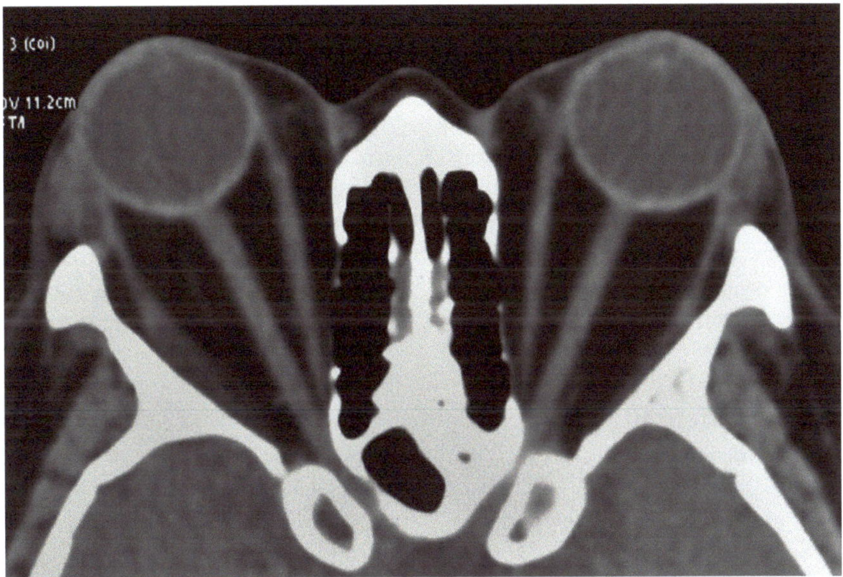

Fig. 3.4 Axial computed tomography scan of the orbit in a case of thyroid eye disease, showing predominantly fat disease. Note the stretching of the optic nerve, indicated by its straightening noted on axial scan

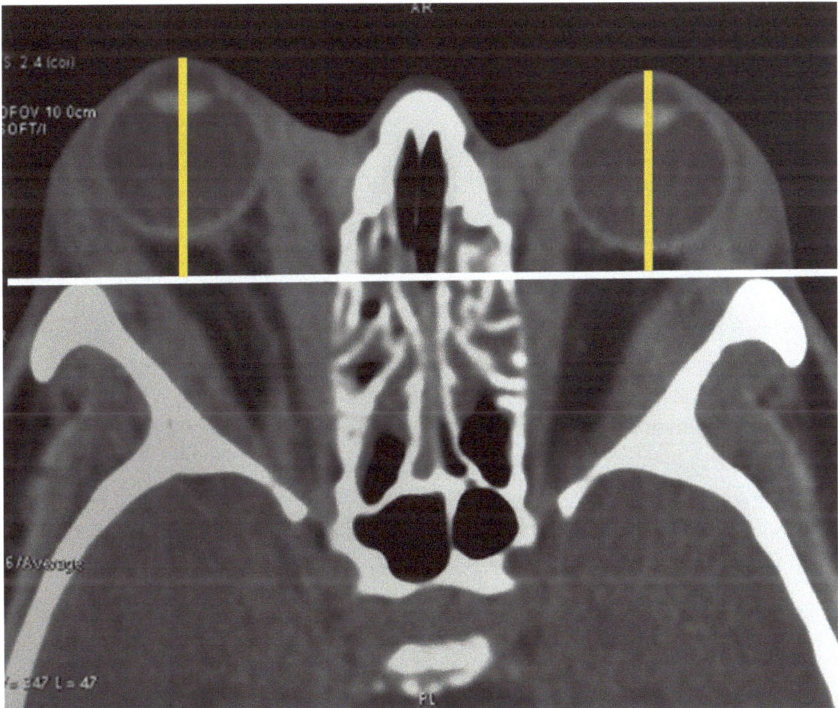

Fig. 3.5 Proptosis can be measured radiologically by the technique described by Hilal and Trokel [19]. A mid-orbital axial scan is chosen, and a line is drawn at the anterior margin of the lateral orbital wall (white line). Another line placed perpendicular (yellow line) measures the distance between the cornea and the inter-zygomatic line. Asymmetry greater than 2 mm or value above 21 mm indicates proptosis

In both these types of TED (muscle disease and fat disease), proptosis is a common feature, and can be radiologically measured by the technique described by Hilal and Trokel [19]. Using a mid-orbital axial scan, a line is drawn at the anterior margin of the lateral orbital wall (Fig. 3.5). Another line placed perpendicular measures the distance between the cornea and this interzygomatic line. Asymmetry greater than 2 mm or value above 21 mm indicates proptosis.

3.4.2 *Rule out* Differential Diagnosis

In unilateral or atypical cases, the diagnosis may be uncertain and hence orbital imaging is advisable [17]. In unilateral TED, imaging can help rule out other causes [20, 21]. Some common differential diagnoses based on the signs of proptosis and motility restriction include orbital myositis, orbital tumors, myasthenia gravis, carotid-cavernous fistula, and progressive external ophthalmoplegia. The important differential diagnosis is myositis. Typically the involved muscle is enlarged including the tendon [22]. Other differential diagnosis of TED include lymphoma, metastasis, and carotid-sinus cavernous fistula [23].

3.4.3 To Assess Disease Activity

During the active inflammatory phase of the disease, muscle enlargement is characterized by cellular infiltration, accumulation of glycosaminoglycans, and edematous changes. A CT scan is unlikely to detect these changes, and would simply show it as muscle enlargement irrespective of edema or fibrosis. On CT scan, intraorbital fat can show stranding and increased density caused by vascular congestion and lymphocytic proliferation [24].

MRI is preferred over CT in the assessment of disease activity, because it can estimate the water content of tissues [11]. MRI is a promising modality to detect disease activity. An increased T2 relaxation time in the extraocular muscles suggests inflammation or a "wet" muscle (Fig. 3.1), thereby predicting the beneficial effect of orbital irradiation or immunosuppressive therapy [25]. High signal intensity in T2 images also indicates disease activity. Early MR studies demonstrated that changes in signal intensity of the EOM on short tau inversion recovery sequences (STIR) correlate with clinical activity score (CAS) [26]. Dynamic contrast-enhanced MRI parameters have also been shown to correlate with disease activity scores and potentially provide a tool for the investigation of EOM microcirculatory changes in TED [27].

3.4.4 To Assess Suspected Compressive Optic Neuropathy

A direct correlation between the degree of muscle enlargement with resultant perineural fat effacement and the clinical severity of optic neuropathy has been repeatedly demonstrated in multiple studies [28–30].

Barrett's muscle index (MI) is measured with a ruler on coronal scans at a point halfway between the posterior globe and the orbital apex [28]. The vertical index is calculated by the sum of the vertical muscle diameters (superior and inferior recti) divided by the height of the orbit along a vertical line through the optic nerve. The horizontal index is calculated by dividing the sum of the horizontal muscle diameters (lateral and medial recti) by the horizontal diameter of the orbit along a horizontal line through the optic nerve (Fig. 3.6). The larger of these two values is taken as the final muscle index. A muscle index >67% is indicative of optic neuropathy with 67% sensitivity.

Optic nerve crowding caused by enlarged extraocular muscles at the orbital apex is assessed on coronal images by *Nugent grading scale* [29]. The effacement of perineural fat planes around the optic nerve was assessed. Grade 0 reflects no effacement of perineural fat planes by enlarged extraocular muscles; grade 1 reflects 1% to 25% effacement; grade 2 reflects 25% to 50% effacement; and grade 3 reflects greater than 50% effacement (Fig. 3.7).

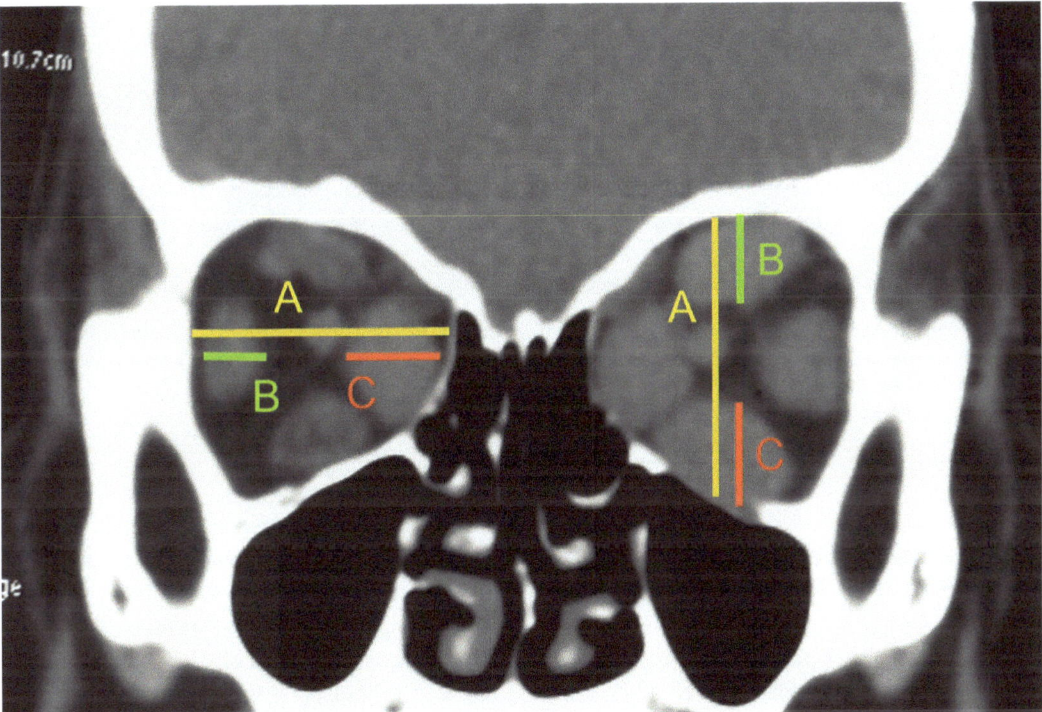

Fig. 3.6 Barrett's muscle index (MI) as a measure of nerve compression. The vertical index is calculated by the sum of the vertical muscle diameters (B + C) divided by the height of the orbit along a vertical line through the optic nerve (A). The horizontal index is calculated by dividing the sum of the horizontal muscle diameters (B + C) by the horizontal diameter of the orbit along a horizontal line through the optic nerve (A). The larger of these two values is taken as the final muscle index. A muscle index >67% is indicative of compressive optic neuropathy

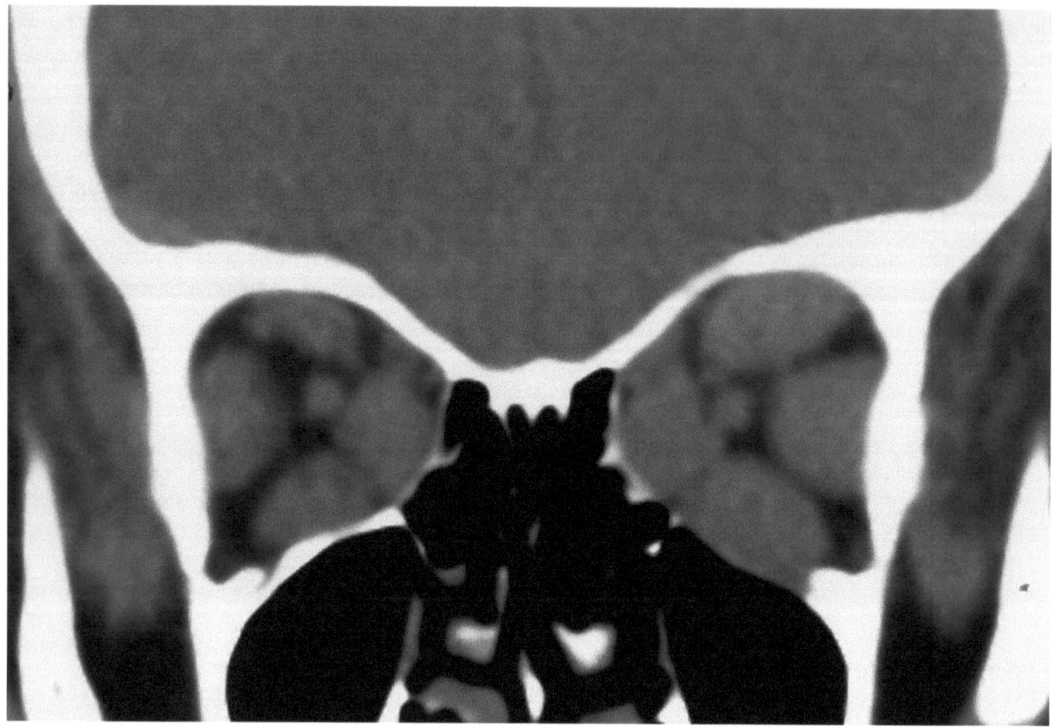

Fig. 3.7 Nugent's grading scale assesses effacement of perineural fat planes around the optic nerve. Assessment is performed at the apex, on coronal scans. The lack of visibility of fat between the enlarged muscle and the optic nerve is assessed, and graded from Grade 0 to 3. In this case both right and left eye is Grade 1 as only medial rectus is touching the optic nerve

3.5 Role of Imaging in Quiescent Phase: Surgical Planning

Imaging in the quiescent phase can be helpful in two ways: to confirm that inflammatory (wet) component within the muscles has resolved (MRI), and for surgical planning prior to decompression (CT).

In this phase, the orbital muscles show reduced edema, increased fibrotic change, reduction in muscle fibers, and fatty infiltration with subsequent loss of elasticity [31]. MRI shows heterogeneity of the muscles on T2-weighted images and the appearance of low signal-intensity regions suggestive of fibrotic changes [32].

In long-standing TED, the chronically increased orbital pressure can displace the thin medial wall medially. When this finding is bilateral, a "spontaneous bony decompression" like picture is noted leading to the so-called "Coca Cola-sign" (Fig. 3.8).

CT scan is the imaging modality of choice when it comes to evaluation and surgical planning of an orbital decompression. A plain CT

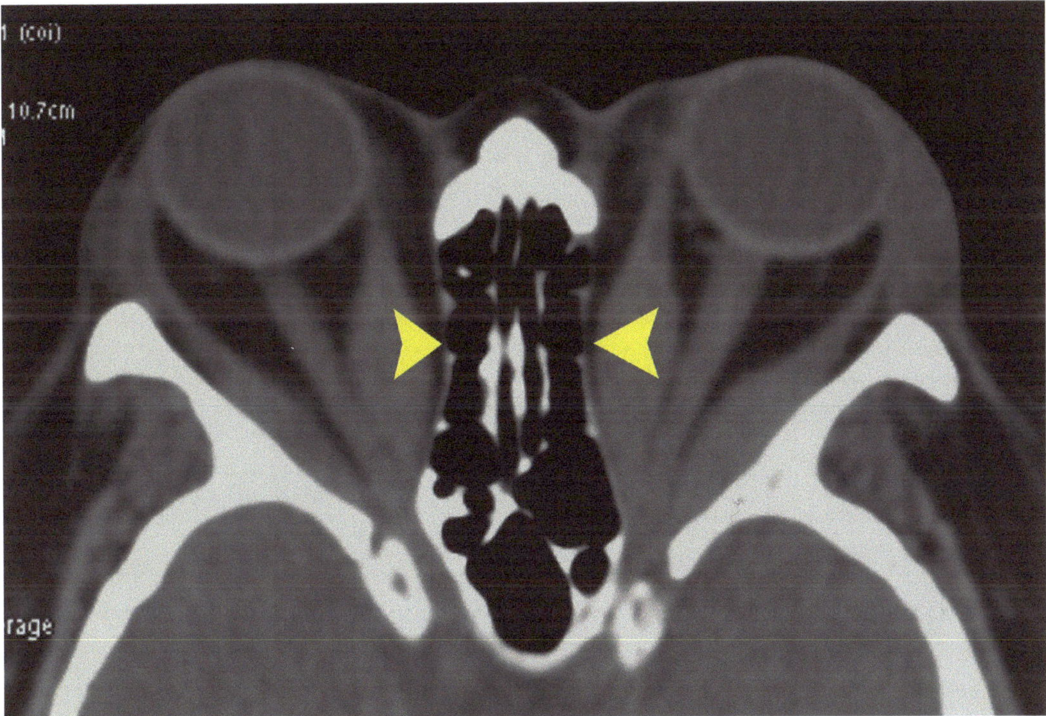

Fig. 3.8 In long-standing thyroid eye disease, the chronic increase in orbital pressure displaces the thin medial wall medially. When this finding is bilateral, a "spontaneous bony decompression" like picture is noted. It is popularly called the "Coca Cola-sign" due to its resemblance to the shape of the coca-cola bottle

scan (axial and coronal) of the orbit is enough if an orbital decompression is being planned. Both soft tissue and bone windows should be requested for better assessment of the anatomy. If the surgery is being performed under navigation guidance, the appropriate navigation protocol has to be obtained on a compact disc (as per the navigation equipment provider's specifications).

The following key information can be looked at when we evaluate a CT scan prior to any decompression: global parameters, medial wall, floor, and lateral wall (Table 3.3).

Table 3.3 Role of imaging in quiescent TED (Surgical planning)

Parameter	Useful radiological signs
Global parameters	1. Disease type (fat, muscle, or mixed) 2. Depth of the orbit (Shallow or deep) 3. 'Coca-cola' sign
Medial wall	1. Ethmoid sinus space (roomy/small) 2. Position of cribriform plate 3. Aeration of fronto-ethmoid sinus complex
Orbital floor	1. Infraorbital canal/groove 2. Position of infraorbital nerve (medial/central) 3. Bone thickness
Lateral wall	1. Bone thickness 2. Trigone volume

3.5.1 Global Parameters

The disease type and the depth of the orbit are two general global parameters that are important. One can classify the *disease type* into predominantly fat, muscle, or a mixed type (Fig. 3.9).

In a purely fat disease, intraoperative retraction and visualization of the anatomy are relatively easy, especially at the depths. Fat disease is also less likely to cause compressive optic neuropathy. On the other hand, a muscle disease is a relatively firm orbit, where visualization can be a challenge. Nerve compression is more likely, so is strabismus. Often, it is a mix of both these types.

Eyeballing the *depth of the orbit* is also important. A deep orbit has enough bony scope for orbital decompression, whereas a shallow orbit would yield limited reduction in proptosis (Fig. 3.10). A case of craniosynostosis is an extreme case of a shallow orbit. Even in TED cases, some orbits may be shallow, and therefore the amount of decompression that can be achieved will be limited.

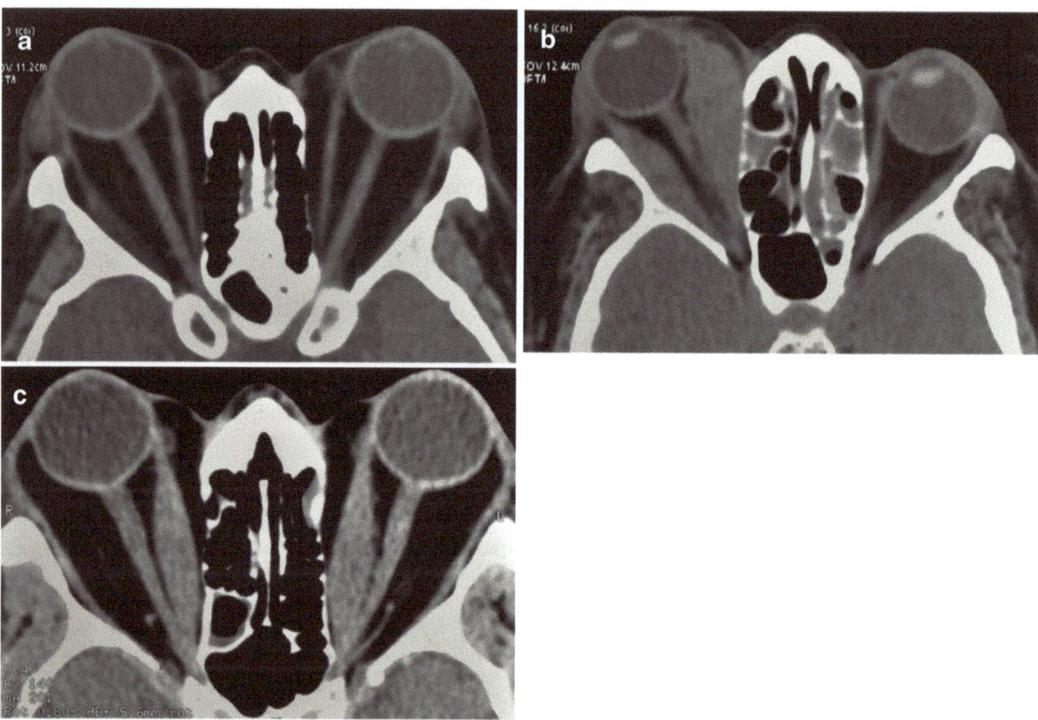

Fig. 3.9 Computed tomography scans showing the three predominant types of thyroid eye disease. The fat predominant type (**a**), the muscle predominant type (**b**) and the mixed type (**c**)

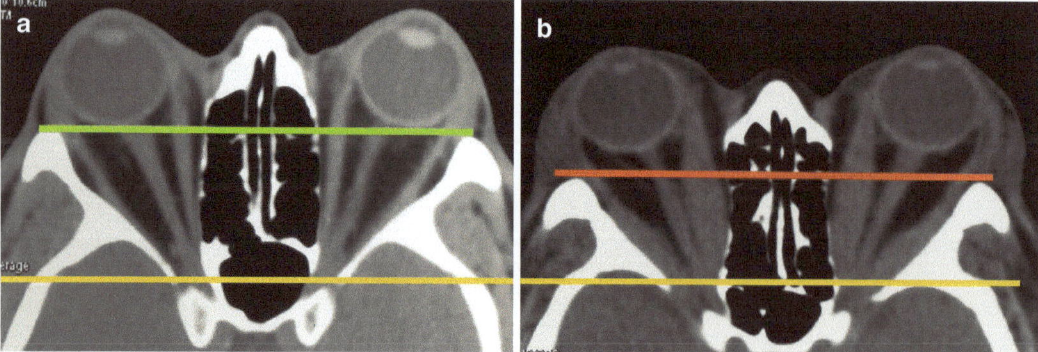

Fig. 3.10 The anteroposterior depth of the orbit can have a bearing on the amount of decompression possible, especially with respect to the lateral wall. A deep (**a**) orbit can allow more decompression than a shallow orbit. (**b**) A case of craniosynostosis is an extreme case of a shallow orbit

3.5.2 Medial Wall

The space available within the ethmoid sinuses can also vary widely. Some are roomy, thereby giving a good advantage of medial wall decompression whereas others will provide very little extra space if decompressed (Fig. 3.11).

Simultaneously, the proximity and position of the cribriform plate should be studied. Some patients have a low cribriform plate, whereas in others, it is well protected by an aerated fronto-ethmoid sinus complex (Fig. 3.12).

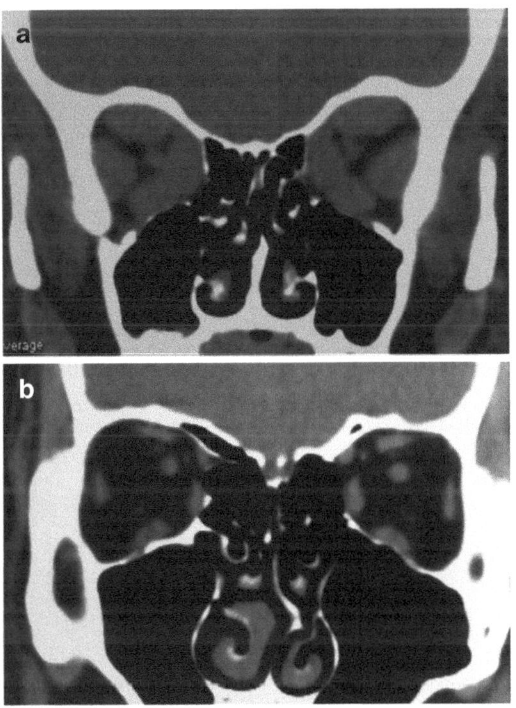

Fig. 3.11 The available volume within the ethmoid sinuses can also vary from patient to patient. Small ethmoids (**a**), provide very little space if decompressed, compared to roomy (**b**) ethmoids. Although difficult to quantify, eyeballing the overall size of available ethmoids helps in surgical planning

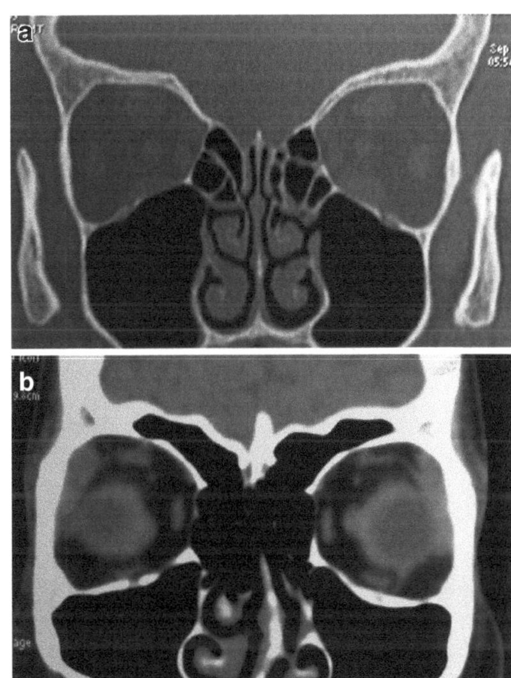

Fig. 3.12 The proximity and position of the cribriform plate should be assessed on coronal scans. A low cribriform plate (**a**) is more at risk of CSF leak during medial wall decompression, than a high cribriform plate that is well protected by an aerated fronto-ethmoid sinus complex (**b**)

3.5.3 Orbital Floor

If floor decompression is being planned, it is good to take a close look at the bone windows and identify the anatomy of the infraorbital nerve: its location, and bony walls. It can be either an infraorbital groove or a canal. Its location too may vary, with some nerves more medially placed than others (Fig. 3.13).

Infraorbital anesthesia is often a troublesome post-operative symptom and paying attention to this aspect helps you prepare the patient for it. In some cases, it also allows you to think ahead, and plan for a piezoelectric floor decompression. Similarly, noting the thickness of the floor would tell you if a mechanical drill would be required, or the bone can be cracked easily for the bone punching (Fig. 3.13).

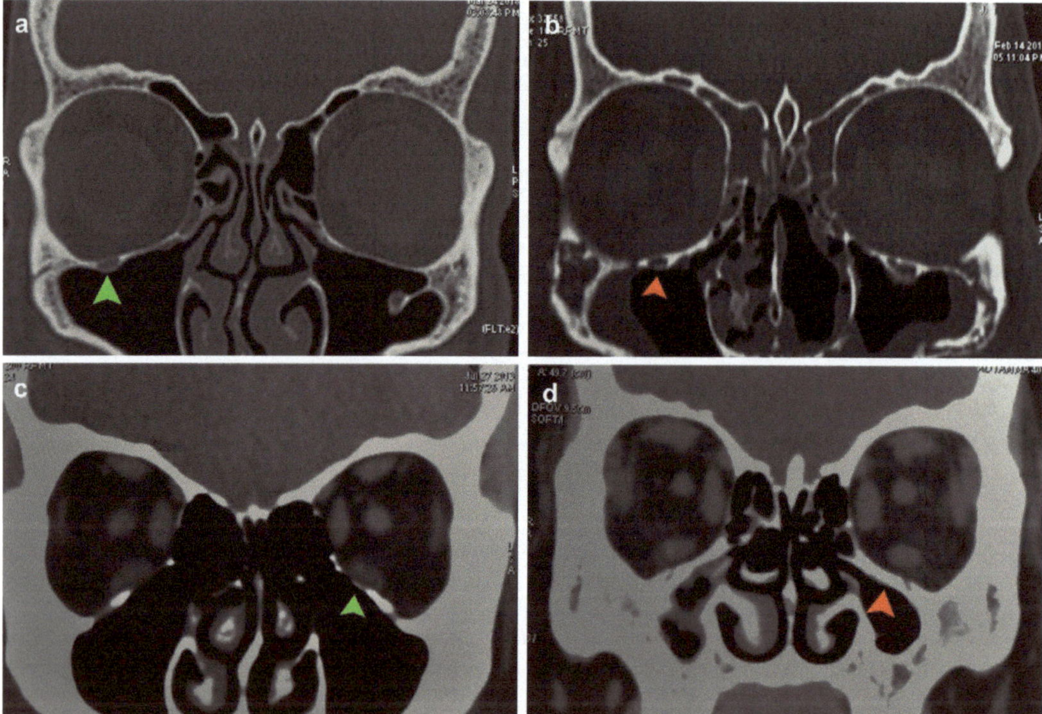

Fig. 3.13 Assessment of the floor on computed tomography scans is important prior to the decompression. Assess the bone windows and note the location of the infraorbital nerve: it could be more lateral (**a**), or medial (**b**). It can be either an infraorbital groove, or a canal. Similarly, note the thickness of the floor. A thin floor (**c**) is easy to crack, and punch with a Kerrison's rongeur. Thick floor (**d**) may need a mechanical drill, or a piezoelectric floor decompression

3.5.4 Lateral Wall

The available bony thickness of the lateral wall, especially the trigone may also vary from patient to patient (Fig. 3.14). Evaluating this would give you a fair idea of the available benefit from lateral wall decompression. In re-surgeries, assessing the bony anatomy is important (for example, part of the orbital rim could be missing), and should be taken into consideration.

In conclusion, imaging has a significant role in the management of TED. Although there is no consensus on the right imaging modality to be used, CT and MRI are most widely preferred. It helps in differential diagnosis from other orbital disorders, assessment of disease activity, diagnosis of compressive optic neuropathy, and in surgical planning.

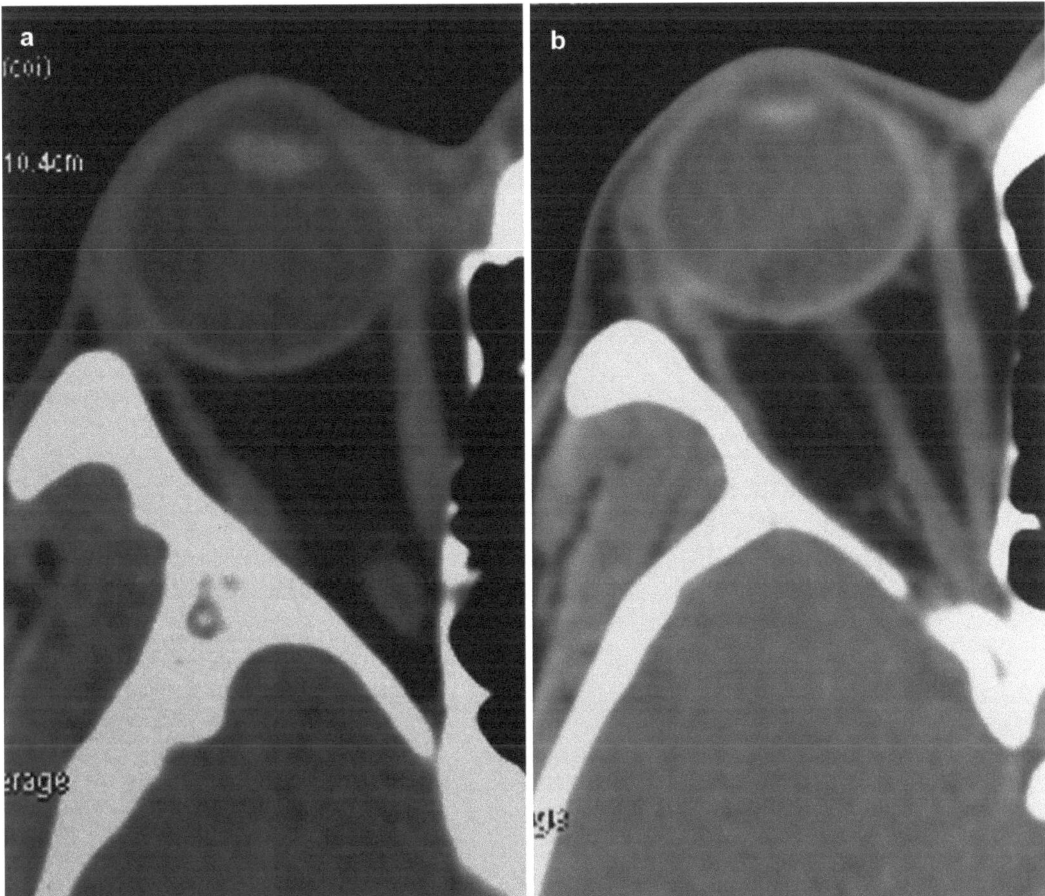

Fig. 3.14 The bony thickness of the lateral wall (trigone) and the greater wing of sphenoid can vary. Some patients have a thicker lateral wall (**a**) compared to others (**b**). Assessment of this bony thickness can give you a fair idea of the available benefit from lateral wall decompression

References

1. Brent GA. Clinical practice. Graves' disease. N Engl J Med. 2008;358:2594–605.
2. Bartalena L, Tanda ML. Clinical practice. Graves' ophthalmopathy. N Engl J Med. 2009;360:994–1001.
3. Naik VM, Naik MN, Goldberg RA, Smith TJ, Douglas RS. Immunopathogenesis of thyroid eye disease: emerging paradigms. Surv Ophthalmol. 2010;55:215–26.
4. Stan MN, Bahn RS. Risk factors for development or deterioration of graves' ophthalmopathy. Thyroid. 2010;20:777–83.
5. Dickinson AJ. Clinical manifestations. In: Wiersinga WM, Kahaly GJ, editors. Graves' orbitopathy: a multidisciplinary approach–questions and answers. 2nd ed. Basel: Karger; 2010. p. 1–25.
6. Müller-Forell W, Pitz S, Mann W, et al. Neuroradiological diagnosis of thyroid-associated orbitopathy. Exp Clin Endocrinol Diabetes. 1999;107:177–83.
7. Bartalena L, Pinchera A, Marcocci C. Management of Graves' ophthalmopathy: reality and perspectives. Endocr Rev. 2000;21:168–99.
8. Weetman AP, Wiersinga WM. Current management of thyroid- associated ophthalmopathy in Europe. Results of an international survey. Clin Endocrinol. 1998;49:21–8.
9. Naik MN, Tourani KL, Sekhar GC, Honavar SG. Interpretation of computed tomography imaging of the eye and orbit. A systematic approach. Indian J Ophthalmol. 2002 Dec;50(4):339–53.
10. Ohnesorge B, Flohr T, Schaller S, et al. Principles and applications of multi-slice CT. Radiology. 1999;11:923–31.
11. Wichmann W. Magnetic resonance imaging (MRI). In: Müller-Forell W, editor. Imaging of orbital and visual pathway pathology. Heidelberg: Springer; 2002.
12. Hosten N, Sander B, Cordes M, et al. Graves'ophthalmopathy: MR imaging of the orbits. Radiology. 1989;172:759–62.
13. Prummel M, Suttorp-Schulten M, Wiersinga WM, et al. A new ultrasonographic method to detect disease activity and predict response to immunosuppressive treatment in graves' ophthalmopathy. Ophthalmology. 1993;100:556–61.
14. Kahaly GJ. Recent developments in graves' ophthalmology imaging. J Endocrinol Investig. 2004;27:254–8.
15. Krassas GE, Kahaly GJ. The role of octreoscan in thyroid eye disease. Eur J Endocrinol. 1999;140:373–5.
16. Förster GJ, Krummenauer F, Nickel O, Kahaly GJ. Somatostatin-receptor scintigraphy in graves' disease: reproducibility and variance of orbital activity. Cancer Biother Radiopharm. 2000 Oct;15(5):517–25.
17. Mourits MP. Diagnosis and differential diagnosis of graves' orbitopathy. In: Wiersinga WM, Kahaly GJ, editors. Graves' orbitopathy: a multidisciplinary approach–questions and answers. 2nd ed. Basel: Karger; 2010. p. 66–76.
18. Peyster RG, Hoover ED. Graves' orbitopathy. In: Peyster RG, Hoover ED, editors. Computerized tomography in orbital diseases and neuro-ophthalmology. Chicago: Year Book Medical Publishers; 1984. p. 97–114.
19. Hilal SK, Trokel SL. Computerized tomography of the orbit using thin sections. Semin Roentgenol. 1977;12:137–47.
20. Strianese D, Piscopo R, Elefante A, et al. Unilateral proptosis in thyroid eye disease with subsequent contralateral involvement: retrospective follow-up study. BMC Ophthalmol. 2013;13:21.
21. Dallow RL. Evaluation of unilateral exophthalmos with ultrasonography: analysis of 258 consecutive cases. Laryngoscope. 1975;85(11 pt 1):1905–19.
22. Flanders AE, Mafee MF, Metal RV. CT characteristics of orbital pseudotumors and other orbital inflammatory processes. J Comput Assist Tomogr. 1989;13:40–7.
23. Kirsch E, Hammer B, von Arx G. Graves'orbitopathy: current imaging procedures. Swiss Med Wkly. 2009;139:618–23.
24. Regensburg NI, Wiersinga WM, Berendschot TT, et al. Densities of orbital fat and extraocular muscles in graves orbitopathy patients and controls. Ophthal Plast Reconstr Surg. 2011;27:236–40.
25. Hiromatsu Y, Kojima K, Ishisaka N, et al. Role of magnetic resonance imaging in thyroid-associated ophthalmopathy: its predictive value for therapeutic outcome of immunosuppressive therapy. Thyroid. 1992;2:299–305.
26. Hoh HB, Laitt RD, Wakeley C, et al. The STIR sequence MRI in the assessment of extraocular muscles in thyroid eye disease. Eye (Lond). 1994;8(pt 5):506–10.
27. Jiang H, Wang Z, Xian J, et al. Evaluation of rectus extraocular muscles using dynamic contrast-enhanced MR imaging in patients with graves' ophthalmopathy for assessment of disease activity. Acta Radiol. 2012;53:87–94.
28. Barrett L, Glatt HJ, Burde RM, et al. Optic nerve dysfunction in thyroid eye disease: CT. Radiology. 1988;167:503–7.
29. Nugent RA, Belkin RI, Neigel JM, et al. Graves orbitopathy: correlation of CT and clinical findings. Radiology. 1990;177:675–82.
30. Birchall D, Goodall KL, Noble JL, et al. Graves ophthalmopathy: intracranial fat prolapse on CT images as an indicator of optic nerve compression. Radiology. 1996;200:123–7.
31. Trokel SL, Jakobiec FA. Correlation of CT scanning and pathologic features of ophthalmic Graves' disease. Ophthalmology. 1981;88:553–64.
32. Yokoyama N, Nagataki S, Uetani M, et al. Role of magnetic resonance imaging in the assessment of disease activity in thyroid-associated ophthalmopathy. Thyroid. 2002;12:223–7.

4 Preoperative Planning for Thyroid Eye Disease Surgery and Preoperative Checklist

Mahasweta Mishra and Suryasnata Rath

Thyroid eye disease (TED) or Grave's ophthalmopathy is an autoimmune process that involves thyroid gland, orbit, and periorbital tissues, sometimes pretibial skin and digits. Merseburg triad including palpitations, goiter, and exophthalmos characterizes the classical description of Grave's disease [1]. The acute progression of TED is an ocular emergency, mostly optic nerve compression and corneal disease as a consequence of constant exposure [2]. Most patients with TED have hyperthyroidism most common cause being Grave's disease, but it may occur in patients who have hypothyroidism (most commonly Hashimoto's thyroiditis) or Euthyroidism [2]. The incidence of TED is 16 per 100,000 females and 2.9 per 100,000 males [3]. Thyroid hormones have a profound effect on multiple systems in the human body and effect of thyroid dysfunction can be manifold thus acutely complicating surgical procedures and post-operative recovery [4]. Optimization of preexisting thyroid dysmetabolism is key to successful surgical outcomes in TED [4].

M. Mishra (✉)
Anaesthesia Services, LV Prasad Eye Institute, Bhubaneswar, India
e-mail: drmahaswetamishra@lvpei.org

S. Rath
Ophthalmic Plastic Surgery and Ocular Oncology Service, LV Prasad Eye Institute, Bhubaneswar, India
e-mail: suryasnata@lvpei.org

4.1 Signs and Symptoms of Hypothyroidism

1. Unexplained weight gain with decrease in appetite
2. Fatigue and depression
3. Constipation
4. Dry hair, skin, and brittle nail
5. Muscle cramps
6. Puffed facies
7. Cardiomegaly and bradycardia
8. Cold intolerance
9. Memory loss and bradykinesia
10. Menorrhagia

4.2 Signs and Symptoms of Hyperthyroidism

1. Weight loss with increased appetite
2. Irritable, nervous, difficulty in sleep
3. Diarrhea, irritable bowel syndrome and dehydration
4. Profuse perspiration, hair loss and soft nails
5. Muscle weakness and osteoporosis
6. Thyroid stare and proptosis
7. Tachycardia and dysrhythmia
8. Heat intolerance
9. Menstrual irregularity
10. Infertility

S. Rath, M. N. Naik (eds.), *Surgery in Thyroid Eye Disease*,
https://doi.org/10.1007/978-981-32-9220-8_4

4.3 Hypothyroidism

The prevalence of hypothyroidism is approximately 10 times higher in elderly population, especially females compared to males [5]. Autoimmune thyroiditis, iodine deficiency, radioiodine ablation, and surgery are the common causes of hypothyroidism [5]. Hypothyroidism may be overt or subclinical (increased TSH with normal FT3 and FT4 levels) [5]. The perioperative period may be the first opportunity to detect underlying hypothyroidism. Presently there is no recommendation for routine screening to detect thyroid disease in patients with previous no history of thyroid dysfunction [5]. A preoperative TSH assessment is required in subjects with suspected thyroid disease or a known case of Thyroid dysmetabolism. [4].

4.4 Preoperative Preparation in Hypothyroidism

- The optimal preparation time before elective surgery can range from 2 to 4 weeks [5].
- Asymptomatic patients with unexplained weight changes, palpitation, tremor, alterations in bowel habits, skin, hair, or eye changes that suggest thyroid dysmetabolism can be screened with TSH titer.
- In patients with clinical signs suggestive of thyroid hypofunction like exophthalmos, weight changes, palpitation, tremor, goiter, abnormal reflexes, hair or skin abnormalities, and bradycardia screening with TSH levels are mandatory [4].
- In patients with known thyroid dysfunction who are on treatment, the thyroid profile including free/total thyroxine (T4), triiodothyronine (T3), and thyrotropin (TSH) titers, needs optimization before surgery.
- Restoration of euthyroid status can be achieved by the administration of Levothyroxine on the day of surgery. Levothyroxine is preferred as it offers the dual benefit of regulating TSH secretion and conversion of T4 to T3.
- A full replacement dose of Levothyroxine is 1.6 μg/kg/day. But patients older than 60 years with coronary disease should not be given a full dose of Levothyroxine. The starting oral dose is usually 25 μg per day with incremental increase every 2–6 weeks until a euthyroid state is reached [4].
- For patients in Myxedema coma who require emergency surgery intravenous Liothyronine is administered [4].
- Patients needing emergency TED surgery have to be individualized with due consideration of the risk-to-benefit ratio. However, when emergency surgery is mandated for organ salvage thyroid hormone levels should be normalized rapidly using intravenous Levothyroxine at loading doses ranging between 200 and 500 μg/day [4].

4.5 Implications of Hypothyroidism for TED Surgery

Patients with hypothyroidism have slower drug metabolism and are at increased risk of developing complications from an overdose of anesthetic agents [6]. Anesthetic agents rather than surgical stress may be considered the main cause of the changes in plasma thyroid hormone concentrations during the intraoperative period [5]. Correction of hypothyroidism, after replacement treatment, usually leads to the regression of pathophysiologic modifications due to low circulating thyroid hormone. Therefore, the achievement of euthyroidism is the goal before elective surgery, in order to prevent the risk of complications. In nonelective surgery, a careful risk–benefit evaluation in hypothyroid patients before surgical treatment is needed [5]. A rare but dreaded complication of surgery in hypothyroid patient is myxedema coma with mortality rates as high as 40% [5]. Myxedema coma is characterized by an altered mental status manifesting as coma and seizure, hypothermia, bradycardia, hyponatremia, congestive cardiac failure, and hypopnea [5]. Precipitating factors include surgery, infection (septicemia), exposure to cold, CVA, congestive cardiac failure, drugs like sedative agents, anesthetics, narcotics, and withdrawal of thyroid supplements [7]. Treatment includes intensive care treatment with ventilator support, appropriate fluid management and correction of hypotension and dyselectrolytemia, aggressive management of precipitating factors, steroid if required, and thyroid hormone replacement [7].

4.6 Preoperative Preparation in Hyperthyroidism

The term thyrotoxicosis refers to a clinical condition resulting from excessive thyroid hormone action in tissues that are generally caused by elevated thyroid hormone levels [8]. Hyperthyroidism, a form of thyrotoxicosis, is the result of an over-synthesis and oversecretion of thyroid hormones [8]. There are several causes of thyrotoxicosis, including Graves' disease, toxic multinodular goiter, toxic adenoma, thyroiditis, and iatrogenic causes. Accurate diagnosis is essential for patients with thyrotoxicosis since its treatment varies according to the cause. Symptoms of thyrotoxicosis are caused by an excess of beta-adrenergic activity and include agitation, tremor, weight loss, sweating, tachycardia, fever, arrhythmia, and heart failure and can lead to death [9]. During the intra-operative and post-operative periods, the patient's cardiac status should be closely monitored along with the potential development of arrhythmias, cardiac ischemia, and congestive heart failure. Patients with thyrotoxicosis presenting for surgery should ideally be made biochemically and clinically euthyroid before surgery, in order to reduce the risk of perioperative thyroid storm. The risk of perioperative thyroid storm is usually higher following an acute event such as surgery, trauma, or infection [9]. Patients with hyperthyroidism who are not adequately clinically prepared for surgery are at serious risk [9]. Elective surgery and treatment should be postponed until the patient becomes euthyroid. Treatment typically lasts for at least 7 to 10 days, according to the half-life of free T4 [9]. For patients with overt hyperthyroidism requiring urgent or emergent surgery, cardiac status must be closely monitored. Cardiac status should be optimized and β-blockers are most commonly used for this purpose. An initial dose of 25 mg daily may be used, often higher doses, such as 50 mg up to more than 200 mg daily, may be required [4]. Calcium channel blockers should be used in patients who cannot tolerate β-blockers. Recommendations for treatment of thyrotoxicosis in cases where thyrotoxicosis is due to the increased synthesis of thyroid hormone, i.e., in the Graves' disease and toxic nodular disease, antithyroid drugs (ATDs) should be used as soon as possible to decrease thyroid hormone levels. Thionamides, including Propylthiouracil (PTU) and Methimazole or Carbimazole, whichever is available [1]. Methimazole may be started in doses of 20 to 30 mg daily and is available in 5, 10, and 20 mg tablets, whereas PTU would generally be administered in doses of 100 to 150 mg every 6 to 8 hours and is only available in 50 mg tablets [4]. For patients who are unable to take oral medications, both drugs can be administered rectally. In addition, it is generally preferred in the first trimester of pregnancy because of its decreased teratogenicity relative to methimazole. Concomitant use of β-blockers and thionamides should adequately prepare most patients for surgery within a few weeks. These agents should be continued throughout the post-operative period to prevent thyroid storm and possibly longer unless the patient is treated with thyroid resection. Iodine may be administered orally, rectally, or intravenously [4]. Commonly administered doses and formulations include 1 drop 3 times daily of a saturated solution of potassium iodide or a dose of 3 to 5 drops of Lugol's solution thrice daily. Glucocorticoids decrease the conversion of thyroxine to triiodothyronine within a matter of hours, so they may be added preoperatively and tapered over 3 days post-operatively. Suggested regimens include Hydrocortisone 100 mg oral or intravenous every 8 hours, Dexamethasone 2 mg oral or intravenous every 6 hours, or Betamethasone 0.5 mg oral, intramuscular, or intravenous every 6 hours [4].

4.7 Preoperative Initial Evaluation of Thyrotoxicosis Patients

According to the 2016 American Thyroid Association Guidelines [10]:

- **Assessment of Disease Severity**: Assessment of thyrotoxic manifestations, especially cardiovascular and neuromuscular complications, elevations of serum levels of free T3/T4, cardiac evaluation like electrocardiogram and echocardiogram (in elderly patients), a comprehensive history and physical examination should be done [10].
- **Thyroid Status Evaluation**: Thyroid size, tenderness, symmetry, and nodularity should be assessed along with pulmonary, cardiac, and neuromuscular function, along with goiter size and obstructive symptoms [10].
- **Biochemical Evaluation**: Serum TSH should be the initial screening test. Serum T3/T4 and Free T3/T4 levels. Thyroid-stimulating immunoglobulin and TSH receptor antibodies (should be done to evaluate hyperthyroidism) [10].

4.8 Thyroid Storm

Thyroid Storm is an, acute, life-threatening hypermetabolic state caused either by an excessive release of thyroid hormones resulting in an adrenergic overdrive or an increased peripheral response to thyroid hormone [11]. Precipitating factors include infection, stress, diabetic ketoacidosis, hypoglycemia, thyroid hormone overdose, parturition, pulmonary embolism, surgery, trauma, and myocardial infarction. Thyroid storm is characterized by high fever, jaundice, goiter, dehydration, and tachycardia. Patients often complain of nausea and vomiting, diarrhea, sweating, and may progress to coma. Management of thyroid storm is aimed at initial resuscitation, reducing the levels of circulating thyroid hormones, obtund the peripheral response of thyroid hormones, treating the precipitating condition and treatment of end-organ dysfunction. These patients require intensive cardiovascular resuscitation and often require mechanical ventilatory support. Significant hemodynamic instability can occur due to tachyarrhythmias, high output cardiac failure, and pulmonary edema. In addition, these patients also require meticulous fluid and electrolyte management, cooling measures, nutritional support, and adequate sedation. Thyroid-specific pharmacological therapy includes specific agents to block synthesis (Methimazole, Propyl thiouracil), release (Lugol's iodine, Lithium carbonate), T4 to T3 conversion (Propranolol, Corticosteroids, high dose Propylthiouracil), beta-adrenergic action of thyroid hormones (Propranolol), and enterohepatic circulation (Cholestyramine) [11]. Extracorporeal plasmapheresis is an additional tool for removing circulating thyroxine in patients who do not respond quickly to conventional standard therapy [12]. Precipitating factors should be scrupulously looked for and aggressively treated as per standard treatment guidelines. Thyroid storm can often cause multiorgan dysfunction and hence organ-specific supportive care has to be initiated at the earliest.

Perioperative care is required in all patients of thyroid eye disease. Based on systemic thyroid status (hypothyroidism or hyperthyroidism), the perioperative care is tailored by the anesthesiologist in consultation with the internist, endocrinologist, and the oculoplastic surgeon. The existing recommendations and guidelines are summarized in the flow chart depicted in Fig. 4.1.

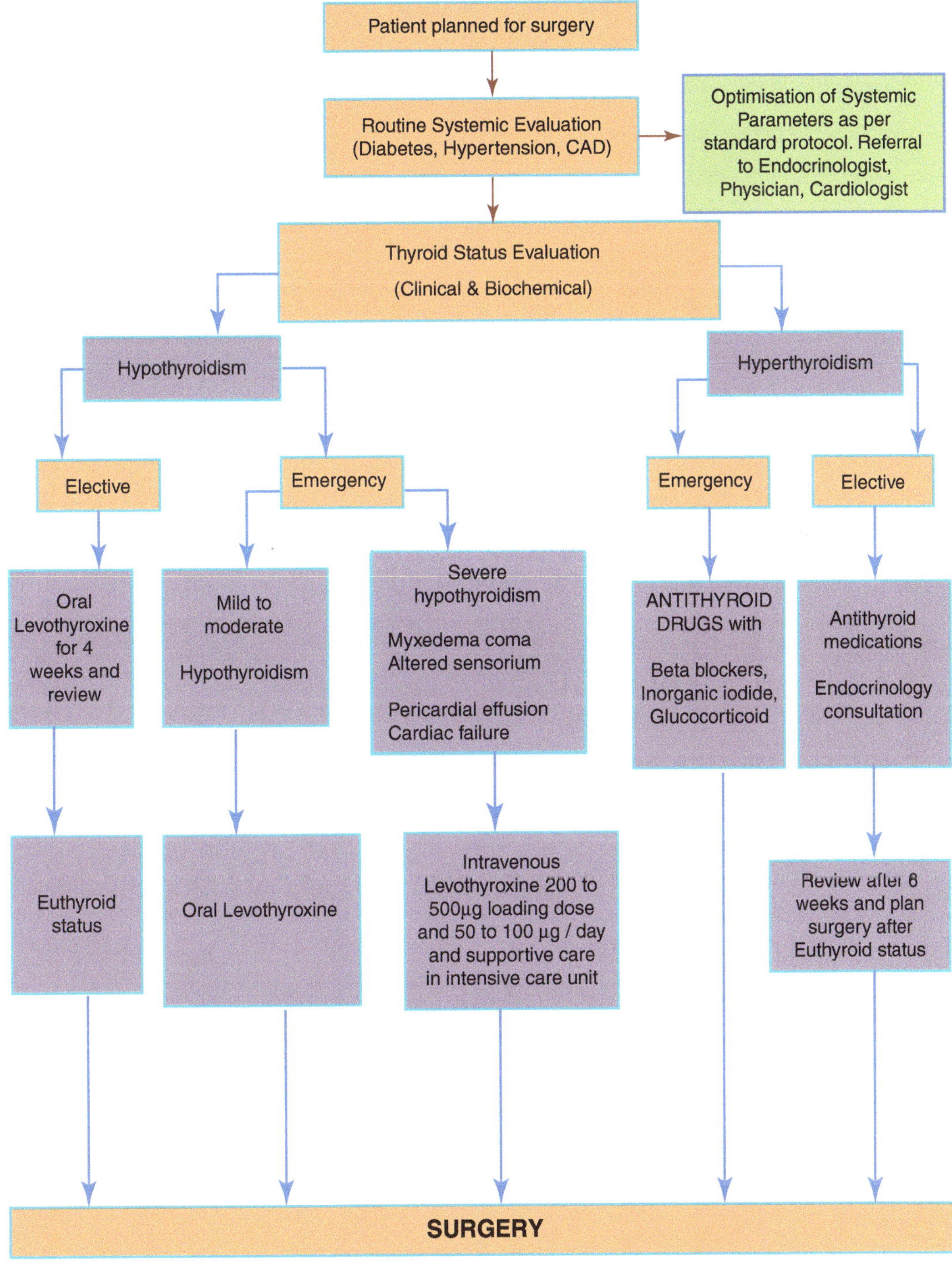

Fig. 4.1 Perioperative management algorithm for patients undergoing surgery for TED

CHECKLIST FOR PATIENTS HAVING THYROID EYE DISEASE :

	YES	NO
• **THYROID STATUS OF THE PATIENT**		
◦ HYPERTHYROID	☐	☐
◦ HYPOTHYROID	☐	☐
◦ EUTHYROID	☐	☐
• **SURGERY**		
◦ ELECTIVE	☐	☐
◦ EMERGENCY	☐	☐
• **ASSOCIATED COMORBIDITIES**		
◦ DM	☐	☐
◦ HYPERTENSIVE	☐	☐
◦ CHRONIC KIDNEY DISEASE	☐	☐
◦ CORONARY ARTERY DISEASE	☐	☐
◦ SEIZURE	☐	☐
◦ ASTHMA/COPD	☐	☐
◦ SMOKER/ALCOHOLIC	☐	☐
• **CURRENT MEDICATIONS**		
◦ ANTIHYPERTENSIVES	☐	☐
◦ ANTICOAGULANTS	☐	☐
◦ ANTICONVULSANTS	☐	☐
◦ ON DIALYSIS	☐	☐
◦ INSULIN THERAPY	☐	☐
• **LABORATORY INVESTIGATIONS**		
◦ T3, T4, AND TSH LEVEL	☐	☐
◦ COAGULATION PROFILE	☐	☐
◦ FBS AND PPBS	☐	☐
◦ SERUM UREA AND CREATININE	☐	☐
◦ SERUM ELECTROLYTES	☐	☐
◦ COMPLETE BLOOD COUNT	☐	☐
• **OTHERS**		
◦ ECG/2D-ECHO	☐	☐
◦ CHEST X-RAY	☐	☐
◦ VIRAL SCREENING	☐	☐

References

1. Piantanida E. Preoperative management in patients with Graves' disease. Gland Surg. 2017 Oct;6(5):476–81.
2. McAlinden C. An overview of thyroid eye disease. Eye Vis (Lond). 2014;1:9.
3. Lazarus JH. Epidemiology of Graves' orbitopathy (GO) and relationship with thyroid disease. Best Practice Res Clin Endocrinol Metabol. June 2012;26(3):273–9.
4. Palace MR. Perioperative management of thyroid dysfunction. Health Serv Insights. 2017 Feb 20;10:117.
5. Vacante M, Biondi A, Basile F, Ciuni R, Luca S, Di Saverio S, Buscemi C, Vicari ESD, Borzì AM. Hypothyroidism as a predictor of surgical outcomes in the elderly. Front Endocrinol (Lausanne). 2019 Apr 24;10:25.
6. Mathew V, Misgar RA, Ghosh S, et al. Myxedema coma: a new look into an old crisis. J Thyroid Res. 2011;2011:493462.
7. Burch H, Cooper D, Jeffrey G, Greenlee M, Klein I, Peter L, McDougall I, Montori V, Rivkees S, Ross D, Sosa J, Stan M. Hyperthyroidism and other causes of thyrotoxicosis: management guidelines of the American Thyroid Association and American Association of Clinical Endocrinologists. Endocr Practice: May 2011. 2011;17(3):456–520.
8. Farling PA. Thyroid disease. BJA: British Journal of Anaesthesia. 2000, 1 July;85(1):15–28.
9. Ross DS, Burch HB, Cooper DS, Greenlee MC, Laurberg P, Maia AL, Rivkees SA, Samuels M, Sosa JA, Stan MN, Walter MA. 2016 American Thyroid Association Guidelines for diagnosis and management of hyperthyroidism and other causes of thyrotoxicosis. Thyroid. 2016 Oct;26(10):1343–421.
10. Carroll R, Matfin G. Endocrine and metabolic emergencies: thyroid storm. Ther Adv Endocrinol Metab. 2010;1(3):139–45.
11. Koball S, Hickstein H, Gloger M, Hinz M, Henschel J, Stange J, et al. Treatment of thyrotoxic crisis with plasmapheresis and single pass albumin dialysis: a case report. Artif Organs. 2010;34:E55–8.
12. Simsir IY, Ozdemir M, Duman S, Erdogan M, Donmez A, Ozgen AG. Therapeutic Plasmapheresis in thyrotoxic patients. Endocrine. 2018;62(1):144–8.

Part II

Surgery in Active Thyroid Eye Disease (TED)

5 Management of Eyelid Retraction in Active TED

Milind N. Naik

5.1 Introduction

Thyroid eye disease (TED) is an autoimmune disease that often leads to facial disfigurement. Graves' Upper Eyelid Retraction (GUER) is one of the most common sign in TED, and has functional as well as cosmetic implications [1, 2]. Surgical correction remains the mainstay for the treatment of eyelid retraction, and shall be separately covered in Chapter 15. However, during the active phase of the disease, a temporary modality for correction is desirable.

Minimally invasive procedures have gained acceptance due to their safety, reversibility, instant results, relatively short downtimes and good patient satisfaction. In this chapter, we shall focus on the use of minimally invasive procedures that can effectively address GUER in the active phase of the disease: Botulinum toxin, Hyaluronic acid and Triamcinolone acetonide injections. Although temporary, these modalities expand our available therapeutic options to improve exposure symptoms and therefore quality of life in patients with TED.

M. N. Naik (✉)
Ophthalmic Plastic Surgery Service, LV Prasad Eye Institute, Hyderabad, India
e-mail: milind@lvpei.org

5.2 Botulinum Toxin in GUER

Botulinum toxin acts on the motor end plates of muscles while preventing local acetylcholine release [3]. It was first approved in 1989 for the indications of strabismus and blepharospasm, followed by its popularity in cosmetic uses [4]. Ptosis, a known complication of periocular Botulinum toxin injection, when deliberately induced, can be a beneficial outcome in patients with TED having eyelid retraction [5].

The two main injection techniques are the trans-cutaneous and trans-conjunctival approaches (Fig. 5.1).

5.2.1 Injection Technique

Trans-cutaneous approach: The trans-cutaneous technique involves entering the superior-anterior orbit in the mid-pupillary plane with a half-inch needle (Fig. 5.1a). The needle is advanced between the globe and the orbital rim, directing it towards the orbital roof. Once the needle hub touches the eyelid skin, and the toxin is injected very slowly, and the needle is withdrawn.

Trans-conjunctival approach: This technique is performed under topical anesthesia (Fig. 5.1b).

S. Rath, M. N. Naik (eds.), *Surgery in Thyroid Eye Disease*,
https://doi.org/10.1007/978-981-32-9220-8_5

The upper eyelid is everted over a Desmarres retractor, and the toxin is injected sub-conjunctivally with a 29 or 30-gauge needle just above the superior tarsal border. The injection can be divided into two point injections, medially and laterally, with more injected laterally.

Botulinum toxin has been reported to successfully reduce exposure symptoms, with effect lasting for 1–6 months in most studies [3, 5–13].

A longer effect is observed in the inactive TED patients [12].

Trans-cutaneous and trans-conjunctival approaches showed similar duration of effect and complications. The trans-conjunctival approach is easier, with less side effect profile (Fig. 5.2). It is possible that trans-conjunctival injection may provide better access to the Müller muscle, and minimise the undesirable weakening of the orbicularis muscle [5].

Table 5.1 details the summary of published articles that reported the use of Botulinum toxin in TED-related eyelid retraction [14]. For Botulinum toxin in GUER, the studies differed in several aspects (brand, dose, site, follow-up, outcome, etc.) making comparisons between them more complex. It is difficult to identify the best dosage of toxin. Ptosis was the most common complication, observed in 16%–75% of the treated eyes in various reports. New onset diplopia or worsening of pre-existing diplopia was the second commonest complication. All studies achieved favourable results with respect to reduction in exposure symptoms suggesting Botulinum toxin as a temporary yet effective treatment for GUER in TED. The results of the injection in the upper eyelid, however, can be unpredictable, and patients must be warned about potential side effects, which are temporary.

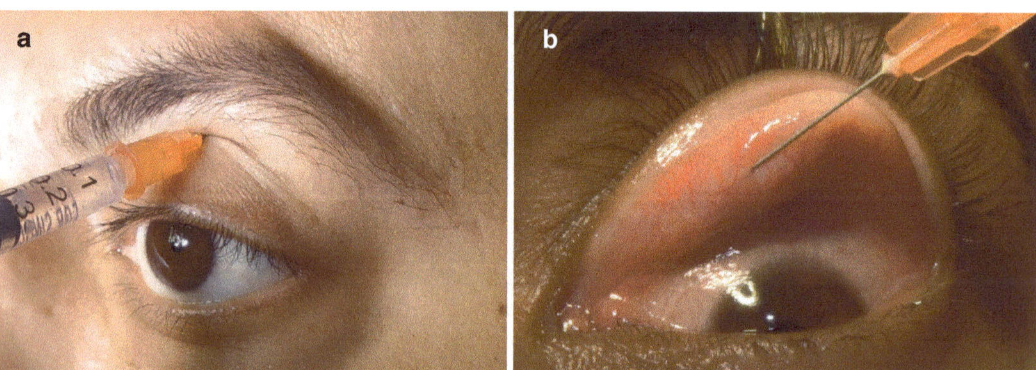

Fig. 5.1 The two techniques of injecting Botulinum toxin for the treatment of eyelid retraction: trans-cutaneous (**a**) and trans-conjunctival (**b**) approaches

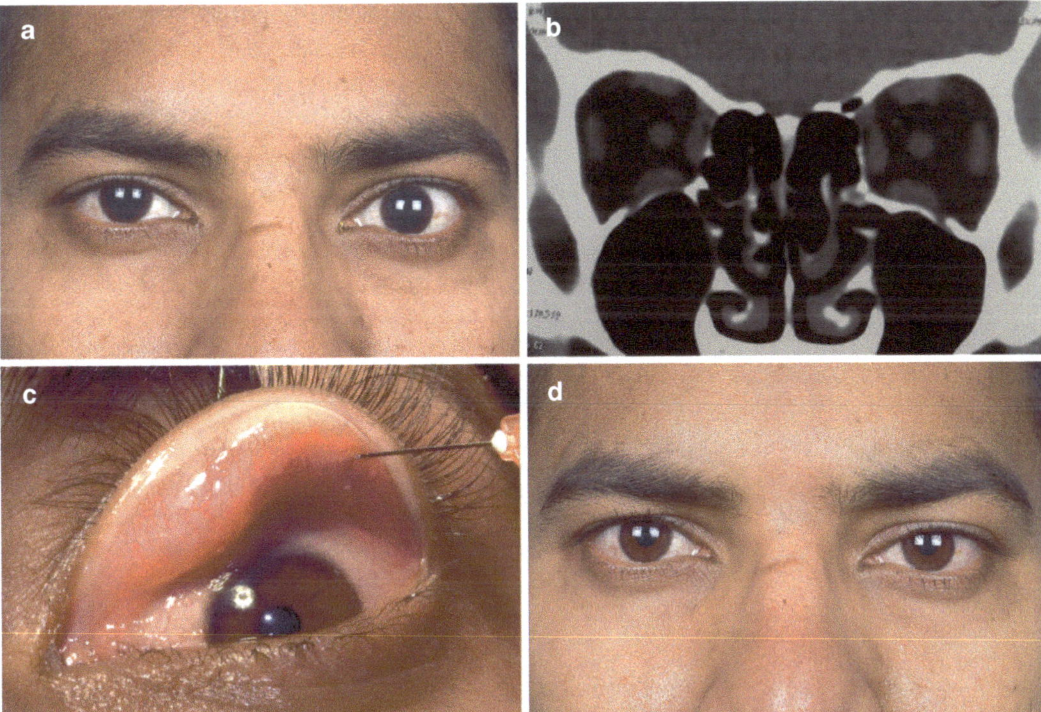

Fig. 5.2 A 23-year-old gentleman with active thyroid eye disease of 3 months duration, with mild left upper lid retraction (**a**). Coronal cut of computed tomography scan of the orbit showing slightly enlarged left superior rectus–levator complex compared to the right (**b**). He received 2.5 units of Botulinum toxin Type A injection by trans-conjunctival approach (**c**). Improvement in the eyelid retraction noted at 2 weeks with resultant improvement in exposure-related symptoms (**d**)

Table 5.1 Published data on Botulinum toxin injection for upper eyelid retraction in thyroid eye disease (*Grisolia ABD* et al)

Author	Number of eyes	Route of injection	Dose	Duration of effect	Mean change in lid position	Complications
Scott	Not specified	Not specified	0.3–10 ng	30 days	Not specified	Levator/superior Rectus paralysis
Ebner	7	Trans-cutaneous	2.5–5 U*	8–32 weeks	1.35 mm	Ptosis
Biglan	4	Trans-cutaneous	5 U*	3–4 months	Not specified	Ptosis
Ozkan et al.	8	Trans-cutaneous	2.5–7.5 U*	3–4 months	6.1 mm	Ptosis
Uddin et al.	16	Trans Subconjunctival	5–15 U*	1–40 months	2.03 mm	Ptosis, diplopia
Traisk et al.	15	Trans-cutaneous	2.5–7.5 U	6–20 weeks	2.61 mm	Diplopia
Morgenstern et al.	27	Trans-conjunctival	2.5–10 U	Not specified	2.35 mm	Ptosis, diplopia
Shih et al.	21	Trans-cutaneous	5–6 U	>2 months	3.09 mm	Ptosis, diplopia
Costa et al.	24	Trans-cutaneous	5–7.5 U	1–3 months	3.05–3.81 mm	Ptosis, Lagophthalmos
Salour et al.	25	Trans-cutaneous	20 U	1–6 months	4.24 mm	Ptosis

*Product name not specified

5.3 Hyaluronic Acid Fillers in GUER

Hyaluronic acid (HA) gel is frequently used in the periocular region due to its reversibility and safety profile [15]. Although more popular for its cosmetic uses, HA gel has been reported in the use of several functional indications in the periocular region [15–21]. Multiple formulations are available, with varying viscoelasticity and cross-linking features. HA is estimated to last 6 to 12 months in the periocular region, which well coincides with the approximate duration of the active phase of TED.

The two main injection techniques are the trans-cutaneous and trans-conjunctival approaches (Fig. 5.3).

5.3.1 Injection technique

Trans-cutaneous approach: The trans-cutaneous technique involves entering the pre-septal region with the filler injection needle. Filler is injected in the sub-orbicularis plane, at the level of the levator muscle (Fig. 5.3a). Pre-tarsal region can also be filled to add weight, however the lid may appear bulky in downgaze. Titration can be done by comparing symmetry in primary gaze.

Trans-conjunctival approach: This technique is performed under topical anesthesia (Fig. 5.3b). The upper eyelid is everted over a Desmarres retractor, and the filler is injected sub-conjunctivally in the plane of the levator. The injection can spread over the extent of the eyelid, and titration can be done by comparing symmetry in primary gaze.

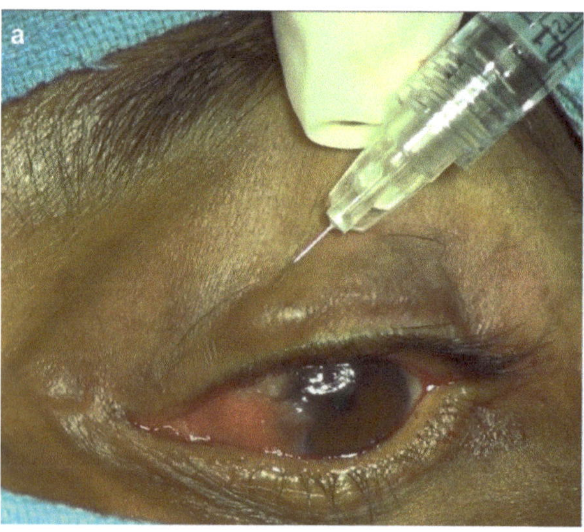

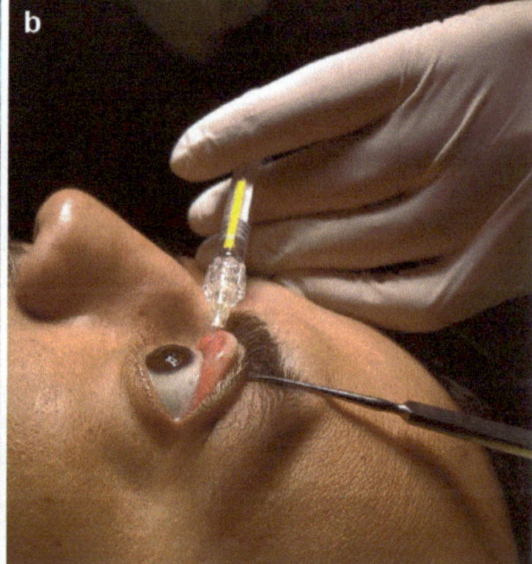

Fig. 5.3 Trans-cutaneous and Trans-conjunctival techniques of injection of Filler for upper eyelid retraction. Following an extreme lateral tarsorrhaphy, Filler is being injected into the pre-septal and pre-tarsal sub-orbicularis planes to lower the eyelid position by it's weight in a case of Graves' upper eyelid retraction (**a**). Another patient with GUER receiving a Filler injection trans-conjunctivally after eversion of the eyelid (**b**). The filler is injected supra-tarsally in the sub-conjunctival plane and along the levator to add weight and to lengthen the eyelid

In the upper eyelid, the aim is to deposit the filler material at the level of the levator to lengthen it, and also to act by adding weight (Fig. 5.4). For the lower lid, injection of filler aims to lengthen the lower lid retractors and provide a scaffold to support the lid against the inferior orbital rim.

Kohn et al. reported the use of trans-conjunctival HA gel injection for unilateral GUER [22]. The site of HA gel placement was in the pre-aponeurotic space, as assessed by Ultrasound. An average of 0.45 mL was required, to achieve a significant reduction in MRD1 by 1 mm lasting up to 15 months. The active TED group showed better results than the inactive group [22].

HA gel has also been used to treat lower eyelid retraction of various aetiologies [23–25]. It can reduce the inferior scleral show, and improve the exposure symptoms (Fig. 5.5). Goldberg et al. reported their experience with 31 patients (of which 8 were TED) with a mean decrease of 0.52 mm in the inferior scleral show after 4 months [26].

Complications of HA injections can be transient, such as oedema, ecchymosis and erythema. Serious complications such as retinal arterial embolisation have not yet been reported with this indication of HA gel, but are possible [27]. The studies that investigated the use of HA as a treatment for eyelid retraction in TED are summarised in Table 5.2 [14].

Although few studies investigated the effect of HA gel in TED patients, these studies indicate that HA may represent a safe, effective and predictable non-surgical alternative for eyelid retraction, especially for poor surgical candidates or medically unstable patients. Further, HA may be more effective in active TED, making it an important tool in the management of ocular exposure symptoms before disease stabilisation. Theoretically, fibrosis may diminish the therapeutic effect of HA, and it may be more beneficial if administered before tissue remodelling has occurred.

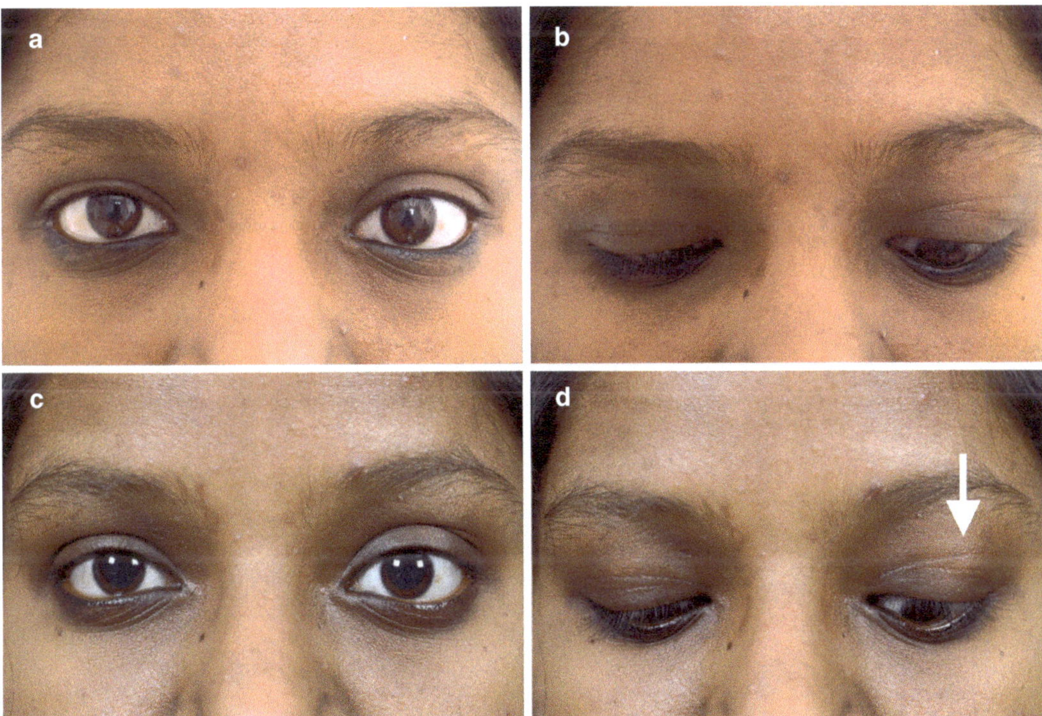

Fig. 5.4 Mild left upper eyelid retraction in a case of active thyroid eye disease with low clinical activity score (**a**, **b**). She received 0.4 mL of Hyaluronic acid gel injection into the levator plane of left upper eyelid. Note the improvement in eyelid retraction 4 weeks post injection (**c**). The downgaze photograph shows minimal fullness (white arrow) in the upper lid due to the presence of the filler (**d**)

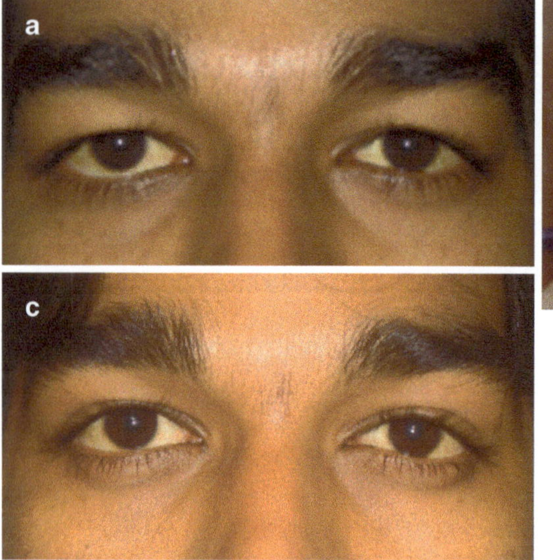
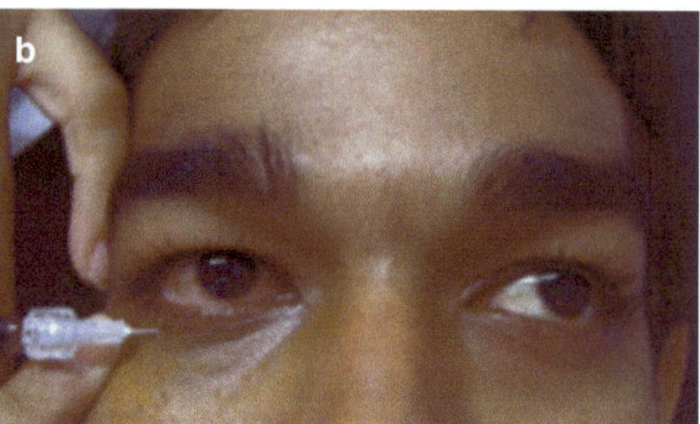

Fig. 5.5 Right lower eyelid retraction in a patient with mild TED (**a**). Filler injection (0.2ml) injected under topical anaesthesia along the plane of lower lid retractors (**b**). Improvement in inferior scleral show noted post-filler injection (**c**)

Table 5.2 Summary of published data on Hyaluronic acid injection for Graves' Upper Eyelid Retraction (*Grisolia ABD* et al.)

Author	Number of TED patients treated with HA filler	Route of injection	Dose (mL)	Follow-up (months)	Mean change in lid position (mm)
Goldberg et al.	8	Trans-cutaneous, lower eyelid	0.9	4.6	1.04
Kohn et al.	8	Subconjuctival, upper eyelid	0.45	1.4	1
Mancini et al.	3	Subconjunctival, upper eyelid	0.2	5.7	0.74

5.4 Triamcinolone Acetonide in GUER

Steroids remain the main treatment for moderate-to-severe TED, promoting a quick reduction in inflammation and related symptoms [28]. Their systemic use (oral or intravenous) is well established, but the local administration of glucocorticoids (subconjunctival or periocular) remains controversial [28–30]. Triamcinolone acetonide (TA) injection has been proposed by multiple investigators as a less invasive treatment for GUER [31–34].

5.4.1 Injection technique

The two main injection techniques are the trans-cutaneous and trans-conjunctival approaches (Fig. 5.6).

The *trans-cutaneous* technique involves entering in the mid-pupillary plane with a half-inch 26 gauge needle (Fig. 5.6a). It is passed between the globe and the orbital rim, directing it towards the orbital roof. The needle is advanced till the hub touches the eyelid skin, and the drug is injected very slowly.

Trans-conjunctival technique is performed under topical anesthesia (Fig. 5.6b). The upper eyelid is lifted off the globe, and Triamcinolone acetonide 1ml is injected with a half-inch 26-gauge needle inserted halfway between the superior tarsal border and the superior fornix. It is directed postero-superiorly towards the orbital rim to deliver it to the levator and Müller's muscle. The injection can be divided into two point injections, medially and laterally.

Chee et al. reported four cases treated with upper eyelid subconjunctival TA injections [31]. Three of the four cases achieved resolution of retraction in 6 to 12 months. Patients with more acute eyelid changes had a better response when compared to patients with chronic changes.

Xu et al. published the results of 21 patients (35 eyes) monthly treated with upper eyelid subconjunctival TA [32]. All the treated patients showed improvement in GUER, compared to only 17.4% in a control group of 15 TED patients who had spontaneous improvement. Thinning of the superior rectus/levator muscle after TA treatment was observed on echography and MRI. Almost half of them had elevation of intraocular pressure. Lee et al. reported 95 patients randomised into subconjunctival TA or observation [33]. Normalisation of GUER was observed in 75% of patients in the TA group versus 57% in the observation group ($p = 0.004$). Lee et al. reported that subconjunctival TA in the active phase was more effective (86.3%) compared to inactive (25%) [34]. Studies that focused on the use of TA for GUER are summarised in Table 5.3 [14].

Current studies indicate that TA injection might be more beneficial for patients with GUER within first 6 months of active disease. It has been suggested that smaller injection volumes, shorter needles and an injection site more distant from the globe could prevent severe IOP elevation [29].

Reduction in the size of levator muscle was observed in patients treated with TA, as previously seen on extra-ocular muscles after intraorbital injection [30]. Since rise in IOP is possible, glaucoma should be considered a contraindication for this therapy. TA injection seems to be an effective alternative to surgical procedures for GUER, although its exact efficacy is difficult to measure. Further studies are required to investigate and compare treatment alternatives.

Comparison of Botulinum toxin, Hyaluronic acid and Triamcinolone acetonide in the temporary correction of eyelid retraction is summarised in Table 5.4.

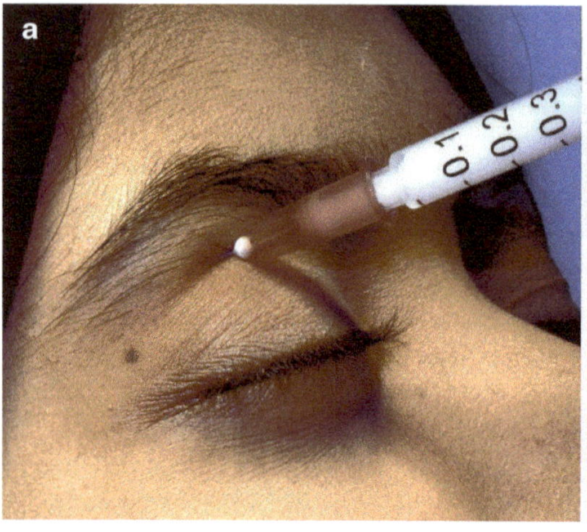

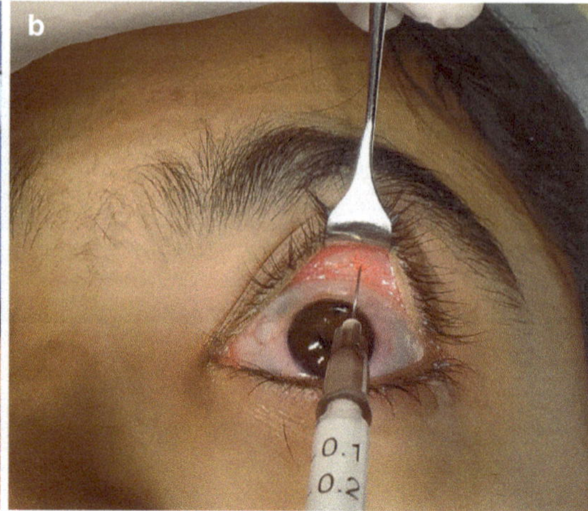

Fig. 5.6 Trans-cutaneous (**a**) and Trans-conjunctival (**b**) techniques of injection of Triamcinolone acetonide (1ml of 40mg/ml concentration) for Graves' upper eyelid retraction in active TED

Table 5.3 Summary of published data on Triamcinolone injection for Graves' Upper Eyelid Retraction (*Grisolia ABD* et al). All studies performed a sub-conjunctival injection

Author	Number of eyes	Duration of eyelid retraction	Average dose	Mean follow-up	Results	Complications
Chee et al.	5	1 month–6 years	20 mg	1 year	Resolved	Not specified
Xu et al.	23	0.5–39 months	20 mg	6–27 months	Mean MRD1 Reduction of 2.19 mm	IOP elevation
Lee et al.	75	≤6 months	20 mg	≥24 weeks	Resolved	IOP elevation
Lee et al.	43	Not specified	20 mg	6 months	Mean MRD1 Reduction of 0.6–1.1 mm	IOP elevation, ptosis

IOP, intraocular pressure; MRD1, margin reflex distance-1; UER, upper eyelid retraction

Table 5.4 Comparison of Botulinum toxin and Hyaluronic acid (HA) gel in the management of eyelid retraction in Thyroid eye disease

Feature	Botulinum toxin	Hyaluronic acid gel	Triamcinolone Acetonide
Indication	Upper eyelid retraction	Upper and lower eyelid retraction	Upper eyelid retraction
Mechanism of action	Relaxation of levator or Muller muscle	Increases weight of the eyelid and lengthens the retractor (levator or lower lid retractors)	Anti-inflammatory effect on levator
Approximate dose	5 Units	0.4–0.5 ml	10–40 mg
Duration of action	6–12 Weeks	6–12 Months	2–4 Weeks
Effectivity	Reported to be more effective in inactive TED	Reported to be more effective in active TED	Reported to be more effective in active TED
Complications	Ptosis Diplopia	Edema, ecchymosis, erythema. Retinal arterial embolization (not reported but possible)	Steroid deposits Steroid induced glaucoma Vascular complication (possible)
Reversibility	Cannot be reversed	Can be reversed with hyaluronidase	Cannot be reversed

5.5 Conclusion

Currently, Botulinum toxin, Hyaluronic acid gel and Triamcinolone acetonide are viable injectable options in the management of GUER in the active phase of TED. HA gel can also be used to improve lower eyelid retraction. These can also be offered in the inactive phase for patients who do not want surgical intervention, and are willing to try temporary measures. Further well-designed studies can assess their therapeutic effects as primary or adjunctive non-surgical treatment modalities in GUER.

References

1. Frueh BR, Musch DC, Garber FW. Lid retraction and levator aponeurosis defects in graves' eye disease. Ophthalmic Surg. 1986;17:216–20.
2. Weetman AP, Disease Grave's *Horm Res* 1835–2002 ;2003(59Suppl1):114–118.
3. Träisk F, Tallstedt L. Thyroid associated ophthalmopathy: botulinum toxin a in the treatment of upper eyelid retraction--a pilot study. Acta Ophthalmol Scand. 2001;79:585–8.
4. Erickson BP, Lee WW, Cohen J, et al. The role of neurotoxins in the periorbital and midfacial areas. Facial Plast Surg Clin North Am. 2015;23:243–55.
5. Morgenstern KE, Evanchan J, Foster JA, et al. Botulinum toxin type a for dysthyroid upper eyelid retraction. Ophthalmic Plast Reconstr Surg. 2004;20:181–5.
6. Scott AB. Injection treatment of endocrine orbital myopathy. Doc Ophthalmol. 1984;58:141–5.
7. Ebner R. Botulinum toxin type a in upper lid retraction of graves' ophthalmopathy. J Clin Neuroophthalmol. 1993;13:258–61.
8. Biglan AW. Control of eyelid retraction associated with graves' disease with botulinum a toxin. Ophthalmic Surg. 1994;25:186–8.
9. Ozkan SB, Can D, Söylev MF, et al. Chemodenervation in treatment of upper eyelid retraction. Ophthalmologica. 1997;211:387–90.
10. Uddin JM, Davies PD. Treatment of upper eyelid retraction associated with thyroid eye disease with subconjunctival botulinum toxin injection. Ophthalmology. 2002;109:1183–7.
11. Shih MJ, Liao SL, Lu HY. A single transcutaneous injection with Botox for dysthyroid lid retraction. Eye. 2004;18:466–9.
12. Costa PG, Saraiva FP, Pereira IC, et al. Comparative study of Botox injection treatment for upper eyelid retraction with 6-month follow-up in patients with thyroid eye disease in the congestive or fibrotic stage. Eye. 2009;23:767–73.
13. Salour H, Bagheri B, Aletaha M, et al. Transcutaneous dysport injection for treatment of upper eyelid retraction associated with thyroid eye disease. Orbit. 2010;29:114–8.
14. Grisolia ABD, Couso RC, Matayoshi S, Douglas RS, Briceño CA. Non-surgical treatment for eyelid retraction in thyroid eye disease (TED). Br J Ophthalmol. 2017 Aug;9
15. Nguyen AT, Ahmad J, Fagien S, et al. Cosmetic medicine: facial resurfacing and injectables. Plast Reconstr Surg. 2012;129:142e–53.
16. Goldberg RA, Fiaschetti D. Filling the periorbital hollows with hyaluronic acid gel: initial experience with 244 injections. Ophthalmic Plast Reconstr Surg. 2006;22:335–41. Discussion 341–333
17. Mancini R, Khadavi NM, Goldberg RA. Nonsurgical management of upper eyelid margin asymmetry using hyaluronic acid gel filler. Ophthalmic Plast Reconstr Surg. 2011;27:1–3.
18. Malhotra R. Deep orbital sub-Q restylane (nonanimal stabilized hyaluronic acid) for orbital volume enhancement in sighted and anophthalmic orbits. Arch Ophthalmol. 2007;125:1623–9.
19. Mancini R, Taban M, Lowinger A, et al. Use of hyaluronic acid gel in the management of paralytic lagophthalmos: the hyaluronic acid gel "gold weight". Ophthalmic Plast Reconstr Surg. 2009;25:23–6.
20. Kwong Q, Malhotra R, Morley AM, et al. Use of dermal filler to improve exposure keratopathy in a patient with restrictive dermopathy. Orbit. 2013;32:70–2.
21. Taban M, Mancini R, Nakra T, et al. Nonsurgical management of congenital eyelid malpositions using hyaluronic acid gel. Ophthalmic Plast Reconstr Surg. 2009;25:259–63.
22. Kohn JC, Rootman DB, Liu W, et al. Hyaluronic acid gel injection for upper eyelid retraction in thyroid eye disease: functional and dynamic high-resolution ultrasound evaluation. Ophthalmic Plast Reconstr Surg. 2014;30:400–4.
23. Romero R, Sanchez-Orgaz M, Granados M, et al. Use of hyaluronic acid gel in the management of cicatricial ectropion: results and complications. Orbit. 2013;32:362–5.
24. Peckinpaugh JL, Reddy HS, Tower RN. Large particle hyaluronic acid gel for the treatment of lower eyelid retraction associated with radiation-induced lipoatrophy. Ophthalmic Plast Reconstr Surg. 2010;26:377–9.
25. Zamani M, Thyagarajan S, Olver JM. Functional use of hyaluronic acid gel in lower eyelid retraction. Arch Ophthalmol. 2008;126:1157–9.
26. Goldberg RA, Lee S, Jayasundera T, et al. Treatment of lower eyelid retraction by expansion of the lower eyelid with hyaluronic acid gel. Ophthalmic Plast Reconstr Surg. 2007;23:343–8.
27. Schanz S, Schippert W, Ulmer A, et al. Arterial embolization caused by injection of hyaluronic acid (Restylane). Br J Dermatol. 2002;146:928–9.

28. Salvi M, Campi I. Medical treatment of graves' Orbitopathy. Horm Metab Res. 2015;47:779–88.
29. Goldberg RA. Orbital steroid injections. Br J Ophthalmol. 2004;88:1359–60.
30. Ebner R, Devoto MH, Weil D, et al. Treatment of thyroid associated ophthalmopathy with periocular injections of triamcinolone. Br J Ophthalmol. 2004;88:1380–6.
31. Chee E, Chee SP. Subconjunctival injection of triamcinolone in the treatment of lid retraction of patients with thyroid eye disease: a case series. Eye. 2008;22:311–5.
32. Xu D, Liu Y, Xu H, et al. Repeated triamcinolone acetonide injection in the treatment of upper-lid retraction in patients with thyroid-associated ophthalmopathy. Can J Ophthalmol. 2012;47:34–41.
33. Lee SJ, Rim TH, Jang SY, et al. Treatment of upper eyelid retraction related to thyroid- associated ophthalmopathy using subconjunctival triamcinolone injections. Graefes Arch Clin Exp Ophthalmol. 2013;251:261–70.
34. Lee JM, Lee H, Park M, et al. Subconjunctival injection of triamcinolone for the treatment of upper lid retraction associated with thyroid eye disease. J Craniofac Surg. 2012;23:1755–8.

6 Tarsorrhaphy in Thyroid Eye Disease

Varshitha Vasanthapuram

6.1 Introduction

"*Tars*" in Greek means *edge of eyelid*, and "*-rrhaphe*" comes from the Greek word meaning to stitch together. Tarsorrhaphy, therefore, means suturing the edges of the eyelids.

Tarsorrhaphy though simple, is a very important and helpful procedure in various stages of Thyroid Eye Disease (TED). It is cardinal to the management of TED with various modifications to suit the indication.

V. Vasanthapuram (✉)
Ophthalmic Plastic Surgery Service,
LV Prasad Eye Institute, Hyderabad, India
e-mail: drvarshithahemanth@lvpei.org

S. Rath, M. N. Naik (eds.), *Surgery in Thyroid Eye Disease*,
https://doi.org/10.1007/978-981-32-9220-8_6

6.2 Indications

The indications may be aesthetic or functional (Fig. 6.1), and are summarized in Table 6.1 [1, 2].

6.3 Types of Tarsorrhaphy

Based on the indication, a tarsorrhaphy can either be temporary (suture tarsorrhaphy) or permanent tarsorrhaphy. A temporary tarsorrhaphy is only held mechanically by the suture, and hence lasts for 2–4 weeks. A permanent tarsorrhaphy involves epithelial freshening of the eyelid margin, thereby forming a permanent biological adhesion between the two lid margins.

Depending upon the site, a tarsorrhaphy can be lateral, medial, central, or paramedian (Fig. 6.1).

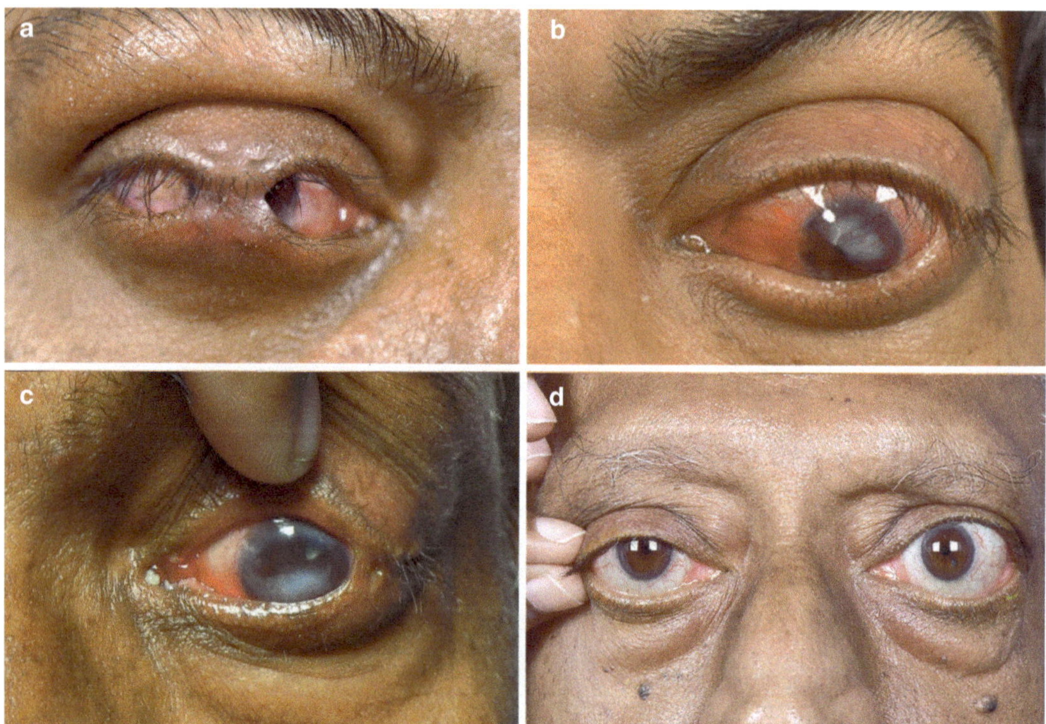

Fig. 6.1 Indications and types of tarsorrhaphy. Functional tarsorrhaphy is primarily for corneal protection, and can be either central (**a**), lateral (**b**), or paramedian (**c**). Cosmetic indications include reduction of scleral show, mild eyelid retraction, or even as an alternative to orbital decompression in mild cases (**d**)

Table 6.1 Indications for Tarsorrhaphy in Thyroid Eye Disease

Role	Indication
Functional	Exposure keratopathy Microbial keratitis Severe conjunctival chemosis
Cosmetic	Scleral show Mild upper and lower lid retraction As an alternative to orbital decompression to reduce the "prominent" appearance of the eye

6.4 Anaesthesia

Tarsorrhaphy is usually performed under local anaesthesia. A mixture of 2% lignocaine with 1:100,000 adrenalin is commonly used. Bupivacaine 0.75% can be added for longer local analgesia. Local infiltration is performed at the eyelid margin, along the intended area for tarsorrhaphy. Infiltrating the posterior lamella allows adequate anaesthesia as these patients can be quite anxious, and have a low pain threshold.

6.5 Temporary Suture Tarsorrhaphy

After local infiltration, the upper lid margin is visualized. A 6–0 Polyglactin (vicryl) or Prolene suture (reverse cutting needle) is used. The needle enters and exits the tarsus, traveling across 2–4 Meibomian gland orifices (Fig. 6.2).

A 3–2 knot is placed to approximate the eyelid margins.

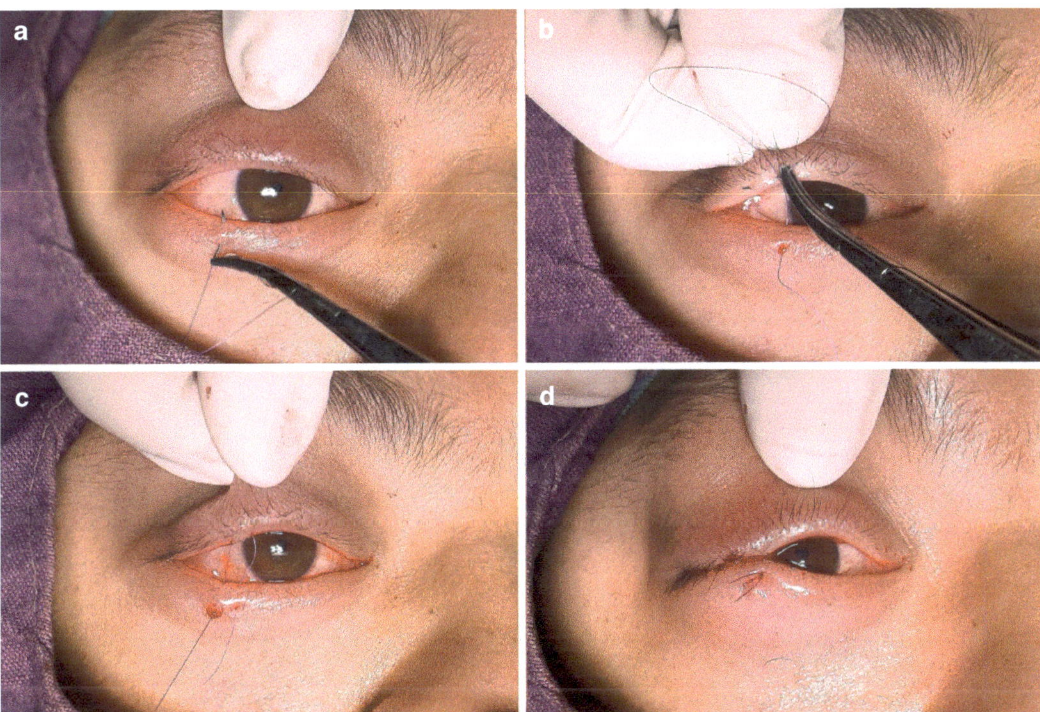

Fig. 6.2 Temporary suture tarsorrhaphy. First, the Vicryl or Prolene 6–0 suture is passed from lower eyelid skin, and brought out at the intermarginal strip through the tarsus (**a**). A posterior lamellar tarsal bite is then passed through the upper lid 4-5 mm wide (**b**). Final pass through the lower eyelid, from intermarginal strip to eyelid skin, 2–4 mm away from the initial entry point (**c**). The suture is finally tied with or without a bolster (**d**)

A horizontal mattress suture can be placed in such a way that the knot can lie at the intermarginal strip (Fig. 6.3a) or on the skin side (Fig. 6.3b).

A Prolene or Silk suture can also be used, and a 4–0 suture may sometimes be required for severe lid retraction. A rubber bolster can also be used to prevent accidental burial of the suture.

A suture tarsorrhaphy can provide corneal protection for 2–4 weeks (Fig. 6.4), and can be performed as a bedside or office procedure.

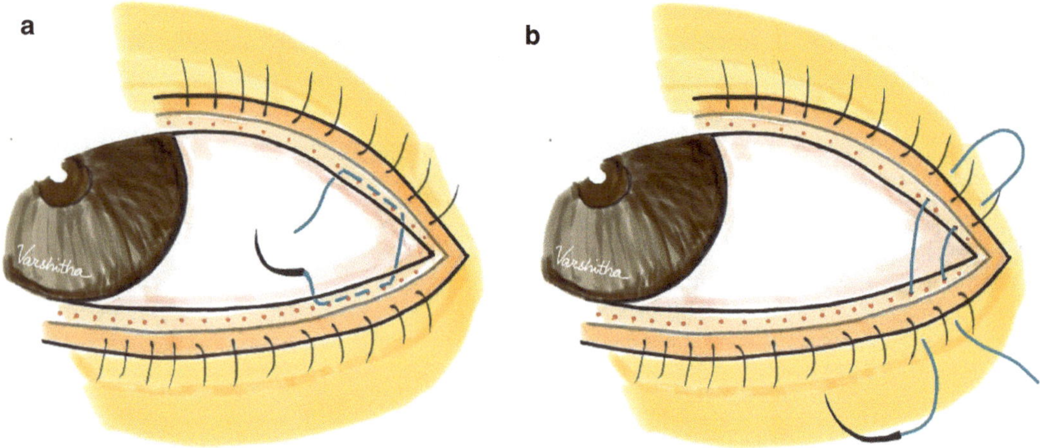

Fig. 6.3 Illustration showing two simple methods of performing temporary suture tarsorrhaphy so as to leave the suture knot either at the intermarginal strip (**a**) or towards the skin side (**b**)

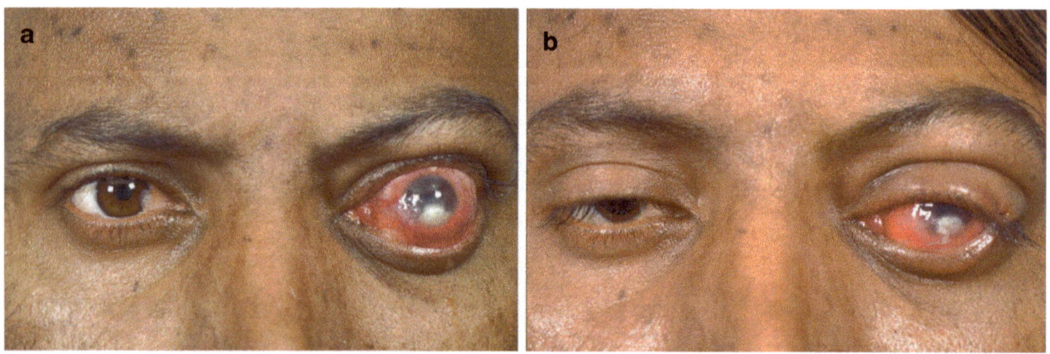

Fig. 6.4 Left active thyroid eye disease with microbial keratitis (**a**), treated with temporary suture tarsorrhaphy (**b**)

6.6 Permanent Tarsorrhaphy

A permanent tarsorrhaphy differs from a temporary suture tarsorrhaphy in that the intermarginal strip is excised, and parts of the opposing lamellae are sutured together to form a permanent bond (Fig. 6.5). With an 11 number Bard-Parker blade, a linear incision is made along the grey line on the lid margin in the area intended for tarsorrhaphy (Figs. 6.6 and 6.7). The incision extends between the anterior and the posterior lamella for a depth of about 2–3 mm. The epithelial lining on the posterior lamella of the lid margin is then undermined and excised with a blade or Westcott scissors (Fig. 6.6). The posterior lamellae of the upper and lower eyelids (tarsal pillars) are sutured together with a horizontal mattress suture, (Fig. 6.7). An additional horizontal box suture with or without bolsters can be placed to approximate the anterior lamella.

A Prolene, Vicryl or Silk suture can be used, and a 4–0 suture may sometimes be required for severe lid retraction. A rubber bolster can also be used to prevent accidental burial of the suture.

The suture can be removed after 2 weeks, following which a permanent tissue adhesion band is formed between the posterior lamella of the two eyelids. This is a quick procedure, easy to perform, and usually lasts for years (Fig. 6.8).

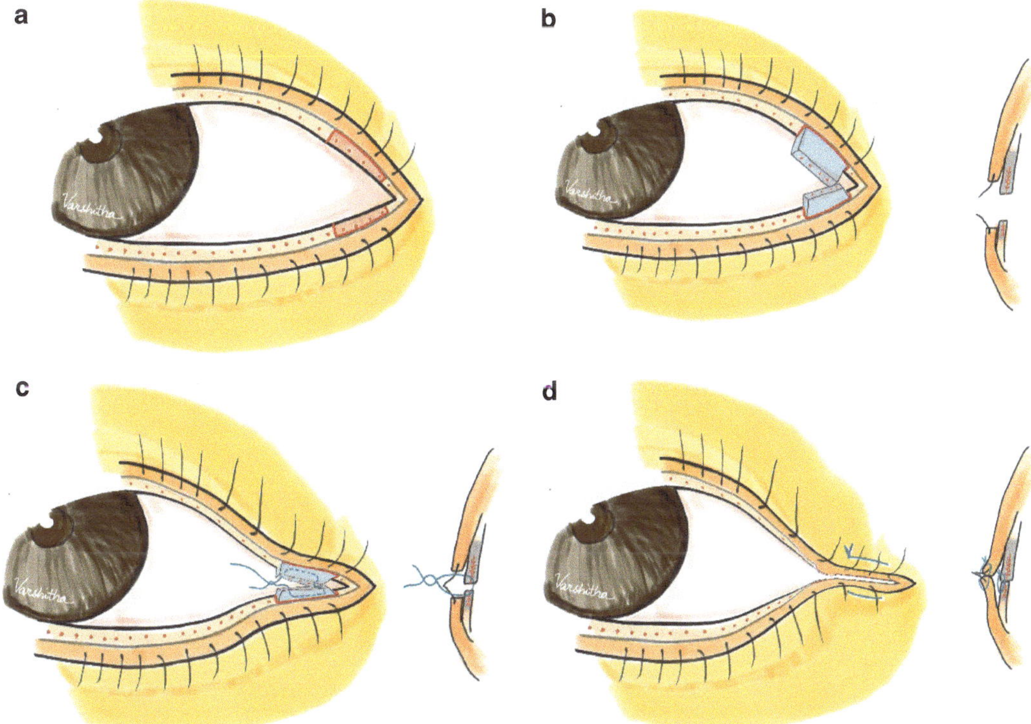

Fig. 6.5 Illustration showing the technique of permanent lateral tarsorrhaphy. Marginal epithelium is excised along the posterior lamella of apposing eyelid tissue (**a**). The two lamellae are split, and raw tarsal plates are brought out for approximation (**b**). A 6–0 or 4–0 Vicryl suture approximates the posterior lamellae (**c**). Anterior lamella is then closed over the approximated posterior lamella with 6–0 Prolene suture (**d**)

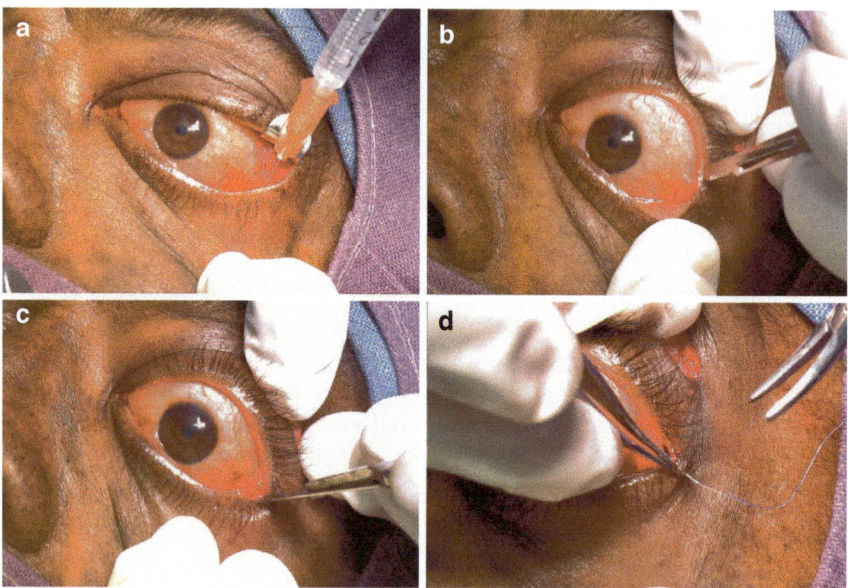

Fig. 6.6 Permanent lateral tarsorrhaphy. Local infiltration along the anterior and posterior lamella (**a**). Lateral 5 mm of intermarginal strip excised from the upper eyelid (**b**) and lower eyelid (**c**). Vicryl 6–0 suture passed from lower eyelid skin, and brought out at the raw intermarginal strip (**d**)

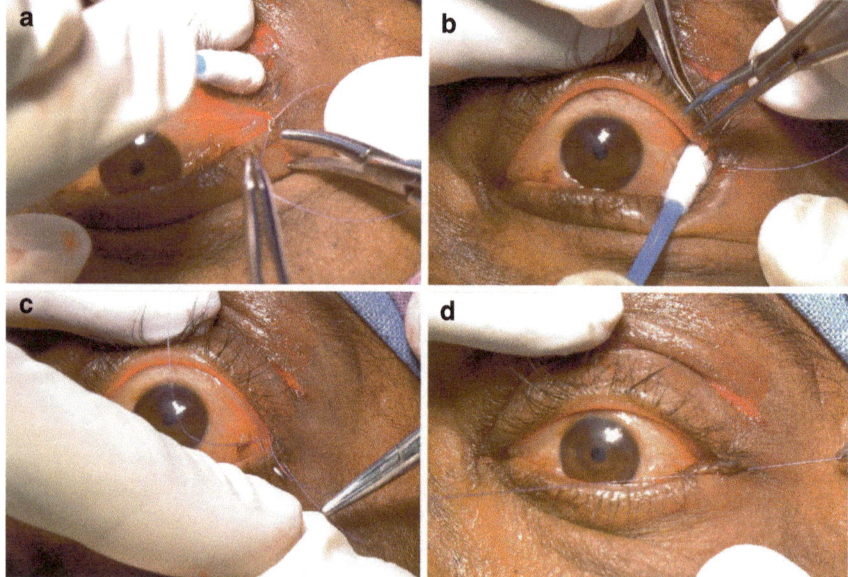

Fig. 6.7 Permanent lateral tarsorrhaphy *continued*. The suture is then passed through the corresponding upper eyelid intermarginal strip, out on the skin (**a**). The needle is then passed through the same exit point, and brought back to the intermarginal strip of the upper eyelid (**b**), and through the lower eyelid, out on the skin (**c**). The suture is then tied with or without a bolster (**d**)

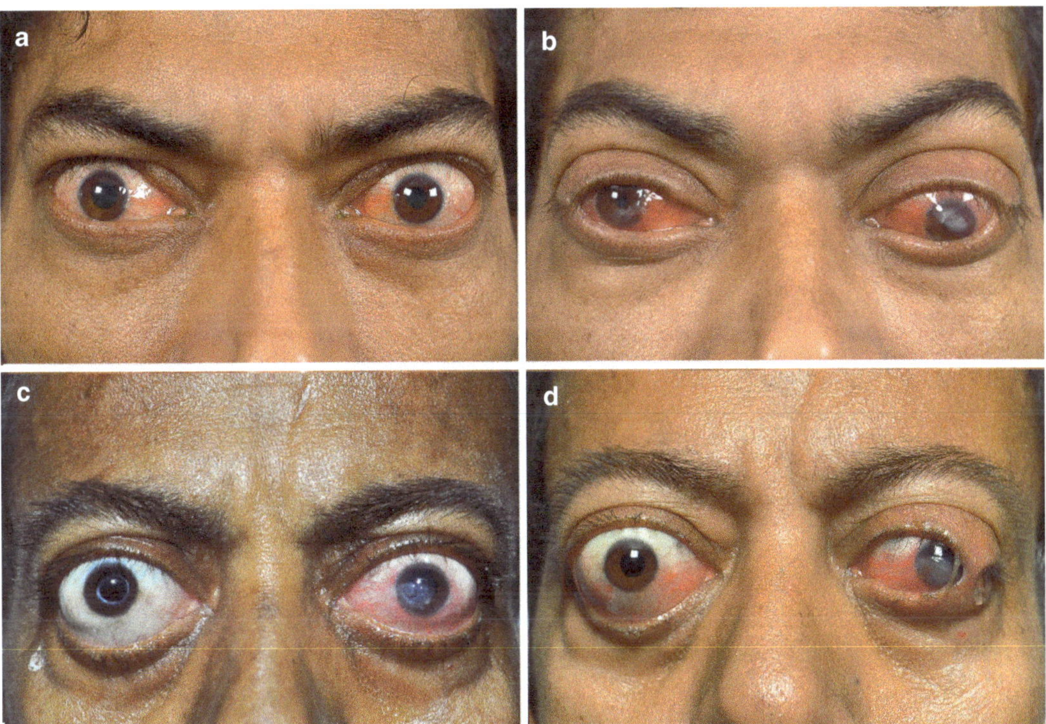

Fig. 6.8 Active thyroid eye disease (**a**, **c**), managed with a lateral (**b**) and a paramedian permanent tarsorrhaphy (**d**) for corneal protection

6.7 Modifications of Permanent Tarsorrhaphy

Don de Silva described a modification of the lateral tarsorrhaphy [3]. This was suggested for inferior scleral show <2 mm. The intended area of lateral tarsorrhaphy is marked, the grey line is split, and anterior lamella is excised. The upper and lower limbs of lateral canthal tendon/lateral ends of tarsal pates are then sutured to reform the lateral canthal angle. This technique avoids an unsatisfactory post-operative appearance of an inferiorly placed lash line at the lateral canthus, since the anterior lamella (lashes) are excised.

The tarsal pillar technique is another modification to achieve the narrowing of the interpalpebral width [4]. The conjunctival-tarsal strip from the upper lid is sutured to the lower eyelid, on either side of the cornea. This technique has the advantages of longevity and the ease of readily severing it.

6.8 Combination with Lid Lengthening Procedures

In severe cases of eyelid retraction, the lid margins simply cannot be brought together to perform a tarsorrhaphy. A tarsorrhaphy in such cases requires to be combined with lid lengthening procedures such as LPS recession or lower eyelid retractor release (Fig. 6.9) [5].

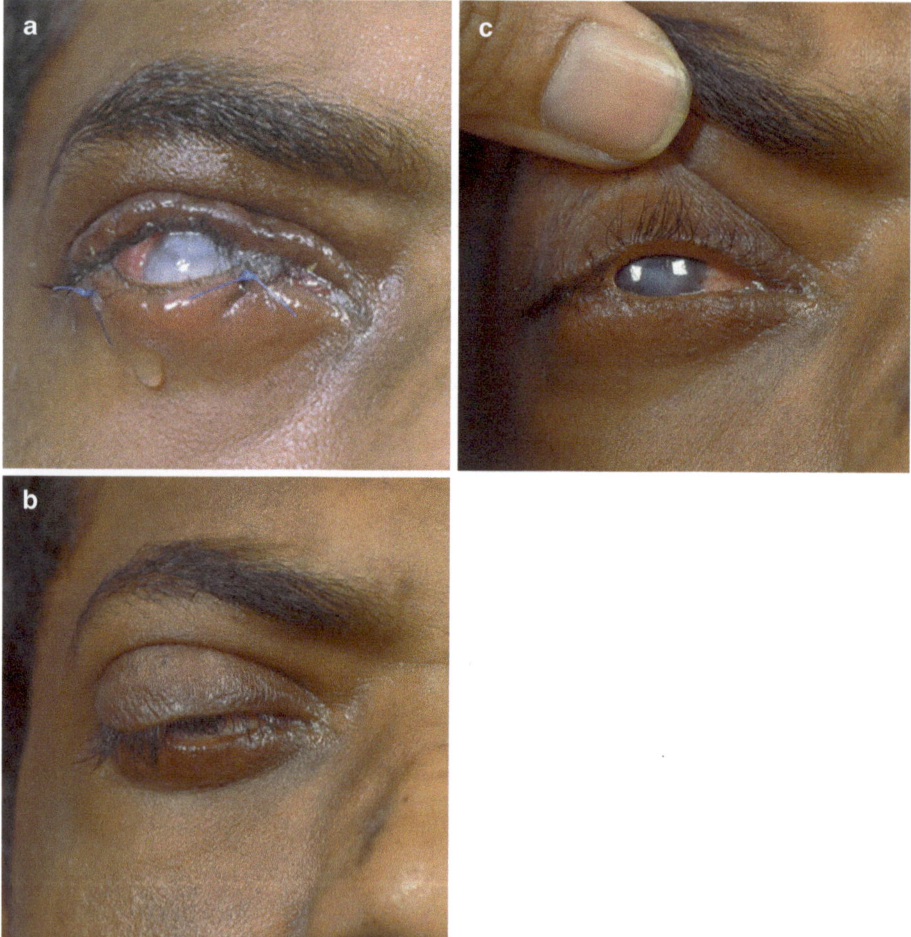

Fig. 6.9 Suture tarsorrhaphy with 4–0 Prolene not holding well due to severe eyelid retraction in a case of active thyroid eye disease with corneal ulcer (**a**). Combination procedure of levator recession and lateral paramedian tarsorrhaphy was performed (**b**), which provided corneal protection to allow healing of the cornea (**c**)

6.9 Summary

In conclusion, tarsorrhaphy is a useful tool in the management of active thyroid eye disease for corneal protection. It reduces the palpebral aperture, protects the cornea, and when performed at the extreme lateral canthus, is cosmetically acceptable to the patient. It can be performed as an office or bedside procedure, is very effective, and can be easily reversed.

References

1. Thaller VT, Kaden K, Lane CM, Collin JR. Thyroid lid surgery. Eye (Lond). 1987;1:609–14.
2. Verity DH, Rose GE. Acute thyroid eye disease (TED): principles of medical and surgical management. Eye (Lond). 2013;27:308–19.
3. de Silva DJ, Ramkissoon YD, Ismail AR, Beaconsfield M. Surgical technique: modified lateral tarsorrhaphy. Ophthalmic Plast Reconstr Surg. 2011;27:216–8.
4. Tanenbaum M, Gossman MD, Bergin DJ, Friedman HI, Lett D, Haines P, McCord CD Jr. The tarsal pillar technique for narrowing and maintenance of the interpalpebral fissure. Ophthalmic Surg. 1992;23:418–25.
5. Naik MN, Vasanthapuram VH, Joseph J, Murthy SI. Microbial keratitis in thyroid eye disease: clinical features, microbiological profile, and treatment outcome. Ophthalmic Plast Reconstr Surg. 2019;35(6):543–8.

7 Surgical Management of Compressive Optic Neuropathy in Active Thyroid Eye Disease

Peter J. Dolman

7.1 Introduction

Dysthyroid optic neuropathy (DON) is a complication of thyroid eye disease (TED) characterized by potentially reversible vision loss from compression or stretching of the optic nerve [1].

Almost 95% of cases are caused by compression of the nerve by enlarged extraocular muscles in the tight confines of the orbital apex (compressive optic neuropathy, CON) (Fig. 7.1) [2, 3]. The remaining 5% of DON results from stretching of the optic nerve (SON) from severe proptosis caused by fat or muscle expansion (Fig. 7.2) [2, 4].

CON occurs in 6–7% of all cases of TED, corresponding to 20% of the higher risk subgroup with myopathic disease [1]. Risk factors for developing CON include advancing age, male gender, smoking, and diabetes mellitus [1, 5].

P. J. Dolman (✉)
Department of Ophthalmology and Visual Sciences, University of British Columbia, Vancouver General Hospital, Vancouver, Canada

S. Rath, M. N. Naik (eds.), *Surgery in Thyroid Eye Disease*,
https://doi.org/10.1007/978-981-32-9220-8_7

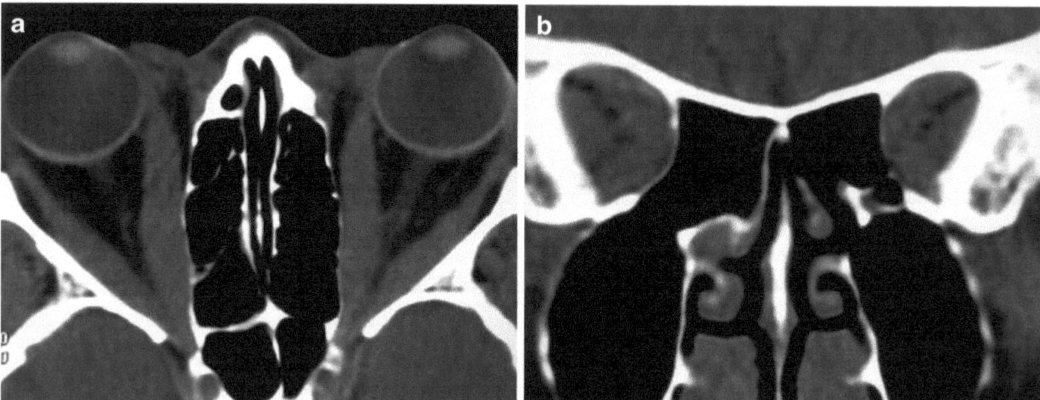

Fig. 7.1 Computed tomography demonstrating compressive optic neuropathy with enlarged extraocular muscles compressing the optic nerve at the orbital apex (**a**). Coronal view showing enlargement of four recti muscles with little fat space visible around the nerve (**b**)

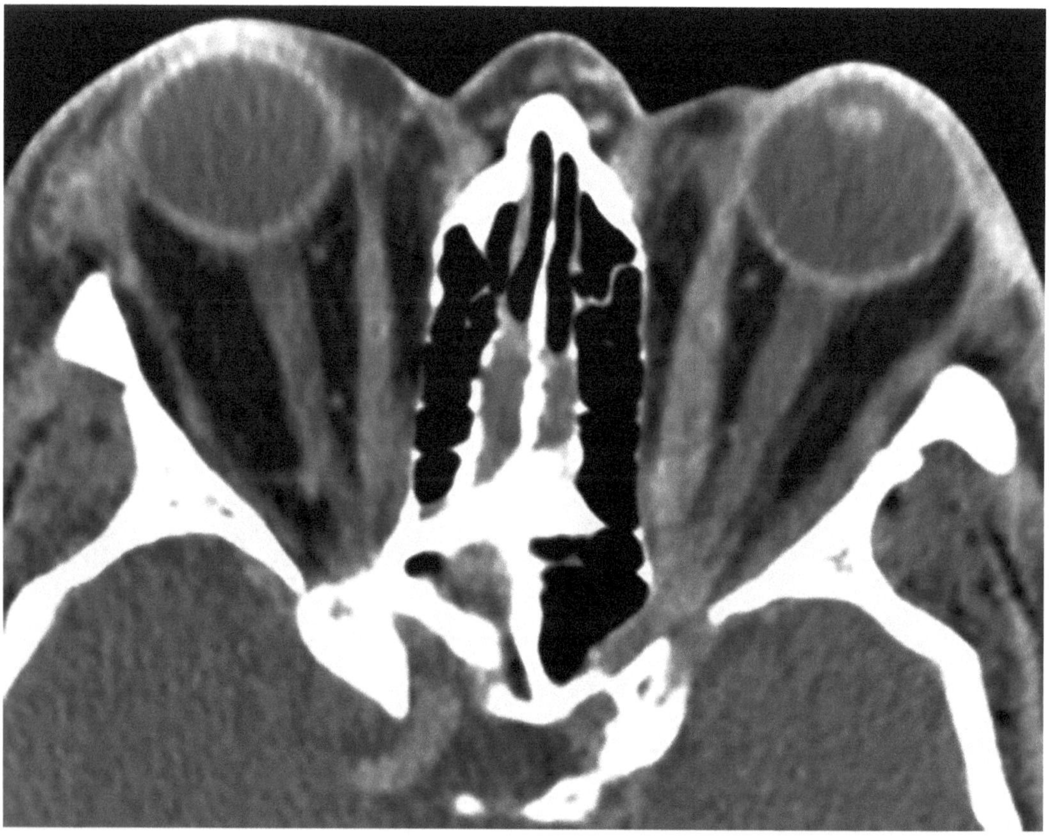

Fig. 7.2 Axial computed tomography scan showing proptotic globes from fat expansion with minimal extraocular muscle enlargement. Optic neuropathy in these cases results from stretching of the optic nerve (Stretch optic neuropathy) rather than apical compression (Compressive optic neuropathy)

7.2 Clinical Features

DON usually develops rapidly in association with obvious features of progressive TED, but occasionally may develop slowly, sometimes with the affected individual being unaware they even have vision loss [1].

The most sensitive clinical features are desaturation of colors or central vision loss [1, 3, 6]. In asymmetric disease, a relative afferent pupil defect may be detected. Optic nerve head findings (edema, congestion, or pallor) are seen in only 15–20% of affected cases; although not a sensitive finding, optic nerve head changes are highly specific for DON [3].

DON is typically diagnosed during the progressive (active) phase and associated with extraocular muscle enlargement. These cases often have periocular edema and injection (reflected by elevated Clinical Activity Score (CAS) or VISA inflammatory scores) and increased prominence of the eyes with restriction of ductions [1, 3, 6]. However, some patients with worsening CON may have little inflammatory soft tissue changes and minimal proptosis. This is particularly common in East Asian individuals and in patients who are started on corticosteroids (CS) for elevated CAS scores but develop CON despite CS therapy (Fig. 7.3a, b) [7–9].

7.3 Investigations and Diagnosis

Visual field defects are documented in 70% of patients with DON and include paracentral partial arcuate and altitudinal defects, with 55% of these located inferiorly [10].

CT scan is the most useful imaging modality [11]. It confirms the diagnosis of DON and helps distinguish between CON and SON. It also allows surgical planning, identifying areas for decompression, and potential hazards such as an inferiorly displaced fovea ethmoidalis that could increase the risk for CSF leaks. Common findings in CON are apical crowding by distended muscles, with an enlarged superior muscle group increasing the incidence of DON (Fig. 7.3b) [11, 12]. Optic nerve stretch with tenting of the posterior globe in the absence of apical crowding occurs in 5% of cases.

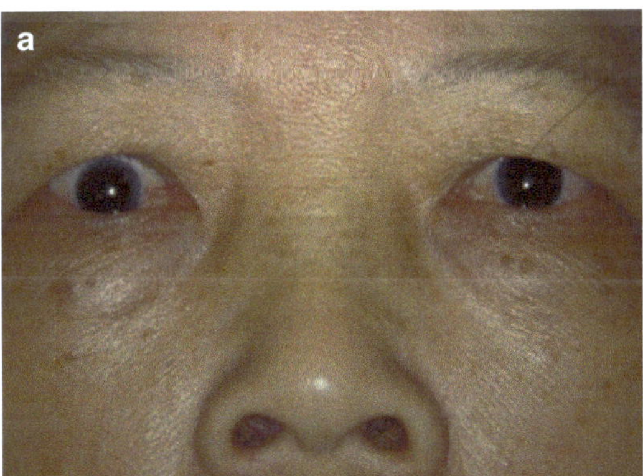

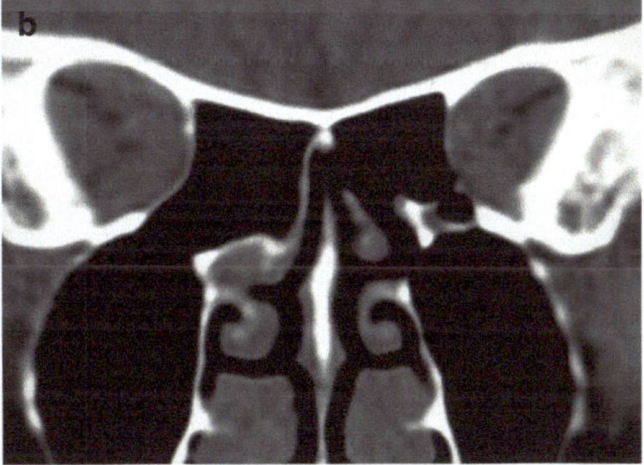

Fig. 7.3 A 67-year-old Asian female with minimal soft tissue signs and no proptosis but with severe bilateral central and color vision loss (**a**). Coronal computed tomography scan shows apical crowding by enlarged muscles (**b**)

7.4 Nonsurgical Management

7.4.1 Medical Options

Oral and intravenous corticosteroids (CS) are the first therapy in active TED and are usually tried in cases of CON identified in the progressive phase [2]. Typical trial doses are oral prednisone 1.5 mg/kg for 3 days or iv methylprednisolone 1 gm three doses for a week to assess for response in central and color vision. Approximately 85% of patients show visual improvement to CS therapy, but this is typically partial and short lived, deteriorating within a day of withholding CS. This therapy may delay or avoid surgery in approximately 25–50% of CON patients [6, 13, 14]. For this reason, the European Group on Graves Orbitopathy (EUGOGO) has recommended a trial of CS prior to orbital decompression (Fig. 7.4a, b).

Two studies have demonstrated that DON may develop even while on standard CS doses that have successfully lowered CAS scores [7, 9]. In one study, 17% of high-risk myopathic TED patients developed DON while on full doses of CS, a rate no better than untreated cases [7].

As CS therapy can elevate serum glucose levels, DON patients on CS must be closely monitored for worsening of DM, a common comorbidity in DON [5].

Intravenous rituximab has been found to both improve or worsen DON in different publications [15].

7.4.2 External Beam Radiotherapy (XRT)

XRT is thought to be helpful in early progressive TED by targeting lymphocytes and fibrocytes. Commonly 2000 Rads (20 Gy) are delivered through a lateral port to the retrobulbar space, fractionated over 10 days. It is avoided in diabetic patients (who also are more likely to develop CON) because of reported worsening of retinopathy in this group [16].

XRT may be helpful in controlling CON in several ways. One report showed that high-risk myopathic TED patients developed the onset of CON in 17% of patients even while on standard doses of CS, but none of this high-risk group developed CON while on combined CS and XRT therapy [7].

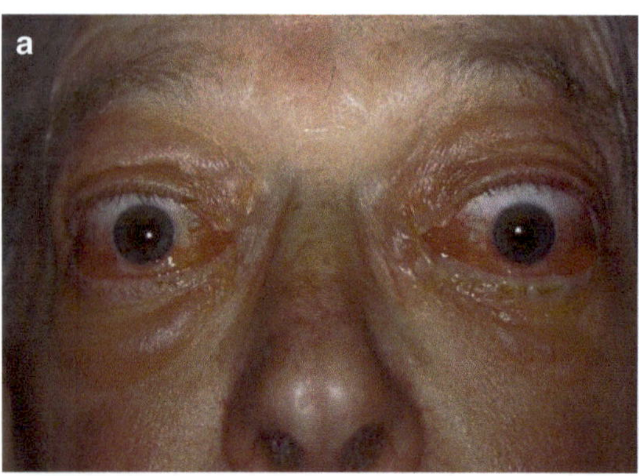

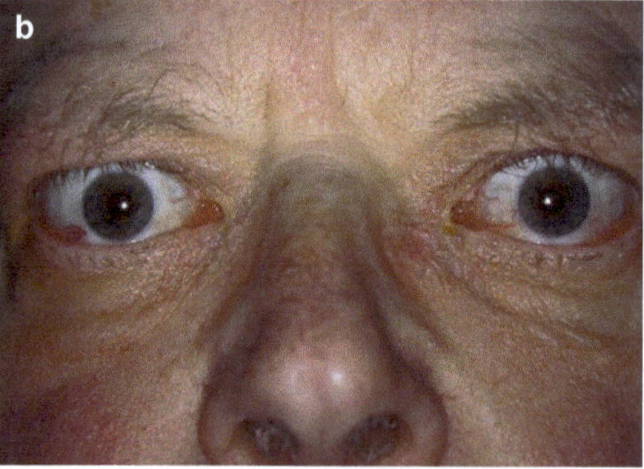

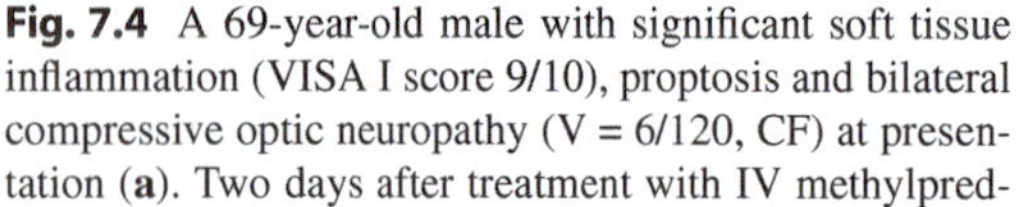

Fig. 7.4 A 69-year-old male with significant soft tissue inflammation (VISA I score 9/10), proptosis and bilateral compressive optic neuropathy (V = 6/120, CF) at presentation (**a**). Two days after treatment with IV methylprednisolone resulted in the reduction of soft tissue inflammatory signs but only partial improvement of vision (V = 6/30; 6/60) (**b**)

Two retrospective studies showed that XRT could delay or avoid the need for orbital decompression surgery in cases of CON [17].

We have found that 20% of individuals who have regained good central visual acuity following orbital decompression for CON subsequently developed recurrent deterioration in vision from progressive enlargement of the medial and/or inferior rectus after surgery. These changes are confirmed on CT scans and are presumed to be progression of active enlarged orbital tissues. These cases all regained vision with a course of XRT. In addition, prophylactic XRT within 2 weeks of orbital decompression for DON found no cases that subsequently developed DON [16].

7.5 Surgical Perioperative Considerations

Surgery is considered when medical options or XRT fail to fully restore vision.

The surgical approach is described to the patient and family with the aid of imaging studies, and the normal post-operative course and possible complications are reviewed.

The goal in CON is to expand the apical space by removing bone from the posterior medial wall and medial floor, allowing displacement of enlarged extraocular muscles into adjoining sinuses. Occasionally the lateral wall can be hollowed into the bone marrow space to provide additional apical decompression [18, 19].

The goal in SON is to relieve globe protrusion and optic nerve stretch by maximal reduction of proptosis, by decompression of fat and multiple bony walls. These procedures are described in subsequent chapters [4, 11–13].

Decompressions are typically performed under general anesthesia, although regional blocks with monitored sedation are possible.

Anticoagulants and antiplatelet agents are generally discontinued several days prior to the surgery assuming this is safe.

Perioperative antibiotics (intravenous cefazolin) are administered prior to the start of surgery. Most cases of DON are in an active phase and likely will already be on intravenous corticosteroids. Local anesthetic with epinephrine may be injected at the intended incision site while cottonoids soaked in cocaine 4% or decongestants may be placed in the nostril for hemostasis. The anesthetist may maintain a lowered blood pressure to limit bleeding in the congested orbit.

7.6 Surgical Technique

7.6.1 Surgical Approaches

The goal in surgical decompression for CON is to relieve pressure on the optic nerve by the enlarged extraocular muscles by expanding the apical space; the bone is fenestrated in the medial wall and floor close to the start of the optic canal as far posterior and superior as possible without entering the cranium [20, 21].

Transantral and transfrontal craniotomies were approaches used in the past but are seldom employed currently because of the indirect route and greater surgical morbidity [20, 22, 23].

Endoscopic transnasal apical decompressions are increasingly popular and allow a magnified direct visualization of the surgical site but require appropriate training to avoid potentially severe orbital trauma [24–26]. Available navigation software allows more precise identification of safe landmarks but the equipment is expensive and its use requires specialized training and a longer surgical time. This approach is presented in Chapter 8.

7.6.2 The Transcutaneous Approach

It is usually performed using a modified Lynch incision. A line is marked running parallel and temporal to the angular vessel (Fig. 7.5a); the area is infiltrated with local anesthesia with epinephrine, and prepped. A scalpel opens the wound and a bipolar cautery is used to control bleeding from the muscle and skin edge and to cauterize the angular vessel if needed (Fig. 7.5b). The nasal wound edge can be retracted with an ophthalmic rake or Desmarres retractor while a monopolar cautery is used to incise through the periorbita (Fig. 7.5c).

A Cottle elevator is used to peel the periorbita temporally over the anterior lacrimal crest to reflect the lacrimal sac temporally (Figs. 7.5d and 7.6a). The periorbita can be relaxed both superiorly (along with disinsertion of the trochlea) and inferiorly behind the lacrimal sac apparatus without widening the cutaneous incision to allow better exposure of the medial wall and floor. Surgical loupes and a headlight are used to visualize the surgical field.

The periorbita is gently peeled off the bony walls using the blunt Freer elevator with a broad ribbon retractor containing the displaced orbital

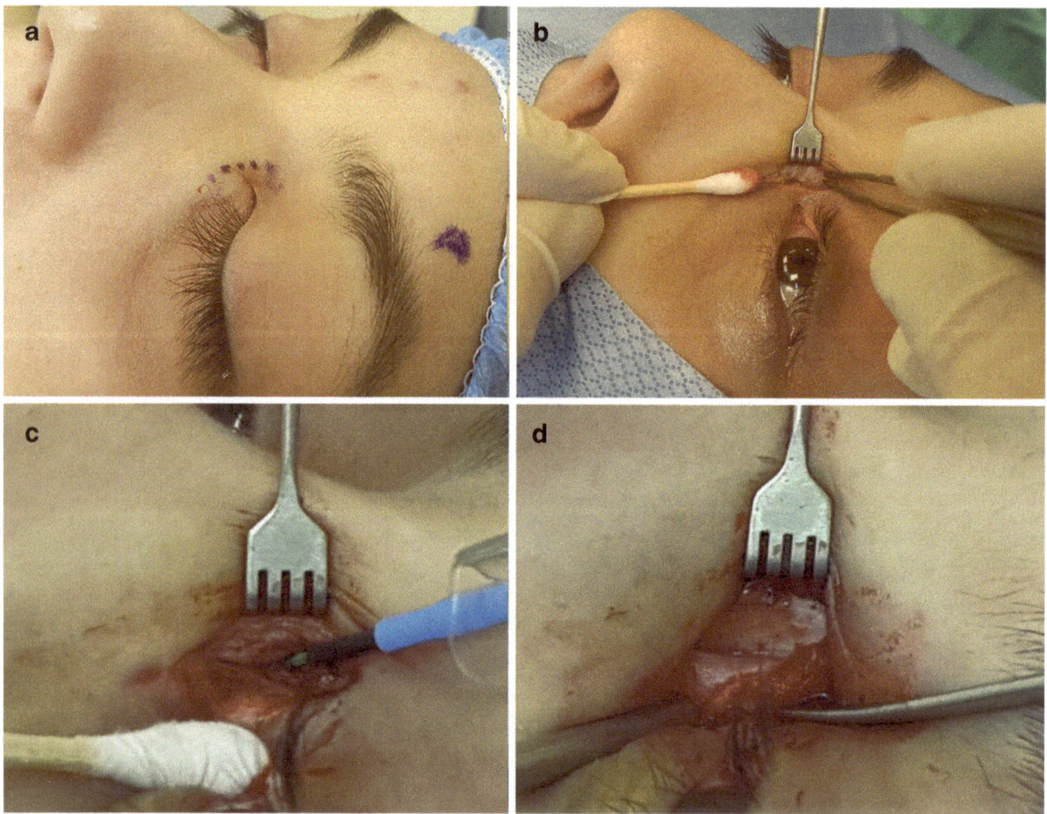

Fig. 7.5 Transcutaneous medial wall decompression. Lynch incision just lateral to the angular vessel (**a**). Bipolar cautery coagulates the angular vessel (**b**). Monopolar cautery cuts periorbita temporal to coagulated angular vessel (**c**). Cottle elevator reflects periosteum from nasal bridge and over anterior lacrimal crest (**d**)

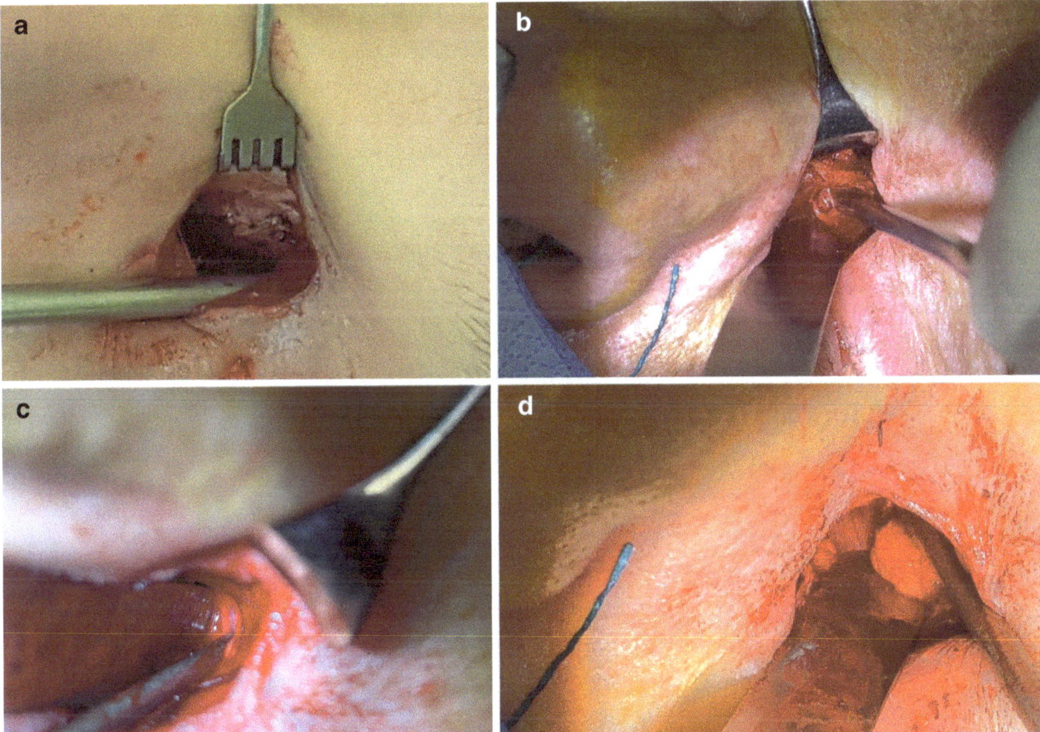

Fig. 7.6 Transcutaneous medial wall decompression continued. Cottle elevator strips the periorbita over the anterior lacrimal crest to expose the lacrimal sac fossa (**a**). Anterior ethmoidal vessels and nerves are exposed along the medial orbit (**b**). Magnified view showing monopolar cautery dividing the ethmoidal vessels (**c**). Periorbita opened exposing orbital fat and medial rectus muscle (**d**)

contents. Care is taken to avoid fracturing the thin bone of the walls or tearing the periorbita, as spillage of orbital fat or enlarged muscle will obscure the view.

The anterior and posterior ethmoidal neurovascular bundles are identified, cauterized, and cut (Fig. 7.6b, c). These provide a landmark for the posterior point of bone exposure (2–3 mm behind the posterior vessel) and the superior aspect of bone removal (at the level of these vessels). Landmarks for bone removal are described below (Fig. 7.6d).

7.6.3 The Transcaruncular Approach

This provides direct access to the medial wall and floor and has the advantage that it bypasses the medial canthal ligament, the lacrimal apparatus, and avoids a cutaneous incision [21, 26]. In the tight congested orbit associated with DON, the view may initially be limited, but the conjunctival incision may be extended inferiorly into the fornix allowing better visualization of the medial floor.

A 4–0 silk suture is passed through the medial upper and lower eyelid margins to expose the caruncle (Fig. 7.7a). Lidocaine with epinephrine is infiltrated into the caruncle just anterior to the plica. A sharp Westcott scissor, Colorado needle or hot-wire cautery is used to incise between the plica and caruncle. Closed Stevens scissors are passed at a 45° angle following the lid margins posteromedially to identify the posterior lacrimal crest behind the lacrimal apparatus. The blades are gently spread vertically to expose the medial wall without releasing the medial orbital fat pocket (Fig. 7.7b). The surgical field is exposed with a rake retractor anteriorly and malleable retractors posteriorly, and a monopolar cautery used to incise the periorbita posterior to the lacrimal sac. A blunt Freer elevator combined with progressively larger ribbon retractors are used to strip the periorbita posteriorly to the leading edge of the optic canal just behind the posterior ethmoidal vessel (approximately 40 mm behind the anterior lacrimal crest), superiorly to the ethmoidal vessels, and inferotemporally onto the medial floor to the edge of the infraorbital canal (Fig. 7.7c, d).

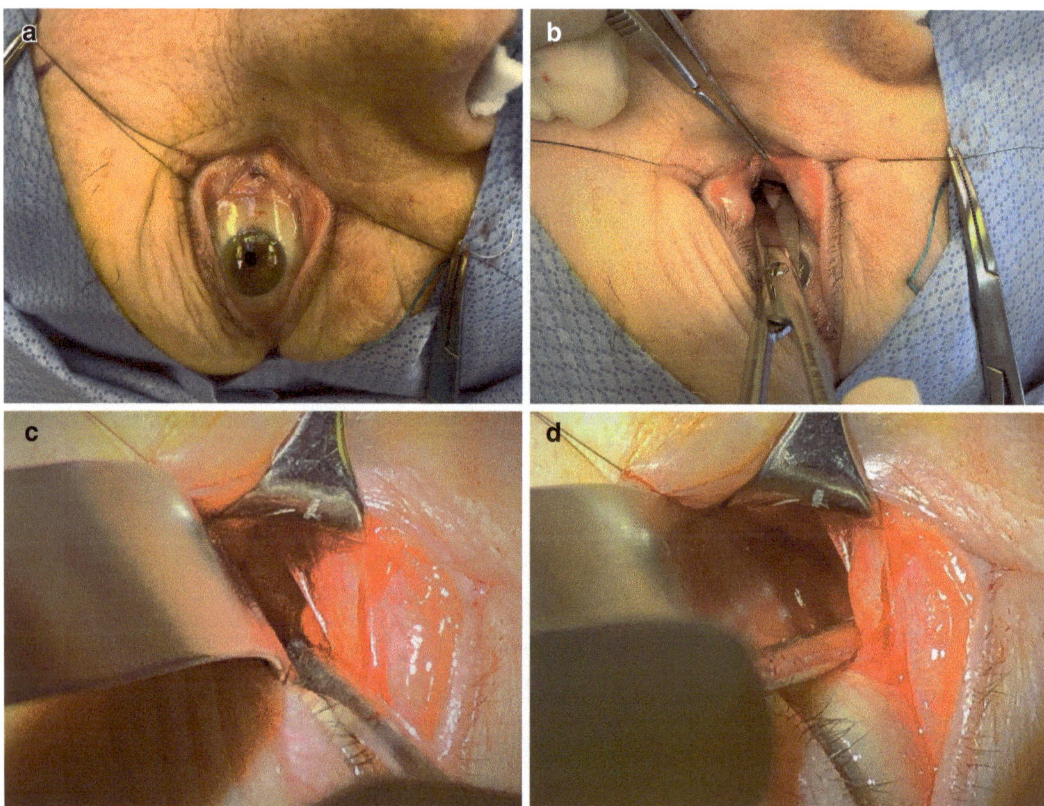

Fig. 7.7 Medial transcaruncular approach: Lids retracted to expose plica and caruncle (**a**). Stevens scissors inserted behind caruncle to posterior lacrimal crest, spread to expose medial bony wall (**b**). Periosteal elevator strips periorbita from medial wall to floor inferiorly (**c**). Periorbita stripped along medial floor to medial margin of infraorbital canal (**d**)

7.6.4 Landmarks for Bone Removal

Following reflection of the periorbita to the planned margins of bone removal, an ethmoidectomy is performed using Weil-Blakesley forceps up to the level of the ethmoidal vessels and posteriorly to the anterior face of the sphenoid sinus, approximately 40 mm from the anterior lacrimal crest. The bony floor is rongeured into the maxillary sinus from behind the lacrimal sac apparatus to the posterior wall of the maxilla and laterally to the medial margin of the infraorbital canal (Fig. 7.8). The orbital strut separating the maxillary and ethmoid sinuses is removed from its midpoint to the face of the sphenoid sinus, leaving a triradiate shape ("Mercedes sign") [21], with the superior arm separating the sphenoid sinus and orbit, the inferolateral arm separating the orbit and maxilla, and the inferomedial arm separating the maxilla and sphenoid sinus (Fig. 7.9).

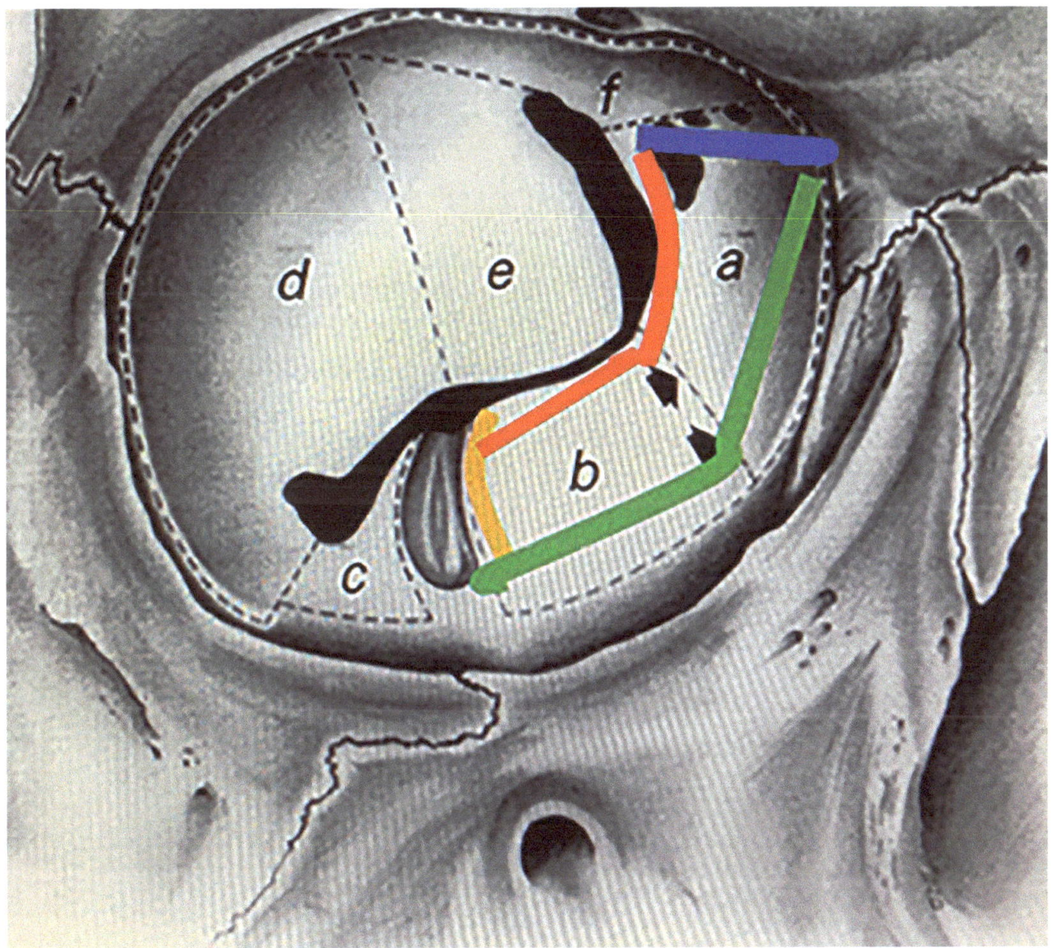

Fig. 7.8 Boundaries of orbital decompression for DON. Green: anterior border follows posterior lacrimal crest medially and just behind anterior rim along floor, Blue: superior border along anterior and posterior ethmoidal foramina; Red: Posterior border from level of posterior ethmoidal foramen (36 mm posterior to anterior lacrimal crest) to posterior wall of maxilla inferiorly; Yellow: lateral extent along infraorbital canal

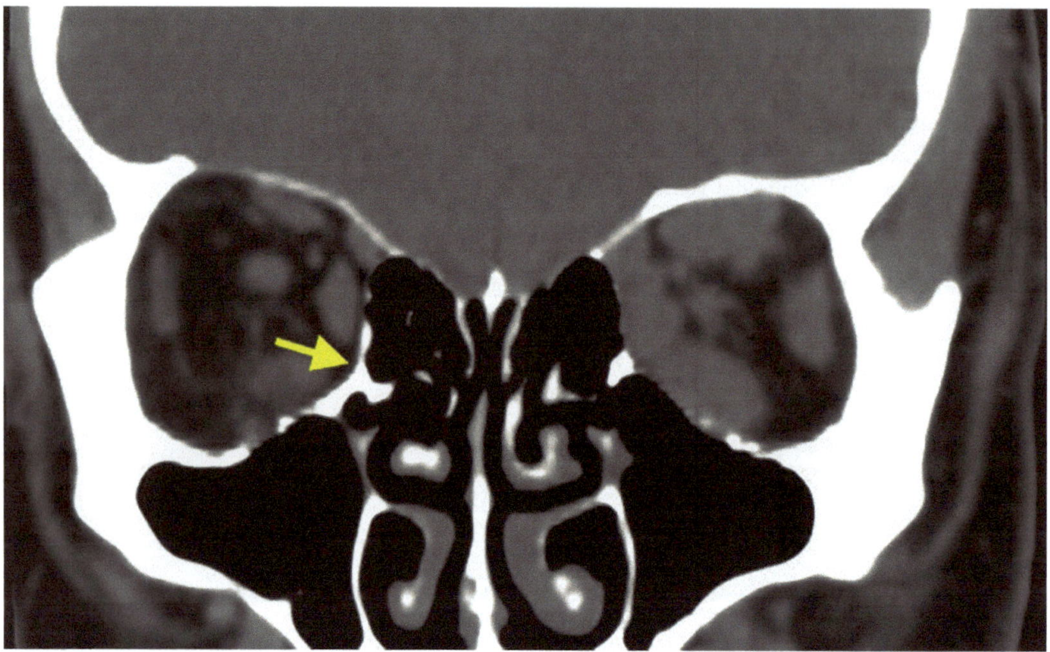

Fig. 7.9 Computed tomography scan (coronal) in the case of asymmetric TED with left DON. Yellow arrow shows optic strut with "Mercedes sign" where bone separates posterior ethmoid/sphenoid sinus, orbit, and maxillary sinus

7.6.5 Opening the Periorbita

The periorbita is punctured near the apex with a #12 blade and advanced anteriorly in two parallel lines above and below the medial rectus muscle. The two incisions are connected anteriorly, and the orbital fat and muscle are allowed to herniate into the ethmoid and maxillary sinuses.

The retrocaruncular conjunctival incision site is closed with a 6–0 gut suture while the Lynch incision can be apposed with 6–0 silk interrupted sutures.

The patient is monitored for retrobulbar hematoma, compartment syndrome, or vision loss over the next 48 hours. Post-operative medications may include 3 days of oral corticosteroids and 5 days of oral broad-spectrum antibiotic (such as cefazolin).

7.6.6 Surgical Outcomes

Surgical decompression is successful in restoring central vision to 20/40 or better in over 80% of our institution's audit of 54 cases over a 15-year period, regardless of the severity of the initial vision loss or the delay to surgery. Occasionally, there is irreversible vision loss but worsening of vision is rare.

Occasionally, vision gains from decompression may be partially reversed from ongoing expansion of muscles adjacent to the decompression site. As mentioned previously, XRT may reverse this vision loss, or can prevent its development if administered shortly after the surgery (Fig. 7.10a, b).

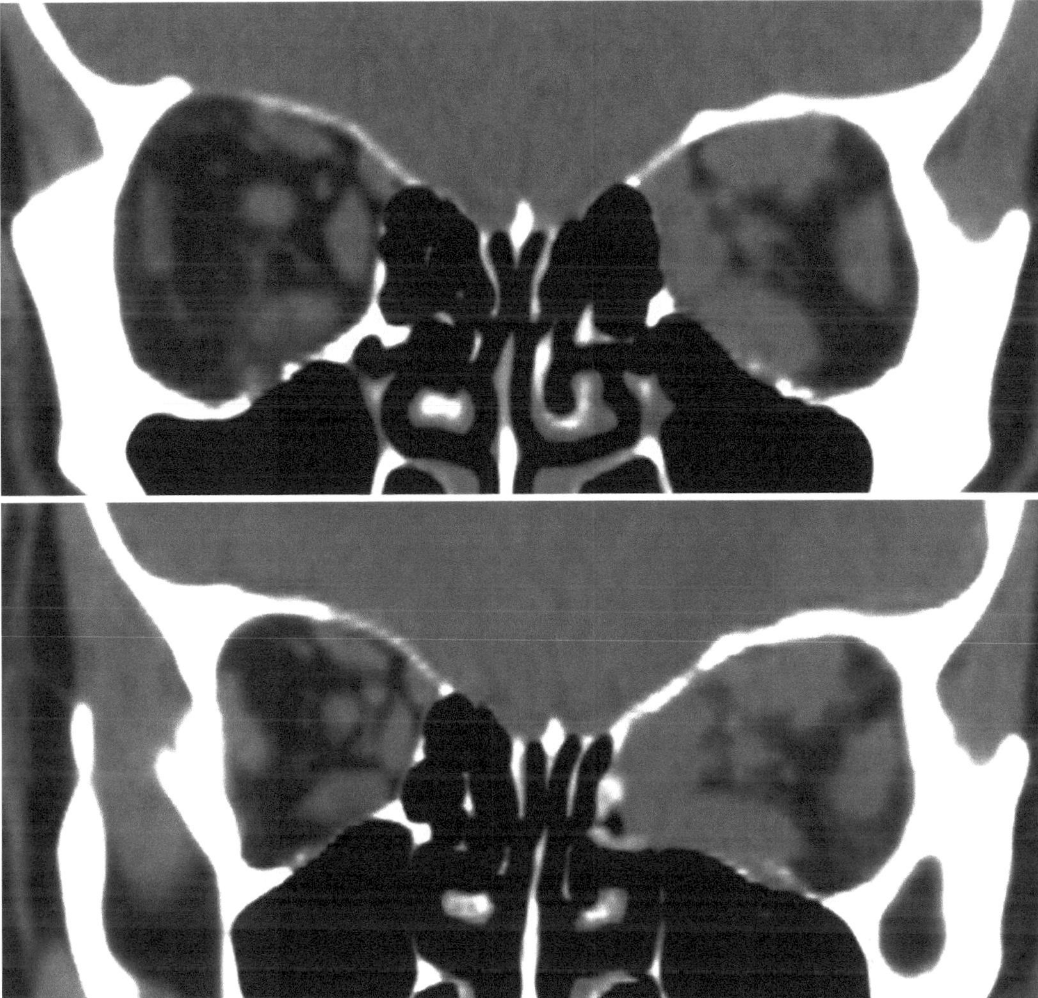

Fig. 7.10 Computed tomography scan in a case of left Dysthyroid optic neuropathy with enlarged extraocular muscles and apical crowding (top). Central vision had reduced to 20/120. Same case following left medial wall and nasal floor decompression (bottom). Vision was restored to 20/20 and then worsened again. Post-operative computed tomography scan shows adequate orbital decompression but secondary further enlargement of the medial rectus muscle. Orbital radiotherapy restored the vision to post-operative level

7.7 Complications

The Lynch incision generally heals well if kept small and lateral to the angular vessel but a webbed scar may occasionally form. The transcaruncular incision avoids this complication (Fig. 7.11a). Care must be taken to avoid trauma to the lacrimal outflow apparatus during the retrocaruncular approach.

A review at our institution found that the incidence of worsening diplopia following medial wall and floor decompression for CON was over 50%. These cases were typically in a progressive phase with inflamed tight muscles, and most would have required alignment surgery eventually regardless of whether decompressive surgery was performed. The tendency in these cases is for esotropia and hypotropia to worsen (Fig. 7.11b) [27].

Temporary anesthesia or paresthesia of the lateral wall of the nose from injury to the ethmoidal nerves usually resolves within several months. Infraorbital anesthesia may be avoided by avoiding the infraorbital canal during bone removal of the orbital floor.

Impaired sinus drainage from anterior orbital strut trauma may lead to fluid retention or frank sinusitis and may require endoscopic sinus surgery (Fig. 7.12).

Injury to the fovea ethmoidalis during removal of the superior bone close to the optic canal can rarely lead to a cerebrospinal fluid leak or intracranial hemorrhage (Fig. 7.13). These serious complications are fortunately rare [28, 29].

Compartment syndrome and vision loss might occur in the first post-operative week from an intraorbital hemorrhage, and patients must be warned to seek immediate help for a lateral canthotomy to treat this [30].

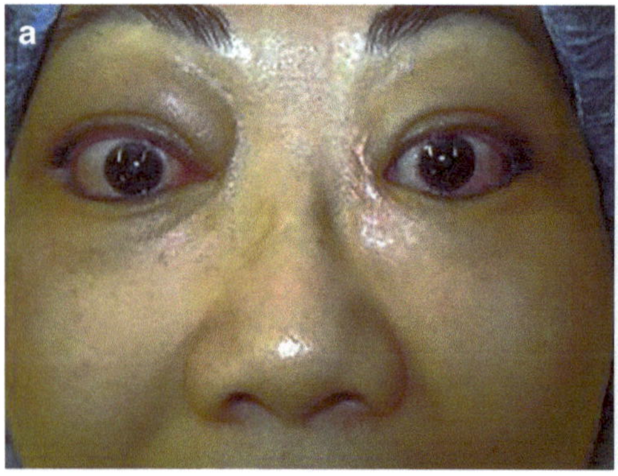
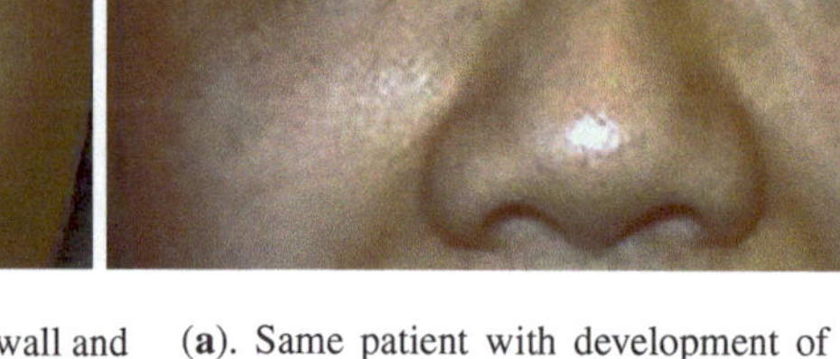

Fig. 7.11 Two weeks following bilateral medial wall and floor decompression for DON. Healing scar from Lynch incision, left eye, and transcaruncular incision right eye (**a**). Same patient with development of consecutive left esotropia from ongoing inflammation and scarring of left medial rectus muscle (**b**)

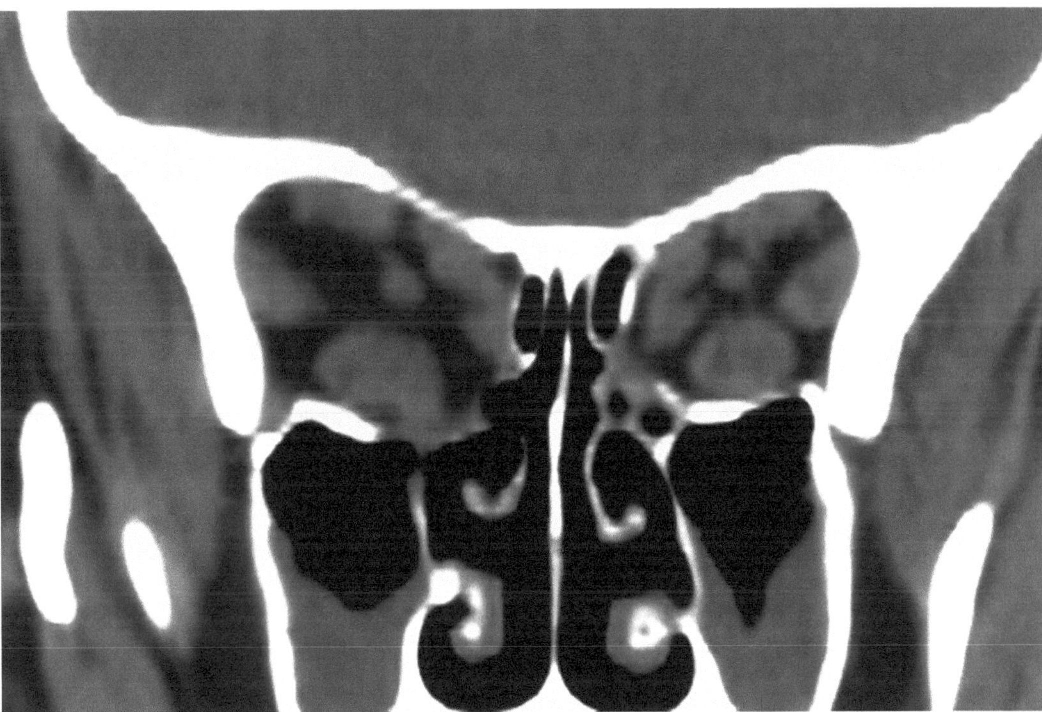

Fig. 7.12 Computed tomography scan showing sinus fluid collection a week following bilateral medial wall and floor decompressions

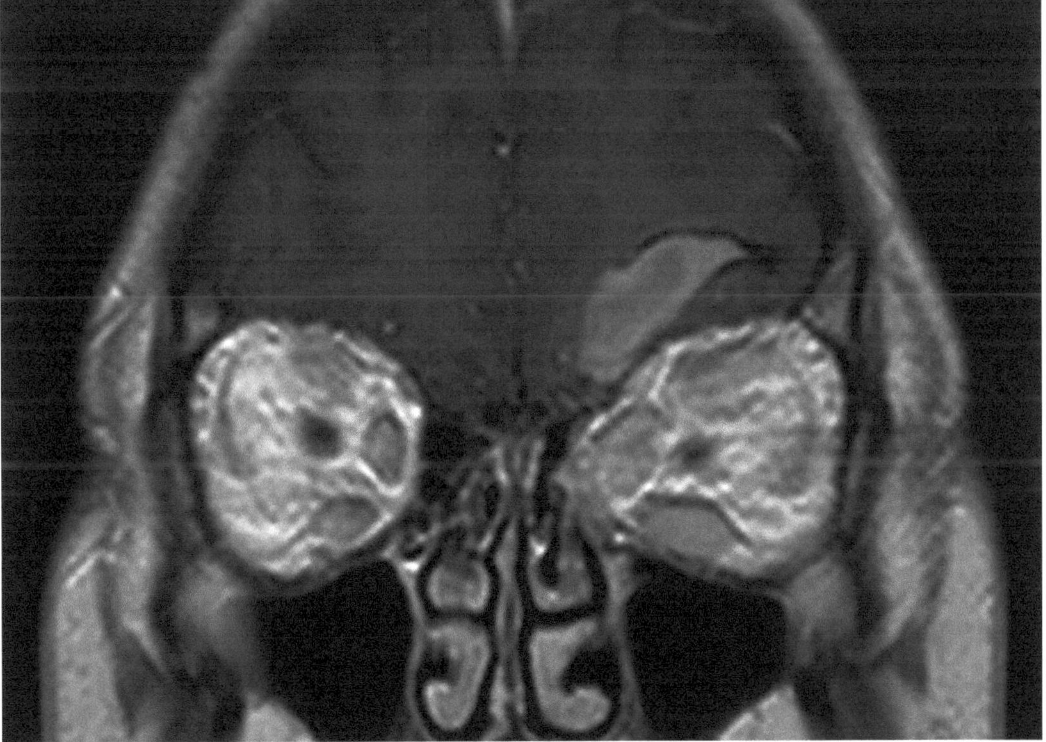

Fig. 7.13 Magnetic resonance imaging, coronal view showing resolving left frontal lobe hematoma following orbital superior apical decompression

References

1. Dolman PJ. Evaluating graves Orbitopathy. Best Pract Res Clin Endocrinol Metab. 2012;26(3):229–48.
2. Saeed P, Tavakoli Rad S, Bisschop PHLT. Dysthyroid optic neuropathy. Ophthalmic Plast Reconstr Surg. 2018;34(4S Suppl 1):S60–7.
3. McKeag D, Lane CM, Lazarus JH, et al. Clinical features of dysthyroid optic neuropathy: a European group on graves' Orbitopathy survey. Br J Ophthalmol. 2007;91:455–8.
4. Kazim M, Trokel SL, Acaroglu G, et al. Reversal of dysthyroid optic neuropathy following orbital fat decompression. Br J Ophthalmol. 2000 Jun;84(6):600–5.
5. Kalmann R, Mourits MP. Diabetes mellitus: a risk factor in patients with Graves' orbitopathy. Br J Ophthalmol. 1999 Apr;83(4):463–5.
6. Wong Y, Dickinson J, Perros P, Dayan C, Veeramani P, Morris D, Foot B, Clarke L. A British ophthalmological surveillance unit (BOSU) study into dysthyroid optic neuropathy in the United Kingdom. Eye (Lond). 2018 Oct;32(10):1555–62.
7. Shams PN, Ma R, Pickles T, Rootman J, Dolman PJ. Reduced risk of compressive optic neuropathy using orbital radiotherapy in patients with active thyroid eye disease. Am J Ophthalmol. 2014;157(6):1299–305.
8. Dolman PJ. Grading severity and activity in thyroid eye disease. Ophthalmic Plast Reconstr Surg. 2018;34(4S):S34–40.
9. Bartalena L, Krassas GE, Wiersinga W. Marcocci C et al; European group on Graves' Orbitopathy. Efficacy and safety of three different cumulative doses of intravenous methylprednisolone for moderate to severe and active graves' orbitopathy. J Clin Endocrinol Metab. 2012 Dec;97(12): 4454–63.
10. Starks VS, Reinshagen KL, Lee NG, Freitag SK. Visual field and orbital computed tomography correlation in dysthyroid optic neuropathy due to thyroid eye disease. Orbit. 2019 May;6:1–7.
11. Giaconi JA, Kazim M, Rho T, et al. CT scan evidence of dysthyroid optic neuropathy. Ophthalmic Plast Reconstr Surg. 2002 May;18(3):177–82.
12. Oropesa S, Dunbar KE, Godfrey KJ, Callahan AB, Campbell AA, Kazim M. Predominant contribution of superior rectus-Levator complex enlargement to optic neuropathy and inferior visual field defects in thyroid eye disease. Ophthalmic Plast Reconstr Surg. 2018 Aug 1;35(3):262–5.
13. Zhao LQ, Yu DY, Cheng JW. Intravenous glucocorticoids therapy in the treatment of graves' ophthalmopathy: a systematic review and meta-analysis. Int J Ophthalmol. 2019 Jul 18;12(7):1177–86.
14. Currò N, Covelli D, Vannucchi G. Campi I et al therapeutic outcomes of high-dose intravenous steroids in the treatment of dysthyroid optic neuropathy. Thyroid. 2014 May;24(5):897–905.
15. Khanna D, Chong KK, Afifiyan NF, Hwang CJ, et al. Rituximab treatment of patients with severe, corticosteroid-resistant thyroid-associated ophthalmopathy. Ophthalmology. 2010 Jan;117(1):133–9.
16. Dolman PJ, Rath S. Orbital radiotherapy for thyroid eye disease. Curr Opin Ophthalmol. 2012;23(5):427–32.
17. Gold KG, Scofield S, Isaacson SR, Stewart MW, Kazim M. Orbital radiotherapy combined with corticosteroid treatment for thyroid eye disease-compressive optic neuropathy. Ophthalmic Plast Reconstr Surg. 2018 Mar/Apr;34(2):172–7.
18. Choe CH, Cho R, Elner VM. Comparison of lateral and medial orbital decompression for the treatment of compressive optic neuropathy in thyroid eye disease. Ophthalmic Plast Reconstr Surg. 2011 Jan-Feb;27(1):4–11.
19. Korkmaz S, Konuk O. Surgical treatment of Dysthyroid optic neuropathy: long-term visual outcomes with comparison of 2-wall versus 3-wall orbital decompression. Curr Eye Res. 2016;41(2):159–64.
20. Tooley AA, Godfrey KJ. Kazim M evolution of thyroid eye disease decompression-dysthyroid optic neuropathy. Eye (Lond). 2019 Feb;33(2):206–11.
21. Jefferis JM, Jones RK, Currie ZI, Tan JH, Salvi SM. Orbital decompression for thyroid eye disease: methods, outcomes, and complications. Eye. 2018;32:626–36.
22. Boboridis KG. Bunce C surgical orbital decompression for thyroid eye disease. Cochrane Database Syst Rev. 2011 Dec 7;12:CD007630.
23. Baldeschi L. Small versus coronal incision orbital decompression in Graves orbitopathy. Orbit. 2010;29(4):177–82.
24. Antisdel JL, Gumber D, Holmes J, Sindwani R. Management of sinonasal complications after endoscopic orbital decompression for graves' orbitopathy. Laryngoscope. 2013;123(9):2094–8.
25. Chu EA, Miller NR, Lane AP. Selective endoscopic decompression of the orbital apex for dysthyroid optic neuropathy. Laryngoscope. 2009 Jun;119(6):1236–40.
26. Liao SL, Chang TC, Lin LL. Transcaruncular orbital decompression: an alternate procedure for graves ophthalmopathy with compressive optic neuropathy. Am J Ophthalmol. 2006 May;141(5):810–8.
27. Dolman PJ. Orbital decompression and its effect on strabismus. Presentation at Oculoplastics SUBDAY, American Academy of Ophthalmology Fall Meeting, Chicago 2014.
28. Badilla J, Dolman PJ. Intracranial hemorrhage complicating an orbital decompression. Orbit. 2008;27(2):143–5.
29. Badilla J, Dolman PJ. Cerebrospinal fluid leaks complicating orbital or oculoplastic surgery. Arch Ophthalmol. 2007;125(12):1631–4.
30. Sellari-Franceschini S, Dallan I, Bajraktari A. Fiacchini G et al Surgical complications in orbital decompression for Graves' orbitopathy. Acta Otorhinolaryngol Ital. 2016 Aug;36(4):265–74.

8 Endonasal Apical Decompression for Compressive Optic Neuropathy

Mohammad Javed Ali

8.1 Introduction

Thyroid eye disease or TED is an autoimmune disorder where organ-specific autoantibodies target the orbits and the periorbita leading to a host of structural and functional disabilities [1–5]. Clinical presentations include erythema and edema of the eyelids, conjunctiva and caruncle, proptosis, extraocular muscle enlargement, restrictive myopathies, and diplopia [1–7]. Rarely dysthyroid optic neuropathy (DON) may be the presenting sign secondary to compression of the optic nerve by enlarged extraocular muscles or stretching of the optic nerve secondary to a gross proptosis. The details of various aspects of TED are covered up in different chapters of this text. The current chapter discusses the indications, surgical techniques, outcomes, and complications of endoscopic approach for orbital decompression in case of compressive optic neuropathy.

8.2 Indications

The indications for an orbital decompression in a case of TED include dysthyroid optic neuropathy, severe proptosis with exposure keratopathy, failed medical therapy, and rehabilitating cosmetic disfigurements [2, 4, 5, 8–12].

A major systematic review [10] of orbital decompressions in TED over nearly a two-decade period showed the most common indications for surgery were cosmesis (42.4%), dysthyroid optic neuropathy (40.6%) and exposure keratopathy (7.9%). The goals of the decompression surgery are to remove medial orbital wall with or without removal of the floor medial to the infraorbital canal. This is followed by removal of the excess fat or simply prolapse of the fat into the newly created recesses in the nasal cavity. Both these would allow expansion of the orbital contents into the paranasal spaces thereby giving more room within the orbit.

M. J. Ali (✉)
Govindram Seksaria Institute of Dacryology,
L.V. Prasad Eye Institute, Hyderabad, India

S. Rath, M. N. Naik (eds.), *Surgery in Thyroid Eye Disease*,
https://doi.org/10.1007/978-981-32-9220-8_8

8.3 Advantages of Endoscopic Approach

There are numerous advantages of performing orbital floor and medial wall decompression via an endoscopic approach [8–13]. The advantages and limitations are summarized in Table 8.1.

Table 8.1 Advantages and limitations of Endonasal Endoscopic approach to Medial wall decompression in TED with dysthyroid optic neuropathy

Advantages	Limitations
Excellent visualization for more bone removal	Endoscopic surgery equipment and expertise
Enhanced safety at crucial anatomical locations	May require additional procedures like septoplasty for better visualization
Better apical decompression	Limited control over intraorbital bleeders (orbital fat space)
Lesser possibility of infraorbital nerve anesthesia	Direct exposure of orbit to the nasal cavity
Lesser possibility of a hypoglobus	
Absence of an external scar	
Enhanced post-operative comfort	
Faster rehabilitation	

8.4 Preoperative Radiological Evaluation

The preoperative clinical evaluation includes detailed clinical examination, proptosis measurements, and grading of severity of inflammation. When an endoscopic approach is planned, a detailed radiologic study is very crucial for successful outcomes [14]. A CT scan of the orbits and paranasal sinuses is the investigation of choice. A good quality scan should be performed at 1-mm intervals in the axial, coronal and parasagittal planes. This helps in seamless assessment of the anatomical structures from one cut to another. All the sections should be printed for the surgeon. The bony windows are of utmost importance for high bony definitions and hence the window width settings should be between 1500 and 2000 Hounsfield units with the window level set at +100 to +300 Hounsfield units. Parameters that should be studied include anatomical details of all the paranasal sinuses, the uncinate process, the maxillary ostium, middle meatal structures, fovea ethmoidalis, frontal recess, 3-dimensional orientation of the frontal sinus pathway, orientation of the ethmoid air cells, sphenoid ostia, optic tubercle, onodi cells, and their relationships with the carotid structures. In addition, the details of the orbital walls, lamina papyracea, infraorbital canal and its course, thickness of the extraocular muscles specifically the medial and inferior recti and their spatial and positional relationships with the walls and adjacent sinuses should be noted. Preanesthetic evaluation is also important to assess the systemic status with special focus on managing the systemic effects of the topical intranasal decongestive agents used during endoscopic approaches.

8.5 Surgical Technique

A standard decongestion and nasal preparation similar to that for any functional endoscopic sinus surgery (FESS) procedure should be carried out. If there is a significant deviated nasal septum, an endoscopic septoplasty should be performed and this procedure, when needed, can notably enhance the comfort of the surgeon as well as the surgical outcome.

The first step to endoscopic medial wall decompression is a good *uncinectomy*, the goal of which would be to expose the natural ostium of the maxillary sinus. The author follows the "Swing-Door" technique as described by Wormald [15]. Sickle-knife is used to incise the superior and inferior ends of the mid-uncinate. A backbiter is gently placed in the middle meatus in a way so as to engage the free edge of the uncinate (Fig. 8.1a). A right-angled ball-probe can help in identifying this free edge if there are any difficulties in doing so. Two to three bites would cut the uncinate sufficiently. Care must be taken not to extend this biting anteriorly, so as to avoid inadvertent injury to the bony nasolacrimal duct [16]. A right-angled ball-probe is then used to pull the uncinate anteriorly and fracture it at its insertion to the lateral wall. An up-biting Blakesley forceps can be used to remove the fractured uncinate (Fig. 8.1b). Subsequently, the footplates of the horizontal process of the uncinate can be separated from the mucosal covering and removed, thereby completely exposing the maxillary sinus ostium (Fig. 8.1c).

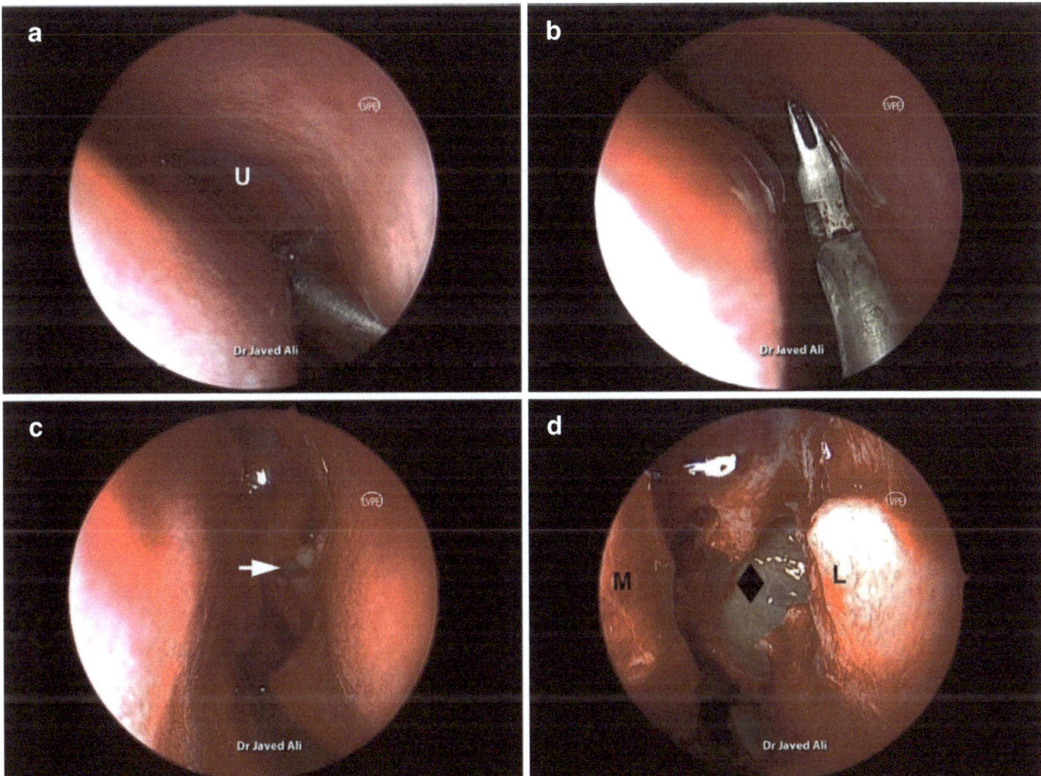

Fig. 8.1 Left endonasal decompression. First, punch in uncinate process (U) using the backbiter (**a**). Uncinectomy in process, using the up-biting Blakesley (**b**). View following a completed uncinectomy. The left maxillary sinus ostium (arrow) is exposed (**c**). Enlarging the Maxillary sinus ostium (black diamond). The middle turbinate (M) and the lacrimal sac area (L) are noted (**d**)

Once the maxillary sinus ostium is exposed, the mucosa is lowered to the insertion of inferior turbinate and a *middle meatal antrostomy* is carried out using a microdebrider and through biting Blakesley forceps (Fig. 8.1d). A large antrostomy should be created to prevent sinus ostium blockage from prolapsed orbital fat following decompression. Maxillary sinus can then be inspected for the location of the infraorbital nerve at its roof (Fig. 8.2) or any other pathologies that can be addressed simultaneously, if needed.

An *axillary flap* is then performed, agger nasi is exenterated, the frontal recess is identified and the frontal sinus pathway is secured (Fig. 8.3). A *complete ethmoidectomy* should now be performed and all air cells of the ethmoids adjacent to the lamina papyracea should be removed (Fig. 8.3b, c). The sphenoid ostium is then identified and enlarged to get a clear view of its contents, specifically the optic canal, carotid tubercle and optico-carotid recess (Fig. 8.4a). The junction of the lacrimal

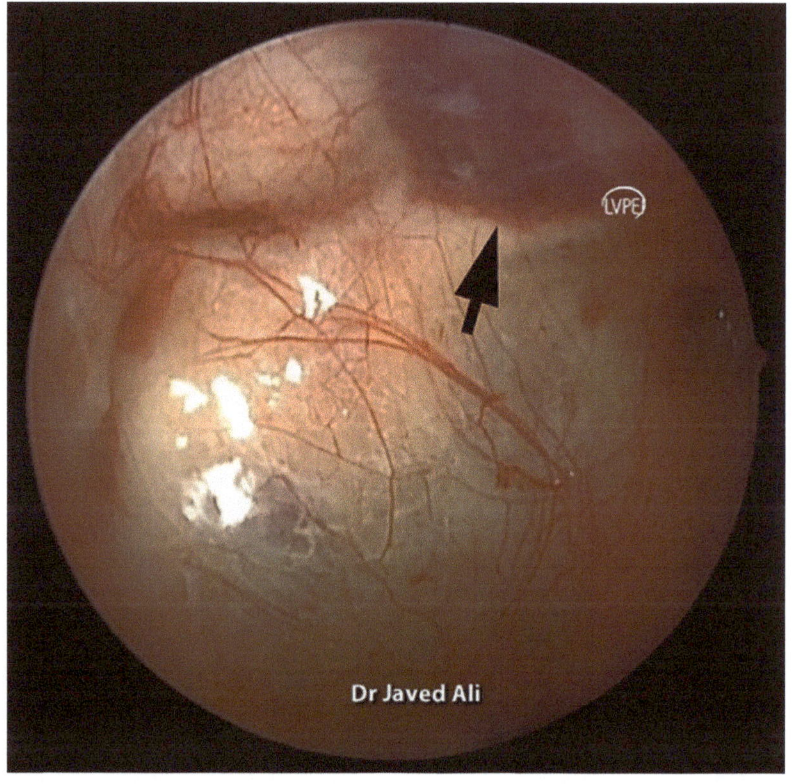

Fig. 8.2 Endoscopic view of the floor of the left orbit. Note the infraorbital nerve hump (black arrow)

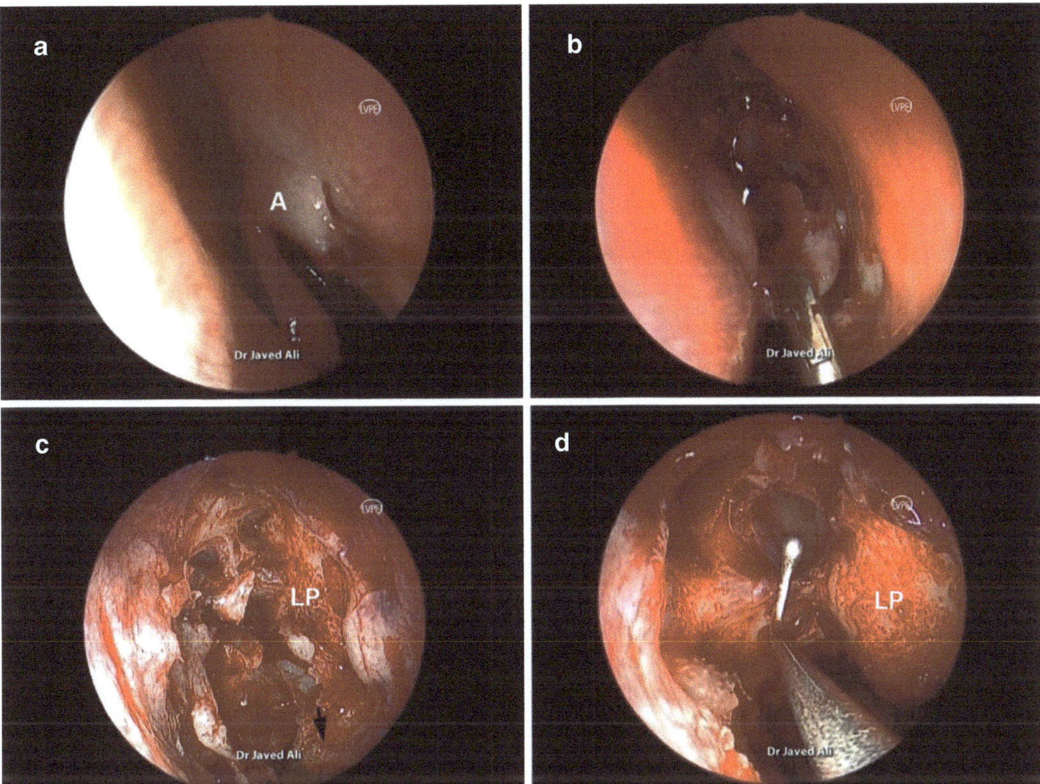

Fig. 8.3 Left endonasal decompression *continued.* Axillary flap (A) creation to initiate ethmoidectomy (**a**). Ethmoidectomy–clearance of ethmoid air cells in progress (**b**). Complete ethmoidectomy up to the posterior ethmoids (**c**); Note the exposed lamina papyracea (LP). Opening up the sphenoid face and frontal sinus ostium above, shown by the ball probe (**d**). Also, note the exposed lamina papyracea (LP)

bone and lamina papyracea is identified and is flaked off the periosteum till the optic tubercle (Fig. 8.4b, c). It is a good idea to leave 1–2 mm of lamina near the frontal sinus opening to prevent the prolapsed fat from blocking its drainage (Fig. 8.3d). If an infero-medial decompression is planned, the thicker portions of the floor, medial to the infraorbital canal can be removed using a Blakesley forceps or Kerrison punches (Fig. 8.4d). Care must be taken to protect the infraorbital nerve (Fig. 8.2).

Once the lamina is removed, the exposed periorbita can be incised to allow the orbital fat to prolapse into the newly created ethmoidectomy area (Fig. 8.5a). Fat can be gently teased out into the sinus to create a desired room within the orbit (Fig. 8.5b). A strip of periosteum, at the mid-level can be retained to help prevent gross prolapse of the medial rectus into the ethmoid sinus thereby lowering the risk of post-operative diplopia. On an average, 4–5 mm of reduction in proptosis can be achieved with an inferomedial decompression.

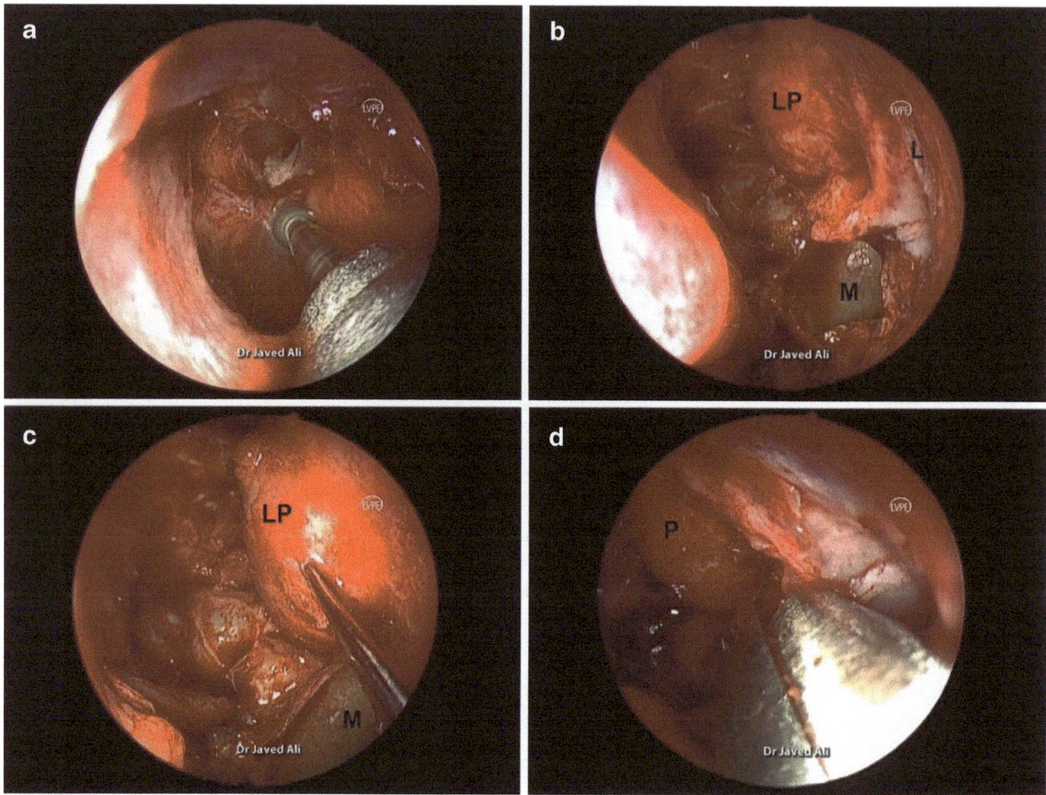

Fig. 8.4 Removal of the thick bone near optic tubercle with a DCR diamond burr (**a**). Periorbita (LP) after complete medial wall removal (**b**). Also, note the enlarged maxillary sinus opening (M) and the lacrimal sac area (L). Removal of the residual thin laminae (LP) overlying the periorbita (**c**). Note its relationship with the maxillary sinus (M). Posteromedial portion of the inferior wall being punched out with a Kerrison punch (**d**). Note its relationship to the exposed periorbita (P)

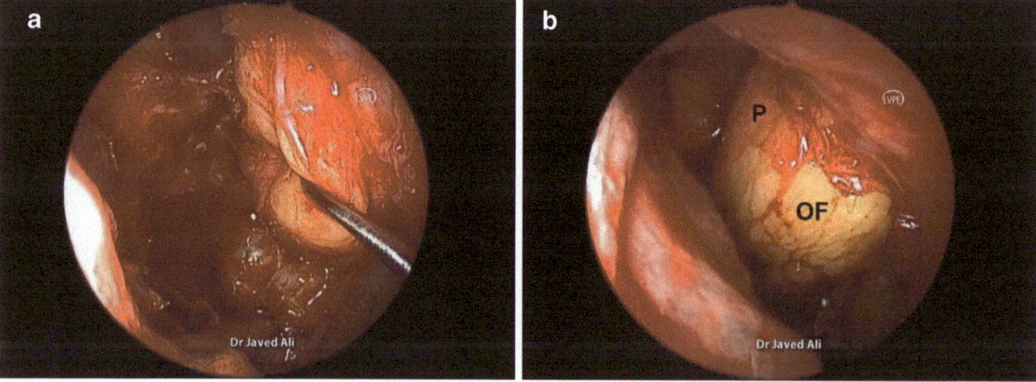

Fig. 8.5 Periorbital incision to prolapse the orbital contents (**a**). Prolapsed orbital fat (OF) into the nasal cavity with residual areas of periorbita (P) are noted (**b**)

8.6 Apical and Optic Canal Decompression

In the event of severe dysthyroid optic neuropathy with a predominant muscle disease, a maximal apical decompression up to the spheno-ethmoidal junction is desirable. Beyond this point, decompression of the optic canal can be achieved. Though not indicated in cases of TED with dysthyroid optic nerve compression, it may be useful in select cases of traumatic optic neuropathy. A good spheno-ethmoidectomy is mandatory for this. Optic tubercle is a thick bone that can be identified at the junction of sphenoid with orbital apex (Fig. 8.6). The posterior end of lamina papyracea can be flaked away from the periosteum but as it reaches the optic tubercle, a dacryocystorhinostomy diamond burr can be used to gently drill it out. Subsequently, the bone over the optic canal is approached and this again can be flaked out because of its thin nature (Fig. 8.6). This would expose the optic nerve sheath clearly. During this entire maneuver, it is very important for the surgeon to be constantly oriented to the crucial anatomical structures in the vicinity like the carotid artery, its genu and branches like the ophthalmic artery (Fig. 8.6). It is very important to understand that optic canal decompression requires a very high level of skill and expertise and should only be performed by well-trained endoscopic sinus surgeons.

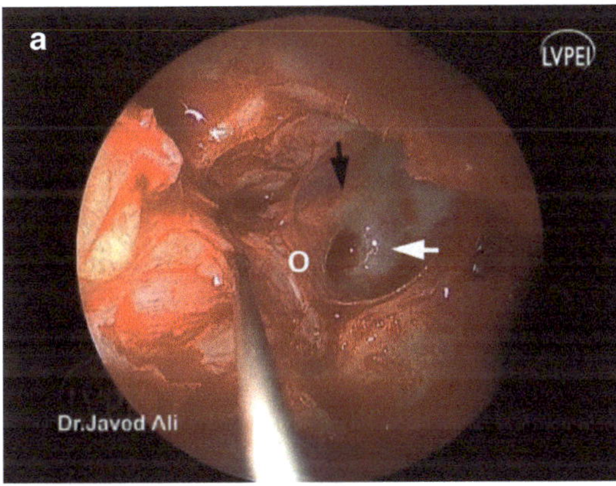

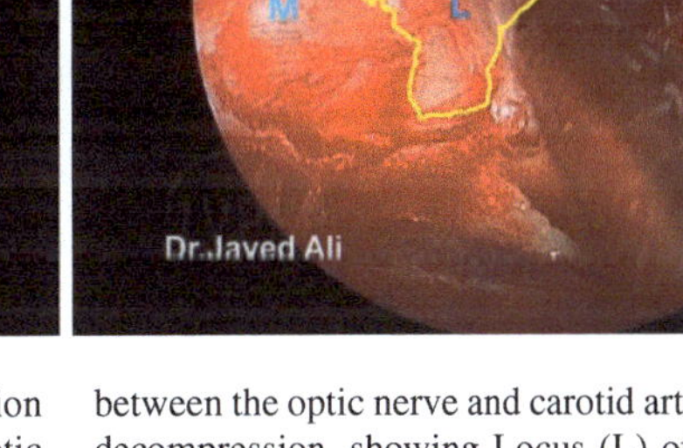

Fig. 8.6 Exposure for right optic canal decompression (different patient). Note the thick optic tubercle (O), optic nerve (black arrow), and carotid artery (white arrow). Also, note the carotico-optic recess, the depression between the optic nerve and carotid artery (**a**). Optic canal decompression, showing Locus (L) of interest (**b**). Note the sphenoid sinus (Sph), area of optic canal (OC), and apical portion of the medial rectus (M)

8.7 Navigation Guided Endoscopic Orbital Decompression

The use of navigation guidance during endoscopic orbital decompression has certain advantages in complex cases that include accurate intraoperative target localization, constant anatomical orientation for the surgeon and enhanced safety (Figs. 8.7, 8.8, 8.9, 8.10, and 8.11) [13, 17–19]. The image guidance allows for more extensive bone removal near the optic tubercle as well as the sphenoid. In addition, it would greatly help in identifying crucial structures like the bony optic canal, onodi cells and the genu of carotid artery and hence has the potential to prevent any inadvertent injuries. Studies on image-guided orbital decompressions have shown that the setup is not challenging and not very different from the routine surgeries. It provides intraoperative accuracy with regard to identifying crucial structures and performing aggressive decompression with lowered risks (Figs. 8.7, 8.8, 8.9, 8.10, and 8.11).

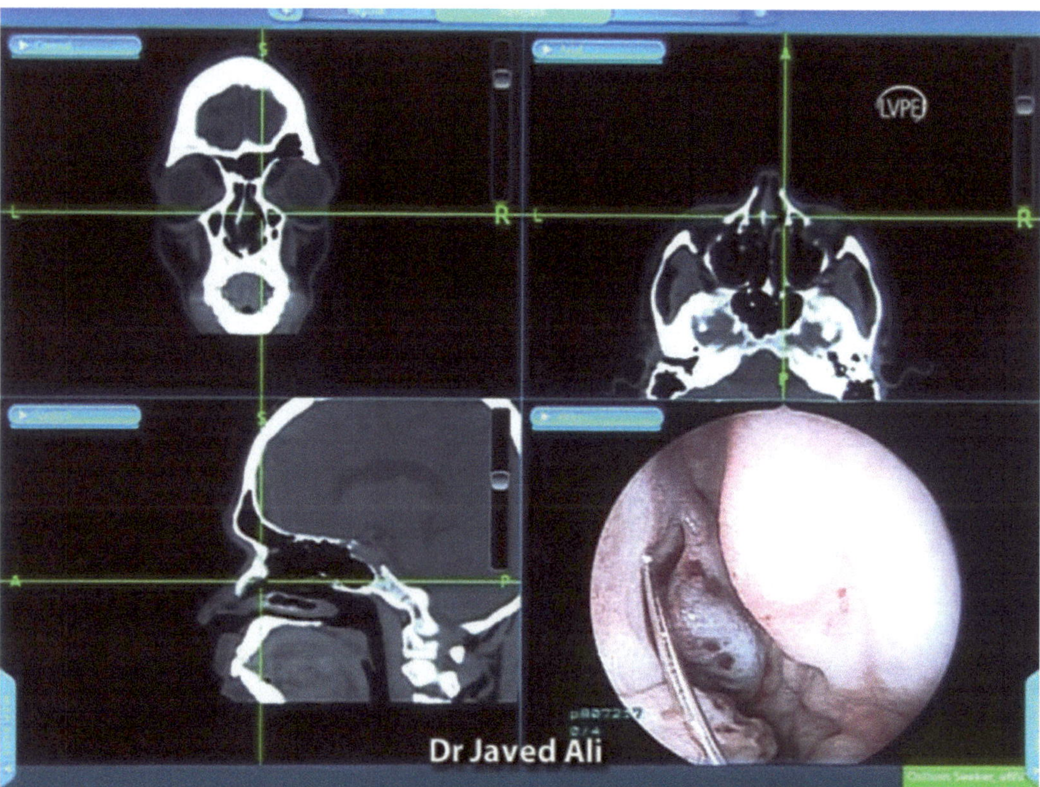

Fig. 8.7 Intraoperative image of navigation guided endoscopic orbital decompression: Note the localization of the maxillary ridge in the coronal, axial, and sagittal planes on the CT scan

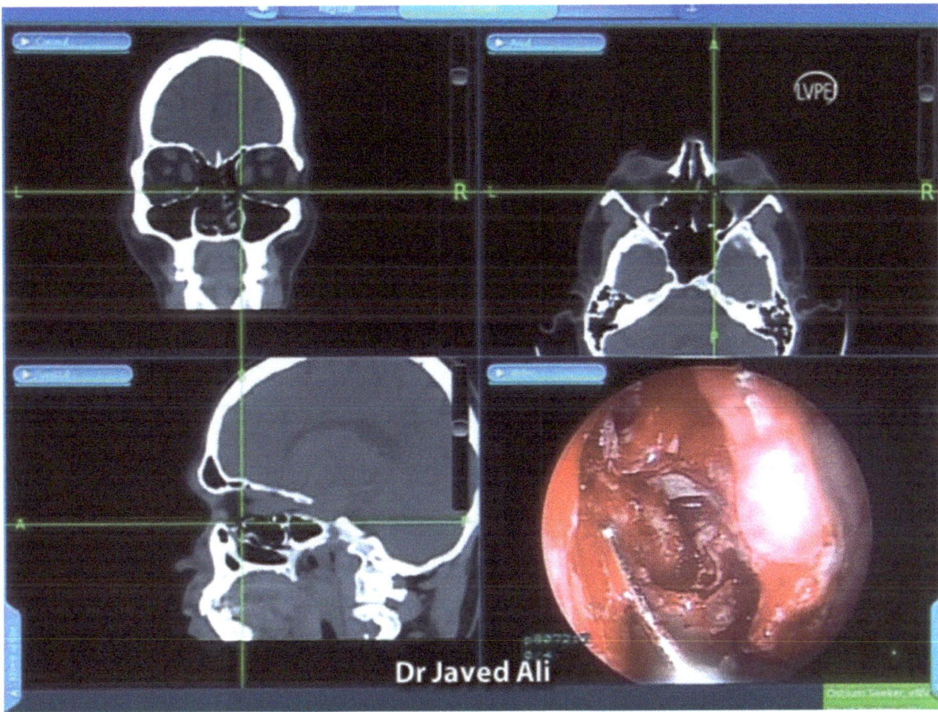

Fig. 8.8 Intraoperative image of navigation guided endoscopic orbital decompression: Note the localization of the lamina papyracea in the coronal, axial and sagittal planes on the CT scan

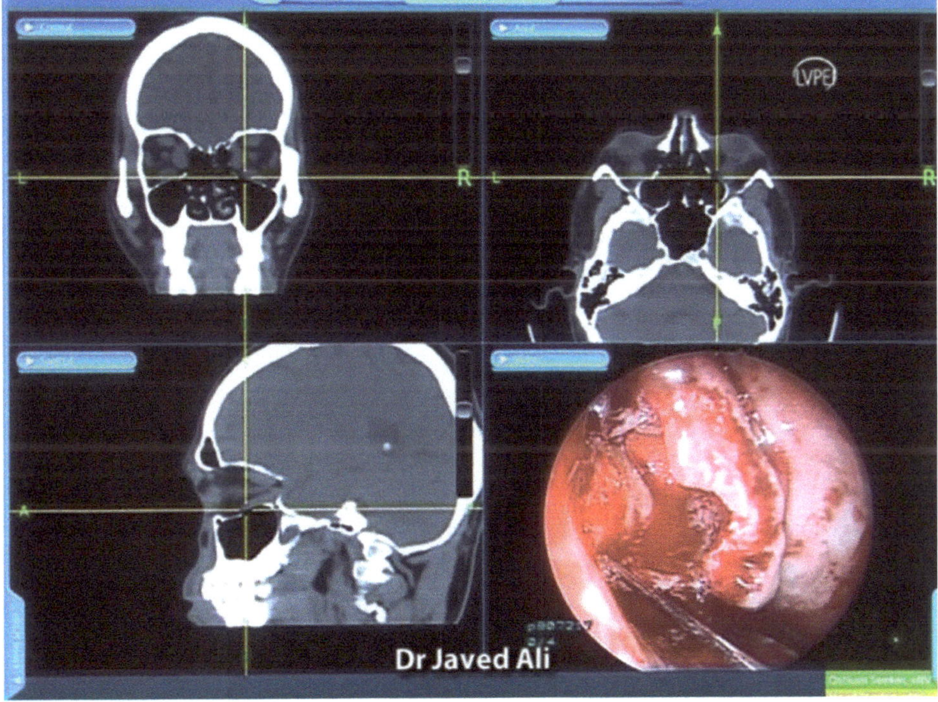

Fig. 8.9 Intraoperative image of navigation guided endoscopic orbital decompression: Note the localization of the middle portion of the inferior rectus following decompression of the orbital floor

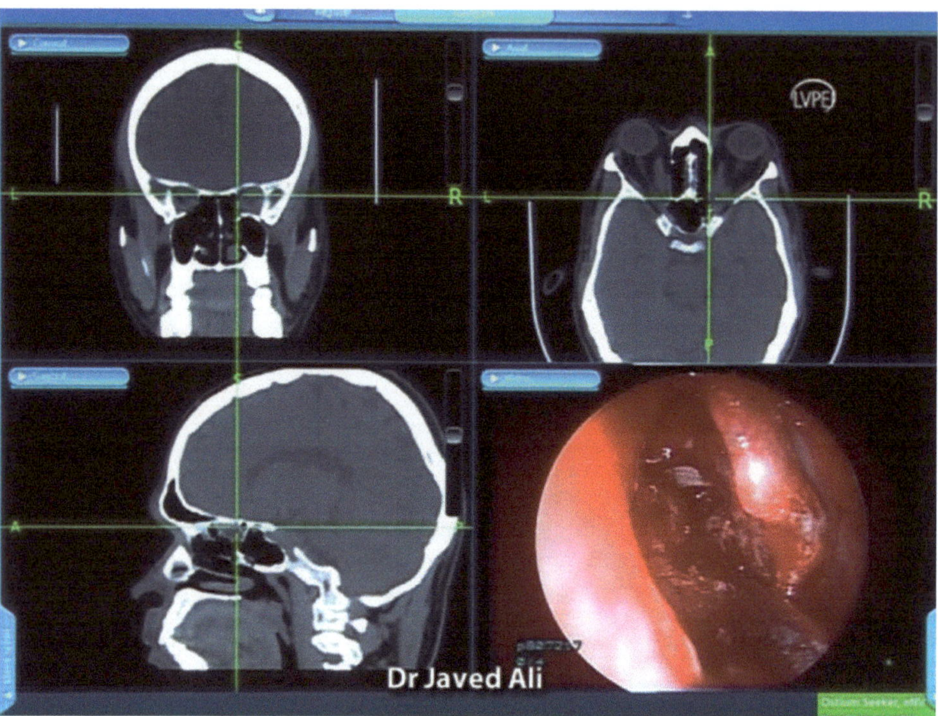

Fig. 8.10 Intraoperative image of navigation guided endoscopic orbital decompression: Note the localization of skull base

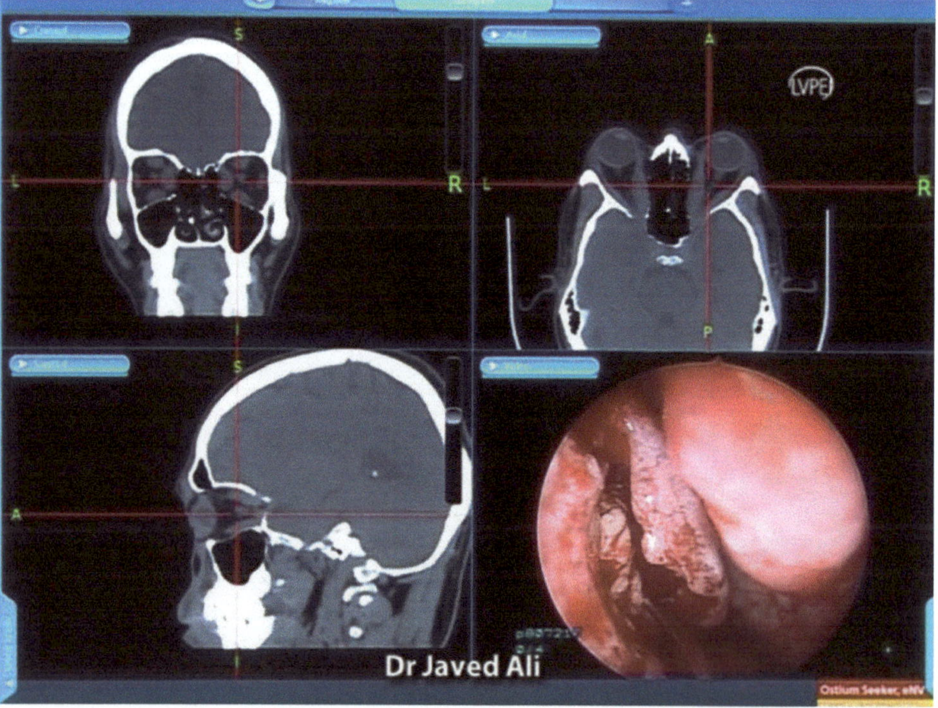

Fig. 8.11 Intraoperative image of navigation-guided endoscopic orbital decompression: Note the localization of the vicinity of optic nerve following fat decompression

8.8 Complications

As with any surgical procedure, endoscopic orbital decompression is not without its own set of complications. However, a complete clinical evaluation, careful patient selection, good surgical training, and the use of navigation guidance where needed can significantly reduce the incidence of complications. The reported complications of endoscopic orbital decompression are summarized in Table 8.2.

8.9 Surgical Outcomes

The surgical outcomes cannot be uniformly measured because of multiple techniques of performing the surgery, heterogenous clinical profiles, and variably documented outcome measures. The overall mean reduction in proptosis appears to be between 4 and 5 mm (range: 1–8 mm) in most studies [8–12, 19, 20]. This is mostly adequate in the setting of compressive optic neuropathy (Fig. 8.12), and additional lateral wall

Table 8.2 Complications of endoscopic orbital decompression reported in the literature

Ophthalmic/Orbital complications	Sinus/Intranasal complications
Decrease in vision (optic nerve injury)	Epistaxis
Postoperative strabismus and diplopia	Acute sinusitis
Infraorbital anesthesia	Sinus mucoceles
Orbital hematoma	CSF rhinorrhea
Orbital cellulitis	
Injury to the nasolacrimal duct	

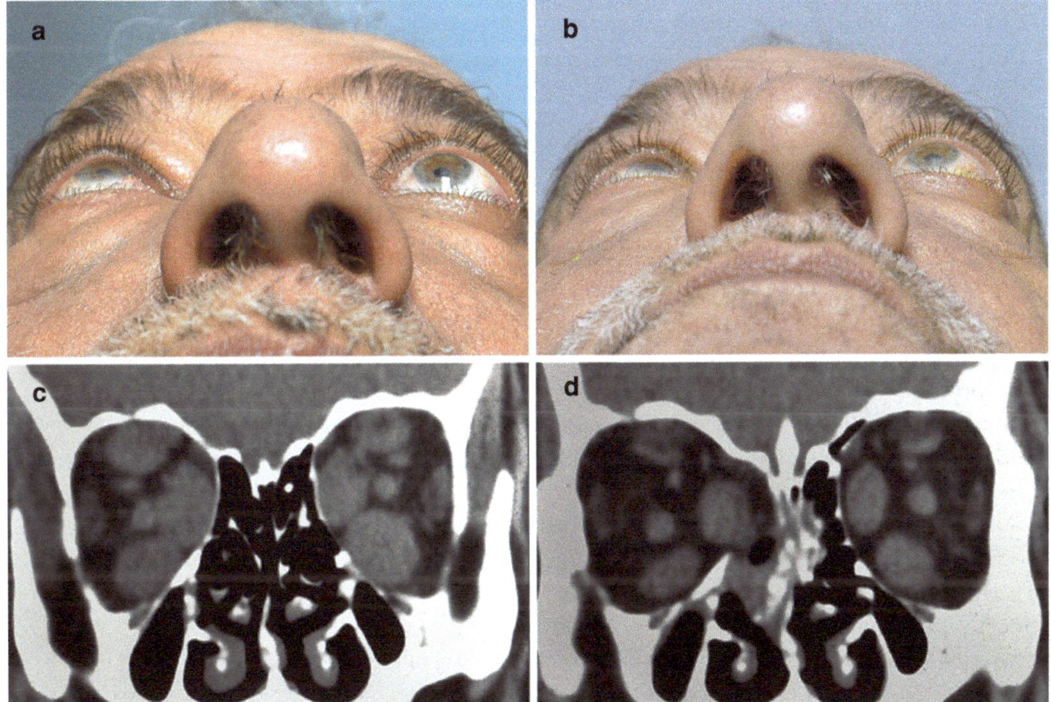

Fig. 8.12 A 60-year-old male with bilateral active TED, with right compressive optic neuropathy before and after endoscopic endonasal medial wall decompression (**a**, **b**) showing reduction in proptosis. Also, note the increase in esotropia of the right eye post-operatively. Computed tomography scan (coronal cuts) of the same patient showing the pre- and post-operative results (**c**, **d**). Note the distance between the optic nerve and the bulky medial rectus before and after the endoscopic orbital decompression

Table 8.3 Reported reduction in proptosis and new-onset diplopia with or without the preservation of infero-medial orbital strut in endoscopic endonasal orbital decompression [11]

Technique	Proptosis reduction (mm)	New-onset diplopia
Endoscopic 2 wall decompressions without IOS preservation	3.06 to 4.7	20 to 50%
Endoscopic 2 wall decompression with IOS preservation	1.64 to 4.6	0 to 47%
Endoscopic balanced 3-wall decompression with IOS preservation	3.4 to 5	0 to 16%
Endoscopic decompression with retained strip of periosteum	5.1	0 to 6%
Endoscopic orbital fat decompression with preserved IOS and strip of periosteum	6.2	Nil
Endoscopic selective decompression for DON	2.2 to 3.1	Nil

decompression can be added if required. The preservation of infero-medial orbital strut (IOS) during surgery and its outcomes is a subject of debate. Variable outcomes have been noted in the literature with regards to this in relation to proptosis reduction, and new-onset diplopia (Table 8.3) [11].

The literature is sparse with regard to long-term outcomes of endonasal decompressions in patients with TED. Gulati et al. [21] studied 37 patients in detail and followed them up to 9 years post-surgery (range: 1–9 years). At a mean follow up of 46 months, they reported improvement in the visual acuity (median pre-op = 0.8, post-op = 1, $p = 0.006$), intra-ocular pressures (median pre-op = 18 mm, post-op = 14 mm, $p < 0.001$), Hertel readings (median pre-op = 22.5, post-op = 19 mm, $p < 0.001$). After the surgery, new-onset diplopia was noted in 19% ($n = 7$) and worsened in 22.5% ($n = 8$). Impaired motility in abduction with or without elevation was noted pre-operatively in 54% ($n = 20$) and this increased to 62% ($n = 23$) following the surgery. More than half of the patients ($n = 22$) required further strabismus surgery. However, at the final follow up, 85% of the patients were totally free of any diplopia. Three patients were treated for sinusitis and all resolved satisfactorily. Taking long-term perspectives into consideration, it would be safe to conclude that majority of patients might need further treatment for diplopia mostly due to a significant increase in the esotropia.

8.10 Conclusion

Endoscopic orbital decompression is a safe and effective surgical modality when used for appropriate indications in patients with thyroid eye disease with apical nerve compression. Navigation guidance can help in certain complex cases for the surgeon to accurately localize crucial anatomical points. Postoperative diplopia is not uncommon, and the patients should be counseled about the possible need for a further intervention for it. An extensive training is of utmost importance before embarking on an endoscopic orbital decompression surgery.

Financial Disclosure Mohammad Javed Ali receives royalties from Springer for the textbook "Principles and Practice of Lacrimal Surgery" and treatise "Atlas of Lacrimal Drainage Disorders."

Conflicts of Interest None.

References

1. Dutton JJ. Anatomic considerations in thyroid eye disease. Ophthalmic Plast Reconstr Surg. 2018;34(4S suppl 1):S7–S12.
2. Uddin JM, Rubinstein T, Hamed-Azzam S. Phenotypes in thyroid eye disease. Ophthalmic Plast Reconstr Surg. 2018;34(4S suppl 1):S28–33.
3. Siakallis LC, Uddin JM, Miszkiel KA. Imaging investigation of thyroid eye disease. Ophthalmic Plast Reconstr Surg. 2018;34(4S suppl 1):S41–51.
4. Saeed P, Tavakoli Rad S, Bisschop PHLT. Dysthyroid optic neuropathy. Ophthalmic Plast Reconstr Surg. 2018;34(4S suppl 1):S60–7.
5. Ediriwickrema LS, Korn BS, Kikkawa DO. Orbital decompression for thyroid-related orbitopathy during the quiescent phase. Ophthalmic Plast Reconstr Surg. 2018;34(4S suppl 1):S90–7.
6. Diana T, Kahaly GJ. Thyroid stimulating hormone receptor antibodies in thyroid eye disease – methodology and clinical applications. Ophthalmic Plast Reconstr Surg. 2018;34(4S suppl 1):S13–9.
7. Dolman PJ. Grading severity and activity in thyroid eye disease. Ophthalmic Plast Reconstr Surg. 2018;34(4S suppl 1):S34–40.
8. Lima WT, Perches M, Cardoso F, et al. Orbital endoscopic decompression in graves ophthalmopathy. Rev Bras Otorhinolaringol. 2006;72:283–7.
9. Metson R, Pletcher SD. Endoscopic orbital and optic nerve decompression. Otolaryngol Clin N Am. 2006;39:551–61.
10. Leong SC, Karkos PD, Macewen CJ, White PS. A systematic review of outcomes following surgical decompression for dysthyroid orbitopathy. Laryngoscope. 2009;119:1106–15.
11. Tyler MA, Zhang CC, Saini AT, Yao WC. Cutting-edge endonasal surgical approaches for thyroid ophthalmopathy. Laryngoscope Investig Otolaryngol. 2018;3:100–4.
12. Boboridis KG, Uddin J, Mikropoulos DG, et al. Critical appraisal on orbital decompression for thyroid eye disease. A systematic review and literature search. Adv Ther. 2015;32:595–611.
13. Servat JJ, Elia MD, Gong D, et al. Electromagnetic image-guided orbital decompression: technique, principles and preliminary experience with 6 consecutive cases. Orbit. 2014;33:433–6.
14. Wormald PJ. Imaging in endoscopic sinus surgery. In: Endoscopic sinus surgery. 3rd ed. New York: Thieme; 2013. p. 13–8.
15. Wormald PJ, McDonogh M. The "swing-door" technique for uncinectomy in endoscopic sinus surgery. J Laryngol Otol. 1998;112:547–51.
16. Ali MJ, Murphy J, Wormald PJ, Psaltis AJ. Bony nasolacrimal duct dehiscence in functional endoscopic sinus surgery: radiological study and discussion of surgical implications. J Laryngol Otol. 2015;129(Suppl 3):S35–40.
17. Klimek L, Mosges R. Computer-assisted surgery in ENT specialty. Development and experiences from the first decade. Larynorhinootologie. 1998;77:275–82.
18. Ali MJ, Naik MN, Kaliki S, et al. Interactive navigation-guided ophthalmic plastic surgery: the techniques and utility of 3-dimensional navigation. Can J Ophthalmol. 2017;52:250–7.
19. Grusha YO, Ismailova DS, Kochetkov PA, et al. Potentials of intraoperative navigation during balanced orbital decompression in thyroid eye disease (preliminary results). Vestn oftalmol. 2016;132:29–34.
20. Yuen APW, Kwan KYW, Chan E, et al. Endoscopic transnasal orbital decompression for thyrotoxic orbitopathy. Hong Kong Med J. 2002;8:406–10.
21. Gulati S, Ueland HO, Haugen OH, et al. Long-term follow-up of patients with thyroid eye disease treated with endoscopic orbital decompression. Acta Ophthalmol. 2015;93:178–83.

Part III

Orbital Surgery in Inactive TED

9 Orbital Decompression: Approaches to the Orbit and Surgical Planning

Milind N. Naik

9.1 Introduction

There are four components of thyroid eye disease (TED) that require attention from the surgical point of view: proptosis, restrictive strabismus, eyelid abnormality (retraction), and cosmetic concerns (fat bags, rhytids, etc). Based on these four components, the surgical management of TED involves four major stages of rehabilitation: orbital decompression, extraocular muscle surgery, eyelid repositioning, and cosmetic soft tissue redraping [1]. Not all patients require all four stages, but one may require more than one stage of surgery. Proptosis is one of the most visible and obvious abnormality of TED that demands treatment. Historically, the inferior and medial walls were removed by the otorhinolaryngologists; and the deep lateral wall by the neurosurgeons. The transantral approach created unbalanced inferomedial decompression with a high incidence of consecutive strabismus, infraorbital anesthesia, and sinusitis [2, 3]. The fourth wall, orbital roof decompression was initially advocated by Naffziger, but is fraught with potentially serious complications, and hence is best avoided except in extreme cases.

9.2 Indications

Traditionally, orbital decompression was performed only for extreme proptosis, or compressive optic neuropathy. There has been a gradual evolution in the indications for orbital decompression [4]. It is increasingly common and accepted to perform orbital decompression not only for extreme vision-threatening proptosis, but also for cosmetically disfiguring proptosis [2, 5]. Though optic neuropathy responds well to surgery, the nerve is resilient, and minor degrees of compressive optic neuropathy are probably not as emergent as we once thought [6, 7]. Proptosis demands treatment not only from a cosmetic standpoint, but also to reduce the symptoms of exposure, and in rare cases, avoid the emergent complication of globe luxation. Earlier, decompression surgery was performed through large incisions and more invasive procedures, with resultant complications such as sinusitis, inferomedial globe displacement, and scarring. Today, advancements in orbital decompression allow new areas of bone removal, an awareness of orbital fat as the “first wall” for decompression, and the use of smaller incisions [8, 9]. Today, all three walls can be reached via hidden incisions and minimally invasive orbital approach by an ophthalmic plastic surgeon [8, 9].

M. N. Naik (✉)
Ophthalmic Plastic Surgery Service, LV Prasad Eye Institute, Hyderabad, India
e-mail: milind@lvpei.org

S. Rath, M. N. Naik (eds.), *Surgery in Thyroid Eye Disease*,
https://doi.org/10.1007/978-981-32-9220-8_9

9.3 Options for Orbital Decompression

There are five anatomic areas that can be targeted to achieve orbital decompression. These include decompression of the fat compartment, the floor, the medial wall, the lateral wall, and rarely the roof. For mild cases (2–3 mm proptosis), decompression begins with orbital fat removal. If additional decompression is required, removal of the bony wall is added as the deep lateral wall, medial wall, and floor in that order (Fig. 9.1). The preference of the available walls for decompression of progressively severe disease may vary from surgeon to surgeon based on the training, access to specialized instruments, and specific factors related to an ethnic group. As a thumb rule, however, each orbital wall would provide approximately 2 mm reduction in proptosis, and fat alone would provide 2 mm reduction.

In this chapter, we shall look at the various *approaches* to each wall, and the *incisions* that can facilitate that approach. A detailed description of technical considerations, advantages, disadvantages, and complications of each approach will be covered in subsequent chapters.

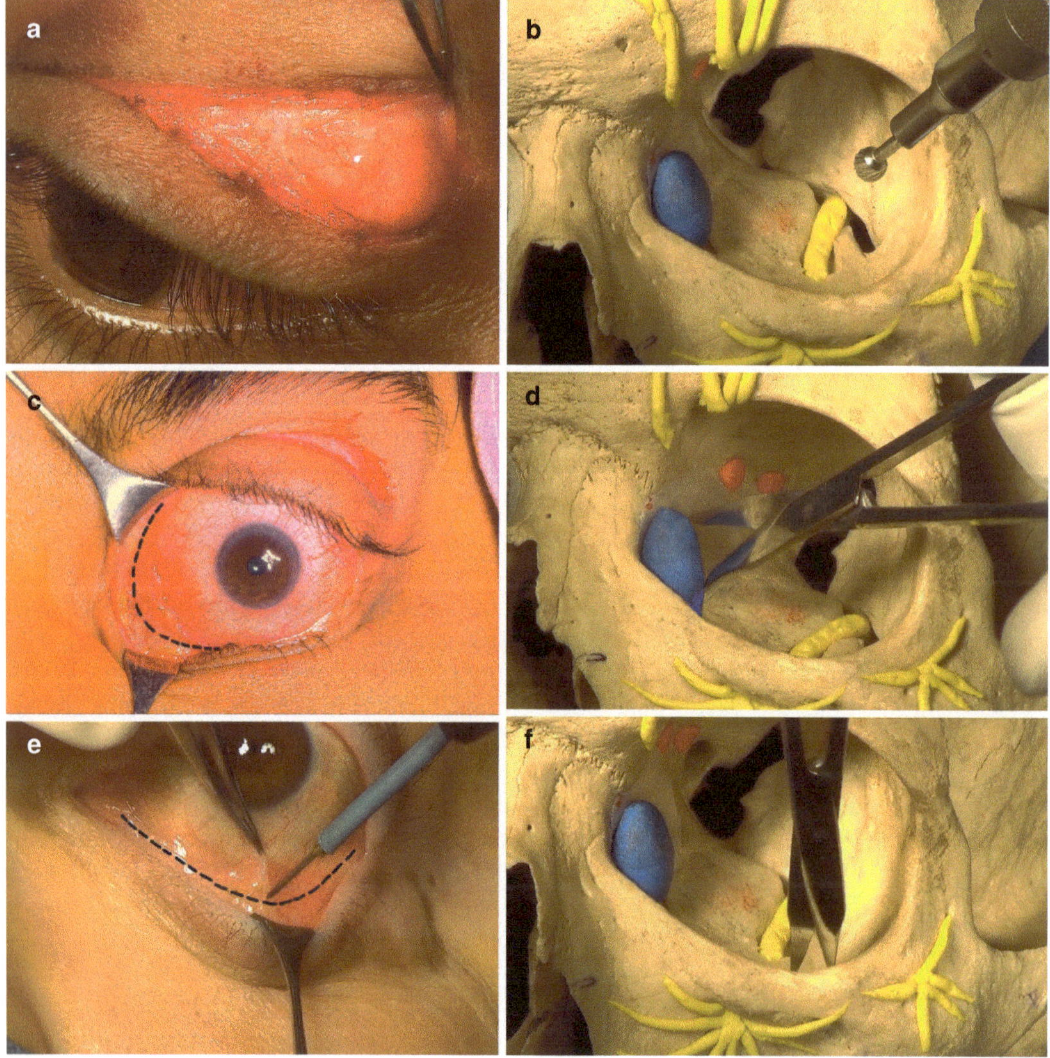

Fig. 9.1 The most popular incisions for transorbital decompression: Eyelid crease incision (**a**, **b**) for the lateral wall, trans-caruncular incision (**c**, **d**) for medial wall, and trans-conjunctival incision (**e**, **f**) for the orbital floor

9.4 Approach Verus Incision

It is important to make a differentiation between approach and incision at this stage. An *approach* defines which anatomic route we take to reach the wall. An *incision*, on the other hand, just represents the starting point of an approach.

Figure 9.2 summarizes the various approaches to the Orbit. The lateral wall can be approached in three ways including the *intracranial* approach, the *ab-externo* approach (from temporal fossa), and the *ab-interno* approach (transorbital). Similarly, the medial wall and floor (clubbed together for convenience) can be approached in three ways: *trans-antral*, *endonasal*, and *transorbital* (caruncular/conjunctival).

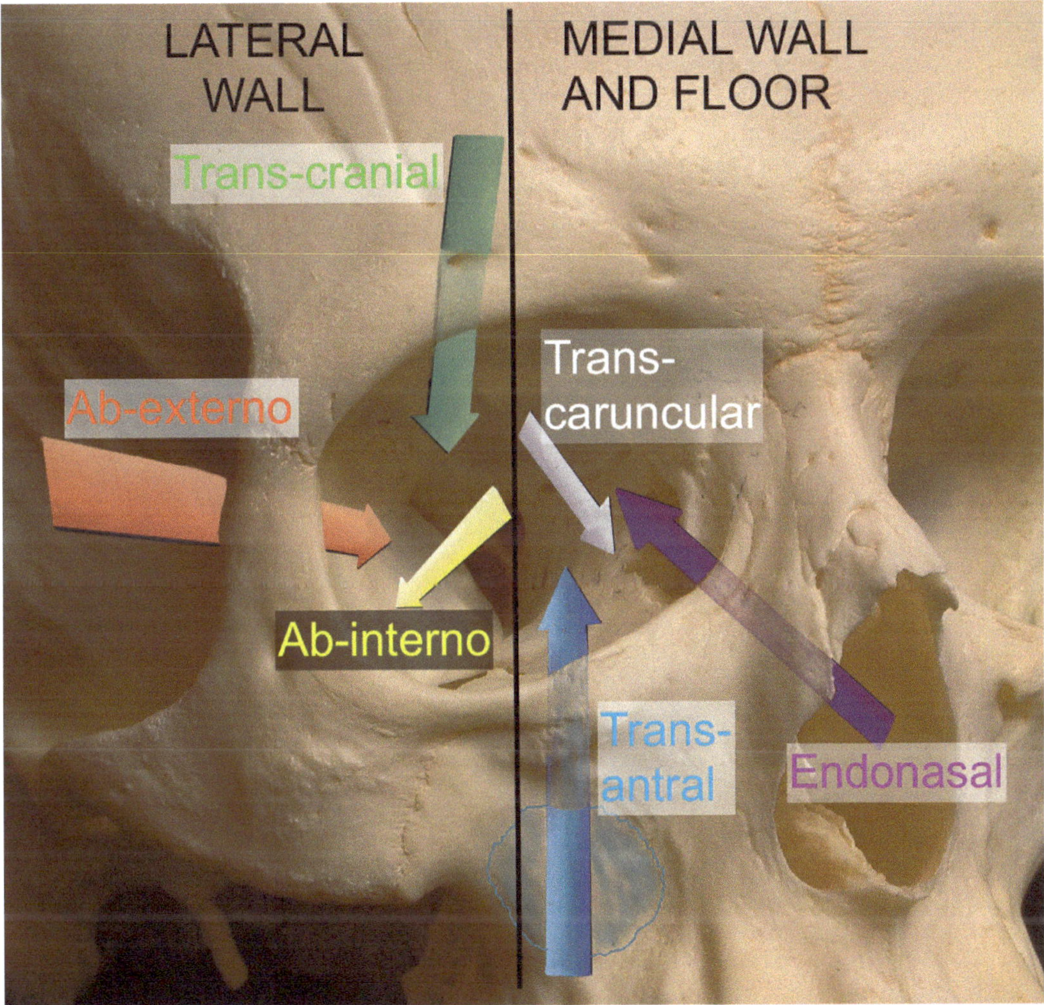

Fig. 9.2 Pictorial representation of the approaches to the lateral wall, floor, and medial wall of the orbit

9.5 Fat Decompression: The Conceptual "First Wall"

Fat decompression essentially means removal of both the intraconal and the extraconal fat from the orbit. First described by Olivari, removal of intraconal fat is the "first wall" for the correction of mild (2–3 mm) proptosis (Fig. 9.3).

9.5.1 Incisions

Orbital fat can be harvested via transcutaneous or trans-conjunctival approaches (Fig. 9.1). For the superior orbit, an eyelid crease incision is most suited to access pre-aponeurotic fat, and also allows removal of skin and excess sub-brow fat if necessary [10]. For the lower eyelid, a transcutaneous approach would be via a sub-ciliary incision. The transconjunctival approach, however, is more popular, either as swinging eyelid or as closed canthal technique (Fig. 9.4) [11, 12].

9.5.2 Technique

Fat is not distributed equally within the orbit. *Inferolateral* fat is the first choice, as it has a greater volume, and there are no important structures in this area (Fig. 9.4a) [11–13] . The *intraconal* fat can also be easily accessed from this space by retracting the inferior and lateral rectus muscle. *Superolateral* fat can be approached through the eyelid crease incision (Fig. 9.4c). *Superomedial* fat is typically of a smaller volume, and inferomedial fat is rarely available for excision.

The advantages and complications of fat decompression are enlisted in Table 9.1.

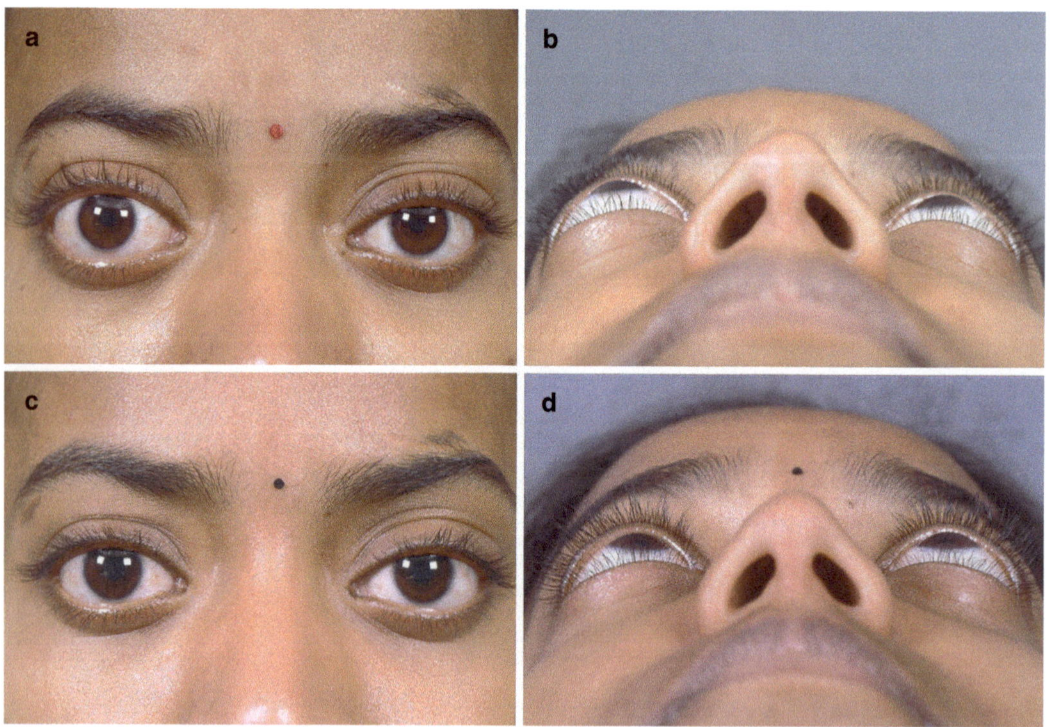

Fig. 9.3 Right proptosis (2mm) in a case of mild inactive TED (**a**, **b**). Inferolateral fat decompression was performed trans-conjunctivally, along with removal of intraconal fat to achieve reduction in proptosis and symmetry (**c**, **d**)

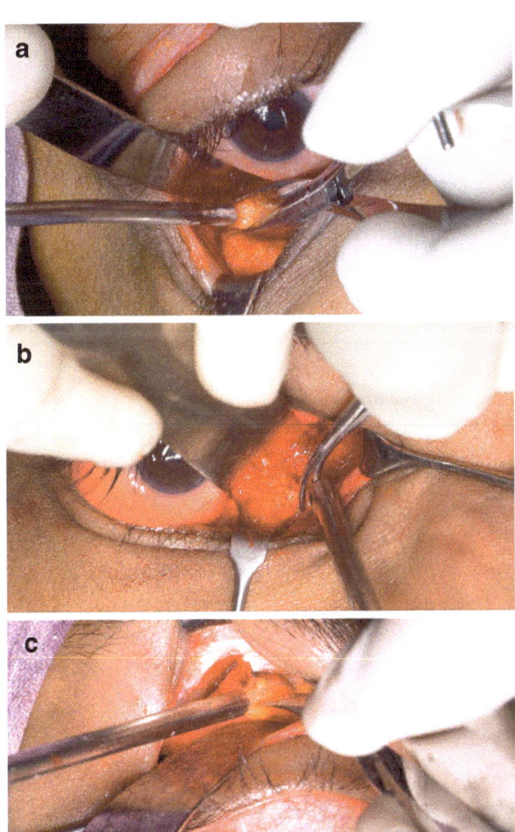

Fig. 9.4 Techniques of orbital fat decompression (conceptual 'first' wall) demonstrated on the right orbit. Inferolateral (**a**), medial (**b**) and supero-lateral (**c**) fat excision is performed by the suction-excision technique while the assistant protects the globe with a malleable retractor and 'prolapses' the fat with right amount of orbital pressure

Table 9.1 Advantages, and complication of orbital 'fat' decompression

	Complications	
Advantages	Intra-operative	Post-operative
Reduction in proptosis (mean 3.5–5.9 mm)	Bleeding	Haematoma and infection
Reduction in intraocular pressure (mean 3.4 mmHg)	Injury to inferior oblique muscle	Supraorbital anaesthesia (due to superomedial fat excision)
Low chances of new onset diplopia	Sectoral pupillary dilatation from injury to ciliary ganglion (aggressive intraconal fat removal via superolateral approach)	Eyelid malpositions (transcutaneous incisions)
		New onset diplopia (0–3%)

9.6 Lateral Wall Decompression

Recently, the lateral wall decompression has emerged as a primary procedure for moderate proptosis [14]. It can be accessed with different incisions, approaches, and instrumentation for bone removal, and provides a significant amount of bony decompression. The zygoma anteriorly and the body of sphenoid posteriorly are the primary bones targeted.

9.6.1 Incisions

Irrespective of the approach (trans cranial or trans orbital), the lateral wall can be reached via any of the following incisions (Fig. 9.5).

1. *Coronal incision*: The use of a coronal flap has been described for access to the lateral orbit (Fig. 9.6) [15]. The widest exposure is obtained through a *coronal* approach, including the deep lateral orbit, even better than a direct lateral orbitotomy. It leaves no visible scar in the presence of adequate scalp hair, and allows performance of a simultaneous upper facelift when desired. Through a coronal approach, the lateral rim can be left intact, or orbital rim onlay implants can be placed [16]. Through the coronal incision, the medial canthal tendon and lacrimal sac can be elevated from their periosteal attachment to expose the medial and inferior orbital walls.
2. *Kronlein incision*: Kronlein is credited with the first direct approach to the lateral orbit described in 1889 via a large curvilinear incision [17].
3. *Stallard–Wright incision*: The incision described by Stallard and Wright is a subbrow incision that extends into one of the lateral canthal folds to give a more acceptable scar (Fig. 9.5) [18].
4. *Berke–Reese incision*: A linear lateral canthotomy incision was proposed by Berke in 1953 (Fig. 9.5) [19].

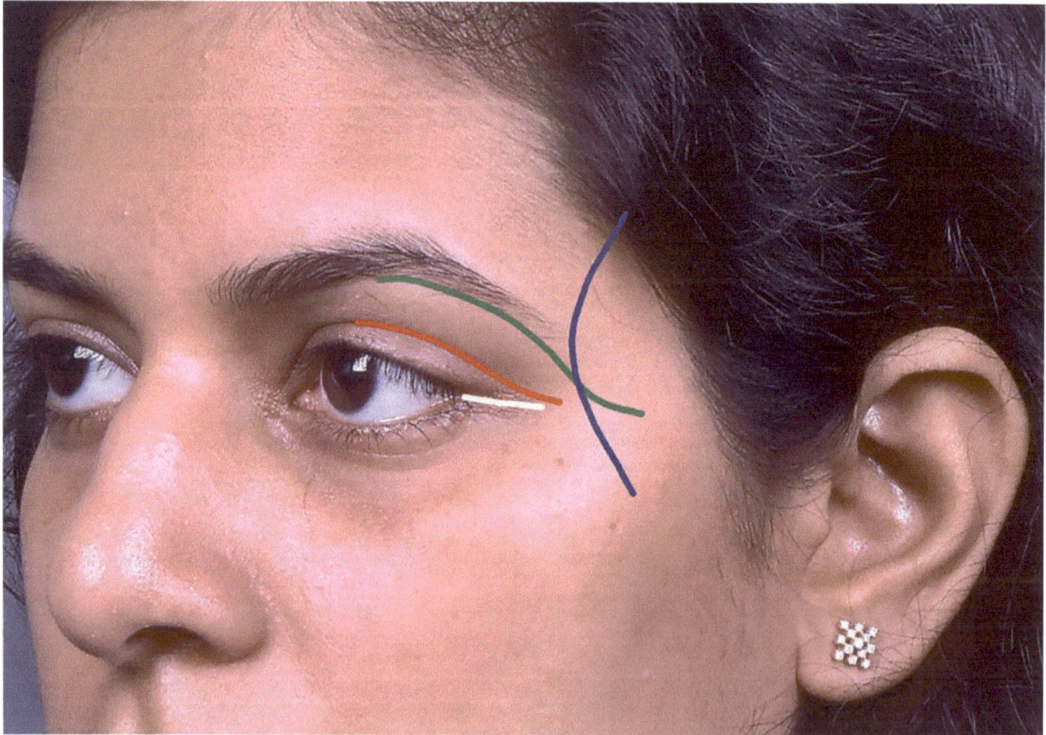

Fig. 9.5 Various incisions to approach the lateral orbital wall. Kronlein (blue), Stallard Wright incision (green), Eyelid crease incision (red), and Berke-Reese incision (yellow)

5. *Eyelid crease incision*: The lateral eyelid crease incision gained popularity in the 1990s and is widely used today (Fig. 9.5) [20, 21]. It provides excellent access to the lateral orbit and hides well in the eyelid crease and crows feet (Fig. 9.7).
6. *Swinging eyelid incision*: Access via a transconjunctival incision has also been reported using a swinging eyelid incision to access the lateral wall and achieve 5.5 mm of proptosis reduction [22].

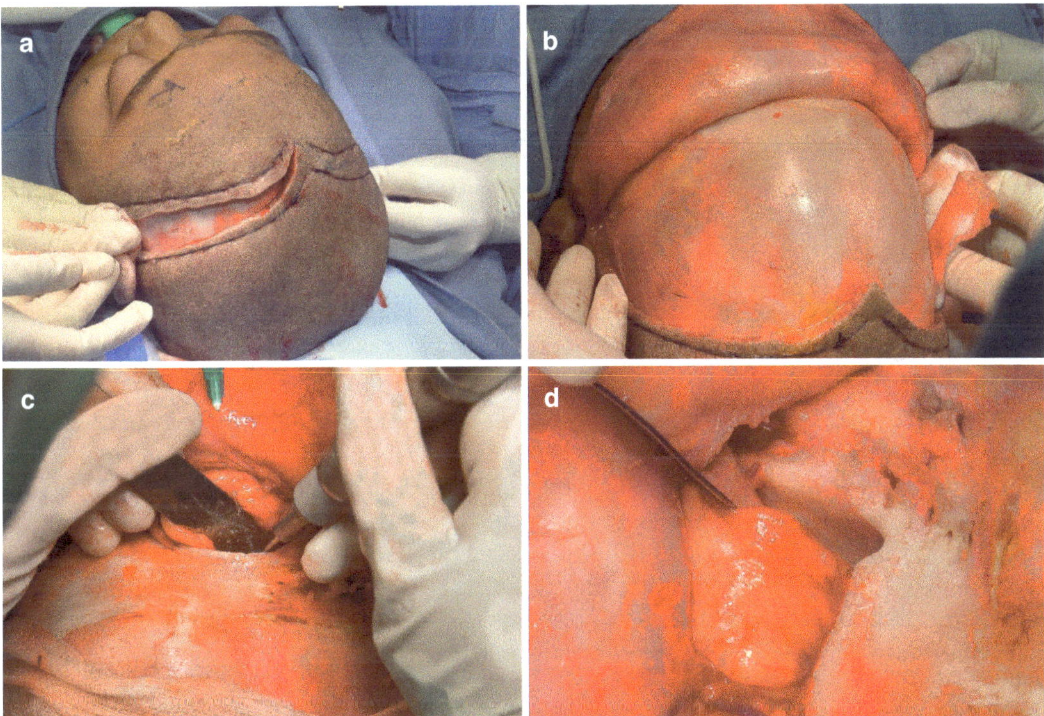

Fig. 9.6 Coronal incision for a bilateral severe proptosis in a case of thyroid eye disease. Placement of the incision (**a**), raising the flap to reach the orbital rim (**b**), drilling the lacrimal keyhole of the right orbit (**c**), good exposure of the lateral orbital wall (**d**) (Photo courtesy Co-surgeon, Dr Gautam Dendukuri, MDS)

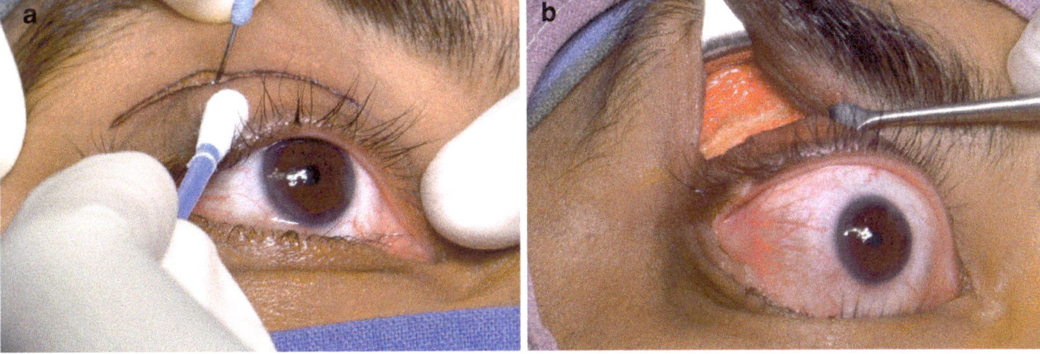

Fig. 9.7 The eyelid crease incision is most popular to expose the lateral wall (**a**). From the eyelid crease, dissection is carried out in the sub-orbicularis plane to reach the orbital rim (**b**)

Most cases do not require maximal bone removal, and the eyelid crease incision is considerably less time consuming than the coronal approach. The eyelid crease incision is well hidden cosmetically and offers excellent exposure to the lateral wall.

9.6.2 Techniques

Irrespective of the incision, the bone removal approaches can be several. Earlier, the lateral orbital rim was removed en bloc as described by Dollinger in 1911 [17, 23, 24]. The deep lateral wall (sphenoid) was originally removed via a neurosurgical approach by Naffziger in the 1930s [25, 26]. The transorbital approach can essentially be of two types: the *ab-interno* approach popularized by Goldberg [14], and the *ab-externo* technique as popularized by Rose (Fig. 9.2) [27].

The lateral wall can also be accessed through the temporalis fossa, without a marginotomy. In this ab-externo approach, the lateral orbital rim is exposed via the temporalis fossa, and the diploic space is then removed from the lateral side. This approach has been reported to produce on average 4.5 mm of proptosis reduction [28].

When accessing the lateral wall, the orbital rim can either be removed (marginotomy) or spared. Decompression with removal of the lateral rim is reported to provide better access, allowing greater reduction in proptosis (5.7 mm) as compared to ab-interno approaches without marginotomy (4.1 mm) [29]. The actual bone removal can be achieved with a curette, mechanized drill, piezoelectric technology or by manual punching with a bone rongeur.

9.7 Floor and Medial Wall Decompression

The orbital floor and medial wall are often decompressed together, as an inferomedial procedure. The approaches to these walls are generally the same and can be grouped together for discussion (Fig. 9.2).

Three main approaches to the floor and medial wall have been described: trans-orbital, trans-antral (Chapter 13), and trans-nasal (Chapter 8). Transorbital floor decompression can be approached via a number of incisions including transcutaneous, transconjunctival, trans-caruncular, swinging eyelid, coronal, and lateral orbital.

9.7.1 Transorbital Approach

The trans-orbital approach involves access to the floor and medial wall via incisions and dissection limited to the orbital cavity. It primarily involves skin or conjunctival incisions to access the extra-periosteal space of the infero-medial orbit, to achieve bone removal.

The floor can be accessed through various trans-cutaneous or trans-conjunctival incisions [30–32].

1. *Sub-ciliary incision*: This is the most popular and cosmetically most appealing skin incision. Once the incision is placed, one can either raise a skin-only flap, or a skin–muscle flap to reach the orbital rim (Fig. 9.8). In the skin-only flap, the dissection from incision to orbital rim is performed in the subcutaneous plane to reach the orbital rim where the orbicularis and the orbital septum are opened together. The skin-only flap approach has a higher incidence of ectropion [32].

In the skin–muscle flap approach, dissection from incision to orbital rim is carried out in sub-orbicularis plane to reach the orbital rim where only the septum is opened.

2. *The mid-eyelid or sub-tarsal incision*: It involves incising the skin and orbicularis in the region below the tarsus and following the orbital septum to the rim, and entering the orbit there (Fig. 9.8) [30–32].
3. *The Orbital rim incision*: This approach involves making an incision directly over the orbital rim through skin, orbicularis, and septum simultaneously (Fig. 9.8). As the incision moves further down from the subciliary region, the scar becomes more noticeable [30].
4. *The transconjunctival incision*: It is made on the palpebral conjunctival surface of the

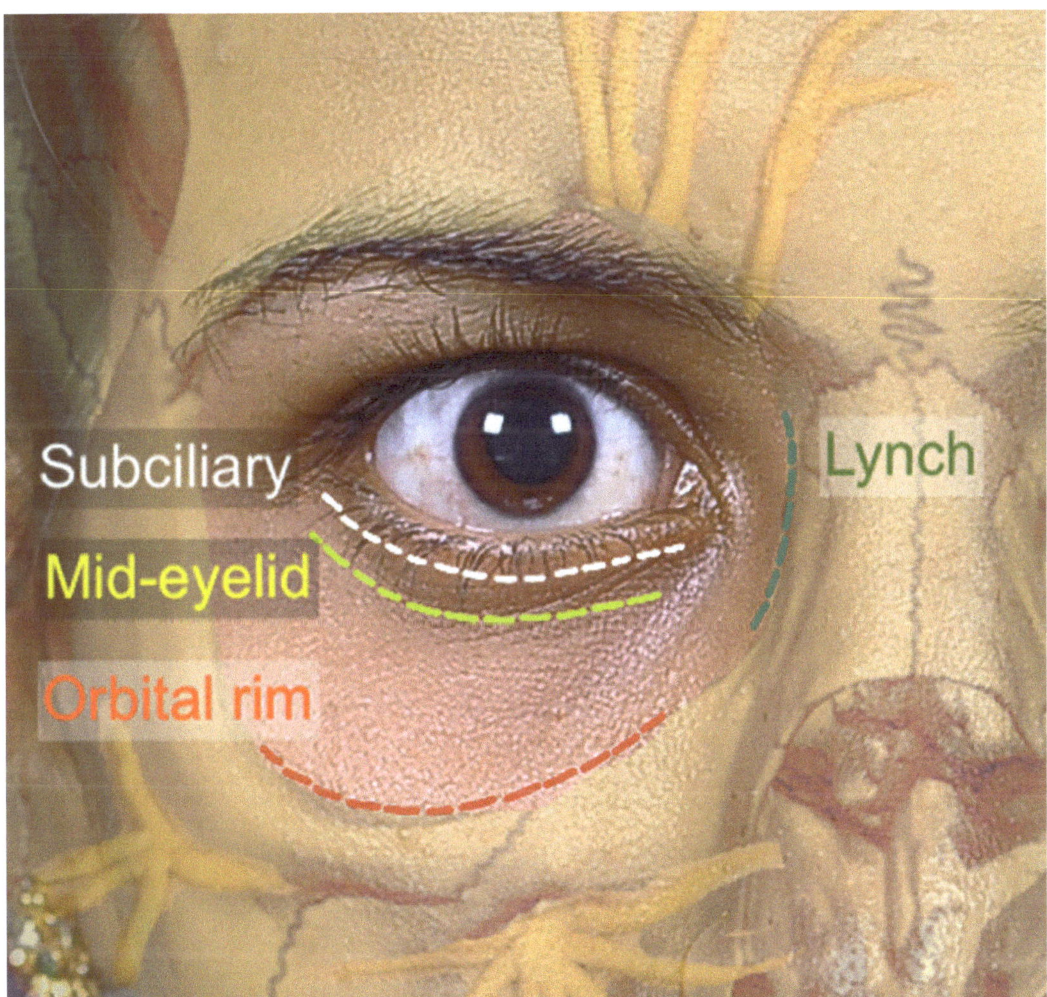

Fig. 9.8 Schematic representation of *transcutaneous* incisions to reach the floor or medial wall. Subciliary incision is the most popular amongst transcutaneous incisions

lower eyelid, between the lower edge of the tarsus and the fornix (Fig. 9.9). This incision may be palpebral (4 mm below the tarsus), or forniceal (closer to the fornix). Beyond the epithelial incision, the transconjunctival approach can be either pre- or post-septal (Fig. 9.9). The palpebral incision allows entry to the bloodless pre-septal plane up to the orbital rim. The orbital septum can then be entered to reach the orbital floor [33]. The forniceal incision allows entry through the post-septal dissection plane, between the orbital fat and the orbital septum [34]. The post-septal dissection is

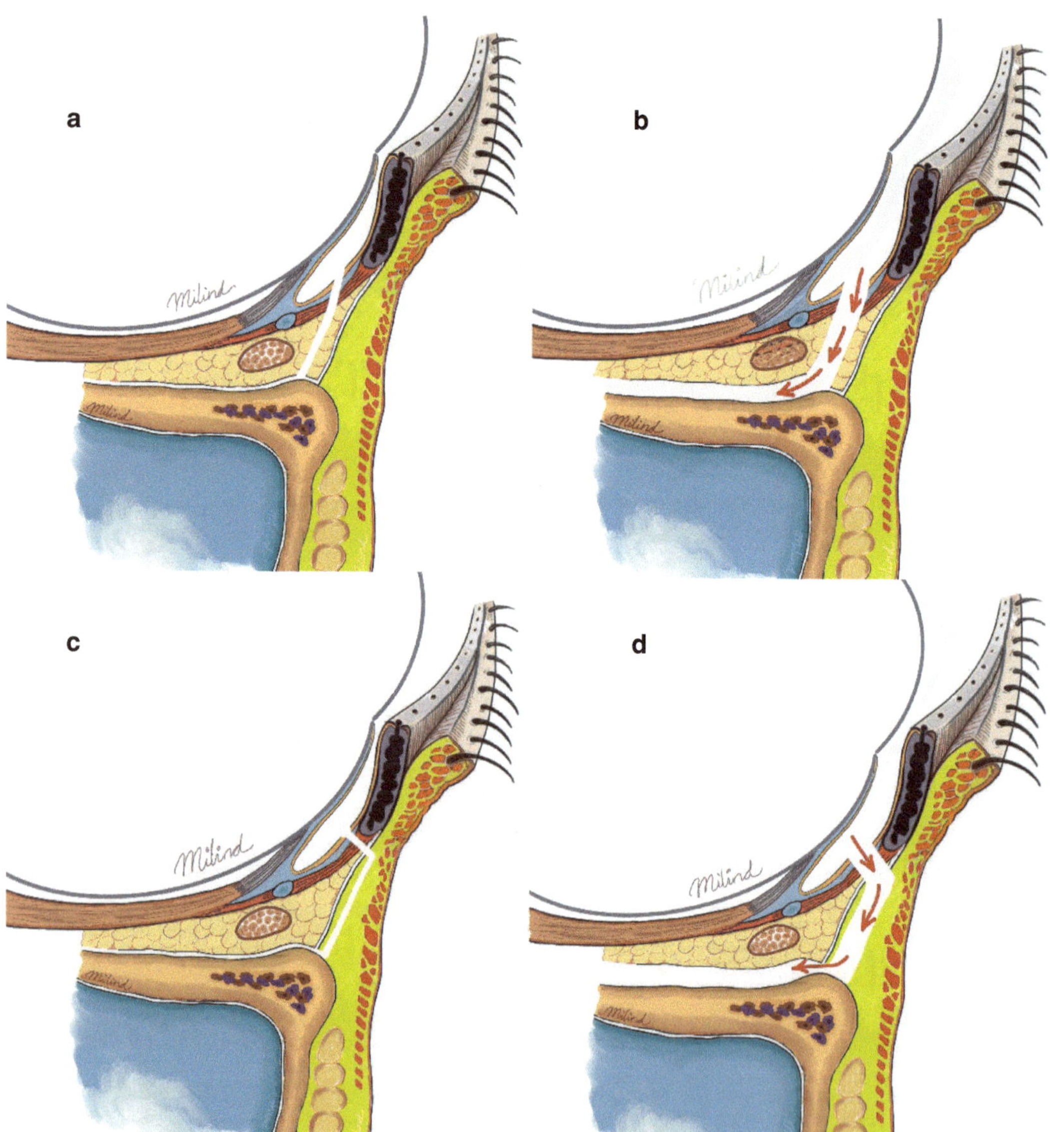

Fig. 9.9 Trans-conjunctival incision to access orbital floor. *Post-septal* incision involves an incision through the conjunctiva mid-way between the lower border of tarsus and the fornix (**a**). The incision travels behind the septum, to land on the floor just within the orbital rim (**b**). *Pre-septal* incision involves a conjunctival incision just below the lower border of tarsus, and traverses in the pre-septal plane to reach the orbital rim (**c**). The periosteum is then incised and raised at the orbital rim to expose the floor (**d**)

quick, and avoids damage to the orbital septum (Fig. 9.10). There is no literature comparing the efficacy and safety of these two dissection planes.

A lateral canthotomy and inferior cantholysis in addition to the conjunctival incision can increase exposure to the floor and inferolateral wall (Fig. 9.11) [35]. This "swinging eyelid"

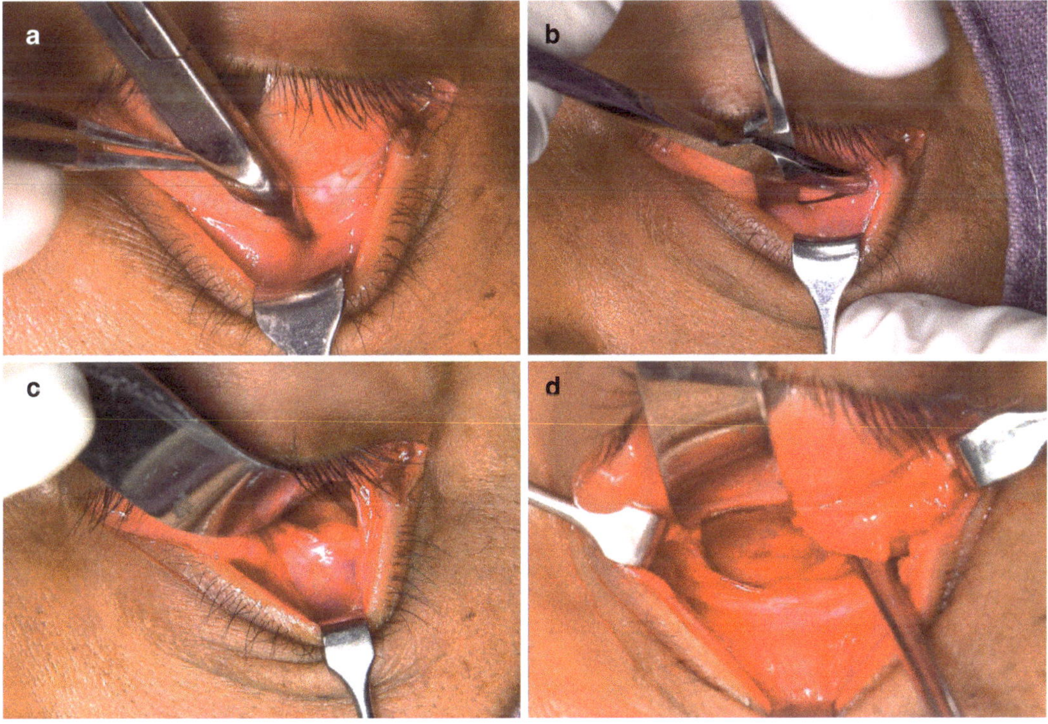

Fig. 9.10 Left trans-conjunctival post-septal incision. Stevens scissors placed just within the orbital rim (**a**). Scissor blades are spread (**b**) and malleable reatractor is inserted (**c**) to land on the orbital floor behind the septum (**d**)

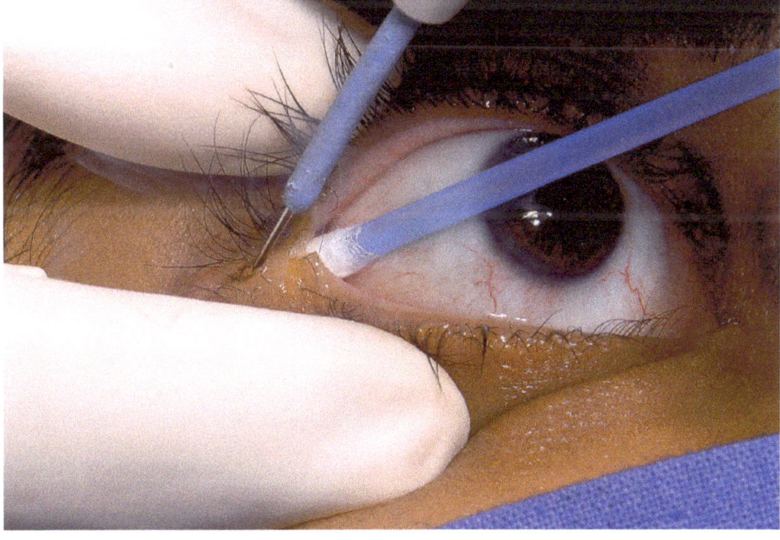

Fig. 9.11 Lateral canthotomy with inferior cantholysis converts a trans-conjunctival incision into a swinging eyelid incision. It improves the exposure and access to the floor, and can even allow limited decompression of the lateral wall

approach has been used extensively for orbital decompression [22, 36].

Transcutaneous and transconjunctival approaches have not been compared in the literature for orbital decompression. Data from the same incisions used for orbital floor fracture repair found the incidence of ectropion to be higher in the transcutaneous group [32].

The medial wall can be accessed via three approaches for transorbital exposure: coronal, lynch incision, and trans-caruncular [37–39].

1. *The Lynch incision*: This incision is midway between the medial canthus and the nasal bridge (Fig. 9.8) [40]. The periosteum is exposed and a plane is developed extra-orbitally. This may involve disinsertion of the trochlea, cauterization of the ethmoidal vessels, as well as retraction of the medial canthal tendon and the lacrimal sac. This approach is now less popular due to external scar and medial canthal scarring [41].
2. *Coronal incision*: The coronal access is best suited for the lateral wall, and is discussed along with the lateral orbitotomy access (Fig. 9.6). The medial wall can also be approached via the coronal incision However, it involves dissection of the supra-orbital nerve, dis-insertion of the trochlea, and management of the ethmoidal neurovascular bundles to access the medial wall and floor. The morbidity of this approach is significant and can include frontal bossing, skin necrosis, alopecia, and anesthesia [42]. Since the transconjunctival approaches are more effective, this incision is rarely used for medial orbital decompression in thyroid eye disease [43].
3. *Trans-caruncular incision*: This approach avoids a visible scar, is quick, and therefore preferred over both coronal and lynch incision techniques to approach medial wall (Fig. 9.12). The caruncle is first split, and the conjunctival incision is then extended inferi-

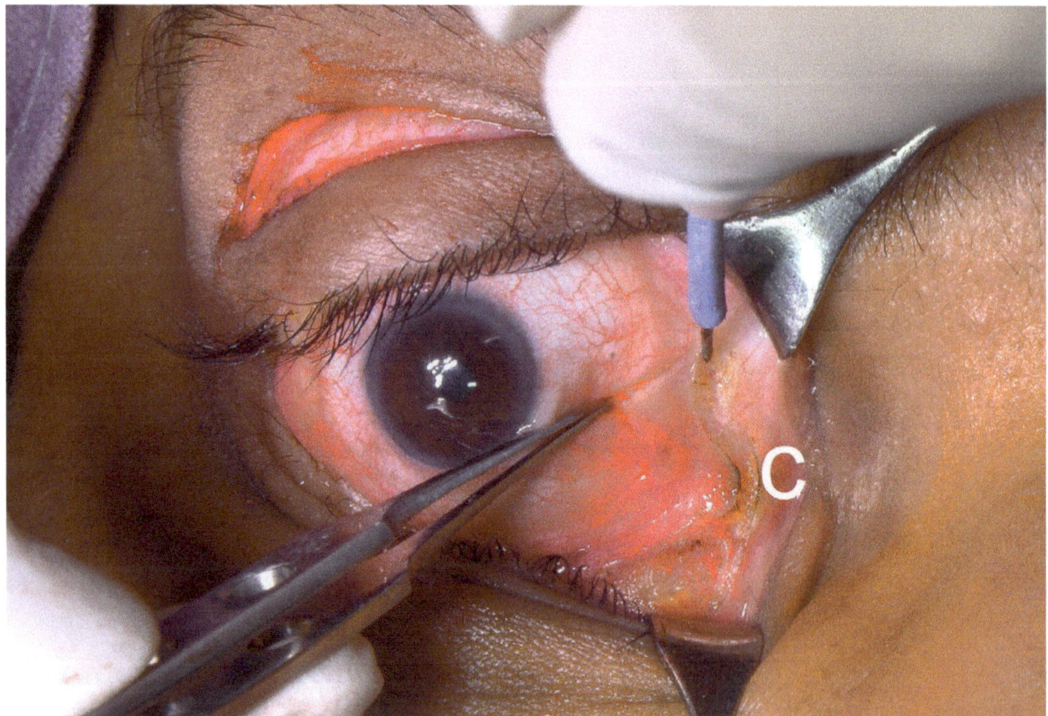

Fig. 9.12 Transcaruncular incision. The caruncle (c) is split with a monopolar cautery to straddle the incision 4–5 clock hours in the medial fornix

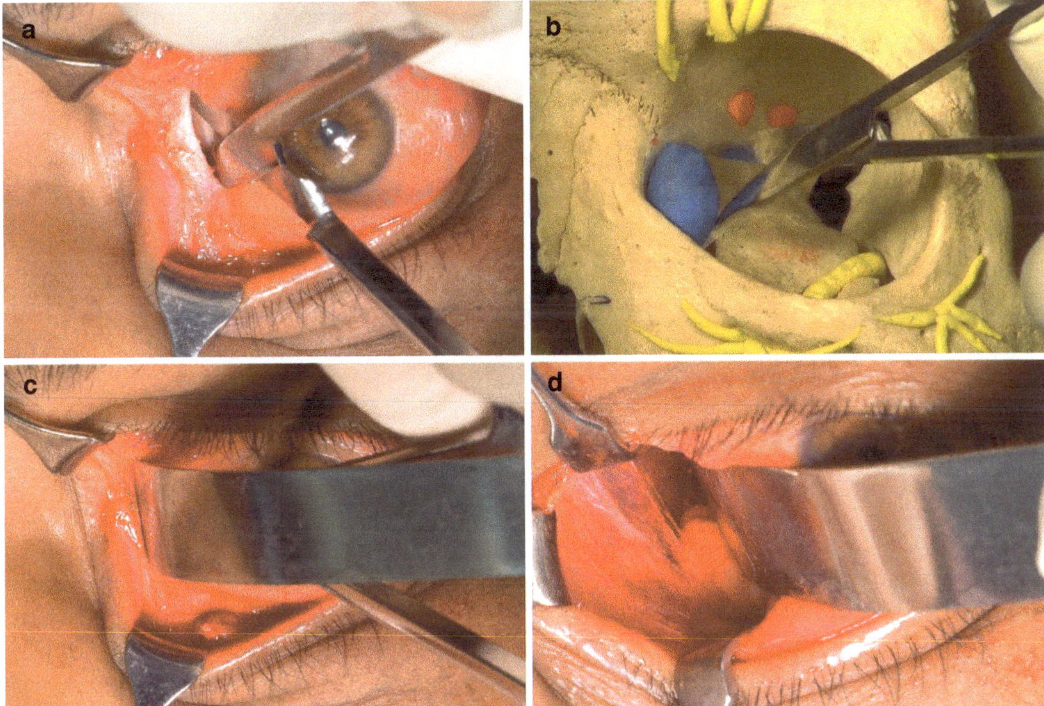

Fig. 9.13 Transcaruncular approach: Stevens scissor is passed postero-medially to palpate the posterior lacrimal crest (**a**). Schematic representation of the orbital anatomy (**b**). The scissors is replaced by a malleable retractor (**c**), to expose the medial wall (**d**)

orly and superiorly to extend over 4–6 clock hours in the medial conjunctival fornix [44]. The incision can be combined inferiorly with transconjunctival swinging eyelid incision for combined access to the floor and inferolateral wall [44]. Medially, the dissection follows a natural plane between the Horner muscle and the orbital septum to reach the posterior lacrimal crest (Fig. 9.13) [44]. Thus, the orbit is entered posterior to the lacrimal sac to avoid damaging this structure [45]. Direct visualization of Horner muscle can aid in the identification of the posterior lacrimal crest and has been described [46]. Both the medial wall and periorbita are extremely thin medially, hence dissection must be carried out with extreme care.

9.8 Transantral Approach

Transantral approach was described by Ogura and Walsh [47]. It involves accessing the maxillary sinus via a Caldwell-Luc antrostomy (Fig. 9.2). An incision is placed in the superior oral sulcus above the canine fossa, up to the periosteum. The periosteum is elevated up to the infraorbital nerve, and the anterior wall of the maxillary sinus is entered with a burr and the ostium is enlarged [48]. The mucosa is stripped to visualize the orbital floor and the anterior ethmoid air cells. The anterior ethmoidal air cells are removed, to expose the medial wall of the orbit.

The advantage of this approach is that it does not produce an external scar. Complications include post-operative paresthesias and anesthesia, oro-antral and gingivo-labial fistulas, and devitalized teeth [49, 50]. A detailed description of this approach is addressed in Chapter 13.

9.9 Transnasal Approach

The transnasal approach involves an uncinectomy and excision of the ethmoid bullae first, which allows entry into the anterior ethmoidal air cells [51–53]. The anterior ethmoid complex is entered, and the medial wall of the orbit is identified (Fig. 9.2). A more detailed description of the trans-nasal approach is discussed in Chapter 8.

9.10 Advantages of Transorbital Medial Wall and Floor Decompression

With the trans-conjunctival and transcaruncular route, the access is quick, and adequate bony decompression can be achieved without complex instrumentation like an endoscope, or mechanized drills. A simple Kerrison's bone punch is adequate to achieve medial wall and floor decompression.

9.11 Orbital Roof Decompression

There are only a few reports of 4-wall decompression. More than 10 mm proptosis reduction has been described with transorbital 4-wall decompression involving the posterolateral roof [54]. A study reported on 8 orbits of 4 patients with recalcitrant dysthyroid optic neuropathy (DON) following steroids, irradiation, and 3-wall decompression where the addition of transcranial orbital roof decompression resolved the compressive optic neuropathy in all cases [55]. One case complained of orbital pulsation after surgery [55]. Another study consisting of 10 patients found 70% response to superolateral decompression via a transfrontal approach after failure of inferomedial decompression [56]. The addition of orbital roof as one more wall is reserved for the extremely severe or recalcitrant cases.

A recent report suggested that the orbit expands into the cranial cavity after transorbital decompression, suggesting a valid basis to perform maximal extradural decompression in the severest of cases [57].

9.12 Summary

There are several options to approach the orbital fat, the lateral wall, medial wall, and floor of the orbit. For orbital fat decompression, transconjunctival incision with inferolateral approach is preferred. For the lateral wall, an eyelid crease incision and an ab-interno approach is preferred. For medial wall decompression, trans-caruncular incision and trans-orbital approach is preferred, whereas for the floor, trans-conjunctival incision and post-septal trans-orbital approach is most popular. The choice of incisions and approaches can vary from case to case, and between surgeons.

References

1. Shorr N, Seiff SR. The four stages of surgical rehabilitation of the patient with dysthyroid ophthalmopathy. Ophthalmology. 1986;93:476–83.
2. Fatourechi V, Garrity JA, Bartley GB, Bergstralh EJ, DeSanto LW, Gorman CA. Graves ophthalmopathy. Results of transantral orbital decompression performed primarily for cosmetic indications. Ophthalmology. 1994;101:938–42.
3. Garrity JA, Fatourechi V, Bergstralh EJ, Bartley GB, Beatty CW, DeSanto LW, et al. Results of transantral orbital decompression in 428 patients with severe graves' ophthalmopathy. Am J Ophthalmol. 1993;116:533–47.
4. Goldberg RA. The evolving paradigm of orbital decompression surgery. Arch Ophthalmol. 1998;116:95–6.
5. Lyons CJ, Rootman J. Orbital decompression for disfiguring exophthalmos in thyroid orbitopathy. Ophthalmology. 1994;101:223–30.
6. Neigel JM, Rootman J, Belkin RI, Nugent RA, Drance SM, Beattie CW, et al. Dysthyroid optic neuropathy. The crowded orbital apex syndrome. Ophthalmology. 1988;95:1515–21.
7. Ben Simon GJ, Syed HM, Douglas R, Schwartz R, Goldberg RA, McCann JD. Clinical manifestations and treatment outcome of optic neuropathy in thyroid-related orbitopathy. Ophthalmic Surg Lasers Imaging. 2006;37:284–90.

8. Naik MN, Nair AG, Gupta A, Kamal S. Minimally invasive surgery for thyroid eye disease. Indian J Ophthalmol. 2015 Nov;63(11):847–53.
9. Rootman DB. Orbital decompression for thyroid eye disease. Surv Ophthalmol. 2018;63(1):86–104.
10. Olivari N. Transpalpebral decompression of endocrine ophthalmopathy (graves' disease) by removal of intraorbital fat: experience with 147 operations over 5 years. Plast Reconstr Surg. 1991;87(4):627e41. Discussion 42–43
11. Wu CH, Chang TC, Liao SL. Results and predictability of fat- removal orbital decompression for disfiguring graves exophthalmos in an Asian patient population. Am J Ophthalmol. 2008;145:755–9.
12. Prat MC, Braunstein AL, Glass LRD, Kazim M. Orbital fat decompression for thyroid eye disease: retrospective case review and criteria for optimal case selection. Ophthalmic Plast Reconstr Surg. 2015;31(3):215–8.
13. Richter DF, Stoff A, Olivari N. Transpalpebral decompression of endocrine ophthalmopathy by intraorbital fat removal (olivari technique): experience and progression after more than 3000 operations over 20 years. Plast Reconstr Surg. 2007;120(1):109–23.
14. Goldberg RA, Kim A, Kerivan KM. The lacrimal keyhole, orbital door jamb, and basin of the inferior orbital fissure. Three areas of deep bone in the lateral orbit. Arch Ophthalmol. 2000;116:1618–24.
15. Stewart WB, Levin PS, Toth BA. Orbital surgery: the technique of coronal scalp flap approach to the lateral orbitotomy. Arch Ophthalmol. 1988;106(12):1724–6.
16. Goldberg RA, Soroudi AE, McCann JD. Treatment of prominent eyes with orbital rim onlay implants: four-year experience. Ophthalmic Plast Reconstr Surg. 2003 Jan;19(1):38–45.
17. Alper MG. Pioneers in the history of orbital decompression for graves' ophthalmopathy. Doc Ophthalmol. 1995;89:163–71.
18. Stallard HB. Evolution of lateral orbitotomy. Trans Ophthalmol Soc U K. 1973;93:3–17.
19. Berke RN. A modified Kronlein operation. Trans Am Ophthalmol Soc. 1953;51:193–231.
20. Harris GJ, Logani SC. Eyelid crease incision for lateral orbitotomy. Ophthalmic Plast Reconstr Surg. 1999;15(1):9–16.
21. Rootman J, Stewart B, Goldberg RA. Orbital surgery: a conceptual approach. Philadelphia: Lippincott-Raven; 1995.
22. Paridaens DA, Verhoeff K, Bouwens D, van Den Bosch WA. Transconjunctival orbital decompression in graves' ophthalmopathy: lateral wall approach ab interno. Br J Ophthalmol. 2000;84(7):775–81.
23. Dollinger J. Die druckentlastung der augenho¨hle durch entfernung der a¨ uberen orbitawand bei hochgradigem exophthalmos (morbus basedowii) und konsekutiver hauterkrankung. Dtsch Med Wschr. 1911;37:1888–90.
24. Lindholm J, Laurberg P. Hyperthyroidism, exophthalmos, and goiter: historical notes on the orbitopathy. Thyroid. 2010;20(3):291–300.
25. Naffziger HC. Progressive exophthalmos following thyroidectomy, its pathology and treatment. Ann Surg. 1931;94:582–6.
26. Naffziger HC. Progressive exophthalmos associated with disorders of the thyroid gland. Ann Surg. 1938;108:529–44.
27. Mehta P, Durrani OM. Outcome of deep lateral wall rim- sparing orbital decompression in thyroid-associated orbitopathy: a new technique and results of a case series. Orbit. 2011;30(6):265–8.
28. Chang EL, Piva AP. Temporal fossa orbital decompression for treatment of disfiguring thyroid-related orbitopathy. Ophthalmology. 2008;115(9):1613–9.
29. Kakizaki H, Takahashi Y, Ichinose A, Iwaki M, Selva D, Leibovitch I. The importance of rim removal in deep lateral orbital wall decompression. Clin Ophthalmol. 2011;5:865–9.
30. Bahr W, Bagambisa FB, Schlegel G, Schilli W. Comparison of transcutaneous incisions used for exposure of the infraorbital rim and orbital floor: a retrospective study. Plast Reconstr Surg. 1992;90(4):585–91.
31. Holtmann B, Wray C, Little GA. A randomized comparison of four incisions for orbital fractures. Plast Reconstr Surg. 1981;67(6):731–5.
32. Wray RC, Holtmann B, Ribaudo JM, Keiter J, Weeks PM. A comparison of conjunctival and subciliary incisions for orbital fractures. Br J Plast Surg. 1977;30(2):142–5.
33. Tessier P. The conjunctival approach to the orbital floor and maxilla in congenital malformation and trauma. J Maxillofac Surg. 1973;1(1):3–8.
34. Converse JM, Firmin F, Wood-Smith D, Friedland JA. The conjunctival approach in orbital fractures. Plast Reconstr Surg. 1973;52(6):656–7.
35. McCord CD. Orbital decompression for graves–diseasedexposure through lateral canthal and inferior fornix incision. Ophthalmology. 1981;88(6):533–41.
36. European Group on Graves Orbitopathy, Mourits MP, Bijl H, Altea MA, Baldeschi L, Boboridis K, et al. Outcome of orbital decompression for disfiguring proptosis in patients with graves' orbitopathy using various surgical procedures. Br J Ophthalmol. 2009;93(11):1518–23.
37. Kalmann R, Mourits MP, van der Pol JP, Koornneef L. Coronal approach for rehabilitative orbital decompression in graves' ophthalmopathy. Br J Ophthalmol. 1997;81(1):41e5.
38. Mourits MP, Koornneef L, Wiersinga WM, Prummel MF, Berghout A, van der Gaag R. Orbital decompression for graves' ophthalmopathy by inferomedial, by inferomedial plus lateral, and by coronal approach. Ophthalmology. 1990;97(5):636–41.
39. Paridaens D, Hans K, van Buitenen S, Mourits MP. The incidence of diplopia following coronal and translid orbital decompression in graves' orbitopathy. Eye (Lond). 1998;12(Pt 5):800–5.
40. Lynch R. The technique of a radical frontal sinus operation which has given me the best results. Laryngoscope. 1921;31:1–5.

41. Esclamado RM, Cummings CW. Z-plasty modification of the lynch incision. Laryngoscope. 1989;99(9):986–7.
42. Baldeschi L. Small versus coronal incision orbital decompression in graves' orbitopathy. Orbit. 2010;29(4):177–82.
43. Cruz AAV, Leme VR. Orbital decompression: a comparison between trans-fornix/transcaruncular inferomedial and coronal inferomedial plus lateral approaches. Ophthalmic Plast Reconstr Surg. 2003;19(6):440e5. Discussion 5
44. Shorr N, Baylis HI, Goldberg RA, Perry JD. Transcaruncular approach to the medial orbit and orbital apex. Ophthalmology. 2000;107(8):1459–63.
45. Seiff SR, Shorr N. Nasolacrimal drainage system obstruction after orbital decompression. Am J Ophthalmol. 1988;106(2):204–9.
46. Rootman J. Orbital surgery: a conceptual approach. 2nd ed. Philadelphia: Wolters Kluwer Health/ Lippincott Williams & Wilkins; 2014.
47. Ogura JH, Walsh TE. The transantral orbital decompression operation for progressive exophthalmos. Laryngoscope. 1962;72:1078–97.
48. Flint PW, Cummings CW. Cummings otolaryngology head & neck surgery. Philadelphia: Mosby; 2010.
49. DeFreitas J, Lucente FE. The Caldwell-Luc procedure: institutional review of 670 cases: 1975–1985. Laryngoscope. 1988;98(12):1297–300.
50. Weisman RA, Osguthorpe JD. Orbital decompression in graves' disease. Arch Otolaryngol Head Neck Surg. 1994;120(8):7–10.
51. Kennedy DW. Functional endoscopic sinus surgery. Tech Arch Otolaryngol. 1985;111(10):643–9.
52. Kennedy DW, Goodstein ML, Miller NR, Zinreich SJ. Endoscopic transnasal orbital decompression. Arch Otolaryngol Head Neck Surg. 1990;116:275–82.
53. Messerklinger W. Endoscopy of the nose. Baltimore: Urban & Schwarzenberg; 1978.
54. Kennerdell JS, Maroon JC. An orbital decompression for severe dysthyroid exophthalmos. Ophthalmology. 1982;89(5):467e72.
55. Bingham CM, Harris MA, Vidor IA, Rosen CL, Linberg JV, Marentette LJ, et al. Transcranial orbital decompression for progressive compressive optic neuropathy after 3-wall decompression in severe graves' orbitopathy. Ophthal Plast Reconstr Surg. 2014;30(3):215e8.
56. Fatourechi V, Bartley GB, Garrity JA, Bergstralh EJ, Ebersold MJ, Gorman CA. Transfrontal orbital decompression after failure of transantral decompression in optic neuropathy of graves' disease. Mayo Clin Proc. 1993;68(6):552e5.
57. Ramesh S, Nobori A, Wang Y, Rootman D, Goldberg RA. Orbital expansion in cranial vault after minimally invasive extradural Transorbital decompression for thyroid Orbitopathy. Ophthalmic Plast Reconstr Surg. 2019;35(1):17–21.

Lateral Wall Decompression 10

Robert Alan Goldberg and Milind N. Naik

10.1 Introduction

Consecutive or worsened strabismus is the most serious complication after orbital decompression surgery. Our interest in the lateral wall of the orbit is precipitated by a continual search for techniques that minimize the risk of new-onset or worsened double vision [1]. Traditional lateral orbital decompression involves removal of the anterior portion of the lateral orbital wall and is limited in the degree of orbital expansion that can be achieved [2]. For more decompression effects, the sphenoid can be drilled to the dura of the middle cranial fossa [3].

10.2 Advantages of Deep Lateral Decompression

Inferomedial orbital decompression via transantral route has high incidence of new-onset diplopia [4, 5]. Balanced decompression and preservation of inferomedial strut may decrease the risk but still can lead to new or worsened diplopia [6, 7]. Recently, the lateral wall decompression has emerged as a primary procedure for moderate proptosis because in minimizes the inferomedial shift of the muscle cone [1].

Removing bone from the deep lateral wall causes less consecutive strabismus, eliminates the risk of sinusitis (as with floor or medial wall decompression), affects faster resolution of post-operative strabismus and is especially useful for woody/fibrotic orbits [1, 8]. A great deal of additional soft tissue expansion can be obtained not only laterally but also posteriorly by removing, with a high-speed surgical drill, the thick areas of bone in the deep portion of the sphenoid wing. The sphenoid trigone forms a "door jamb" which severely limits the lateral expansion of the orbit. When it is removed back to the cortical bone overlying the middle cranial fossa and lateral to the anterior cranial fossa, the orbit obtains considerable lateral and posterior expansion. Thinning of the greater wing of sphenoid directly posterior to the orbit may allow proptosis reduction in cases of "woody" orbits that have little ability to enlarge their shape laterally but may move as a unit directly posteriorly.

R. A. Goldberg (✉) · M. N. Naik
Stein Eye Institute, UCLA, Los Angeles, CA, USA
e-mail: goldberg@jsei.ucla.edu

S. Rath, M. N. Naik (eds.), *Surgery in Thyroid Eye Disease*,
https://doi.org/10.1007/978-981-32-9220-8_10

10.3 Surgical Steps

10.3.1 Approach

The lateral wall can be accessed either intracranially, or trans-orbital by the ab-interno or ab-extero techniques (Fig. 9.2). The trans-orbital approach has much less morbidity, and is the most preferred technique [9].

10.3.2 Incisions

The deep lateral wall (sphenoid bone) can be accessed through either a coronal, eyelid crease, Berke-Reese, or a swinging eyelid incision (Fig. 10.1).

Although we now use it only rarely for maximal bone removal, the widest exposure is obtained through a *coronal* approach (Fig. 9.4)

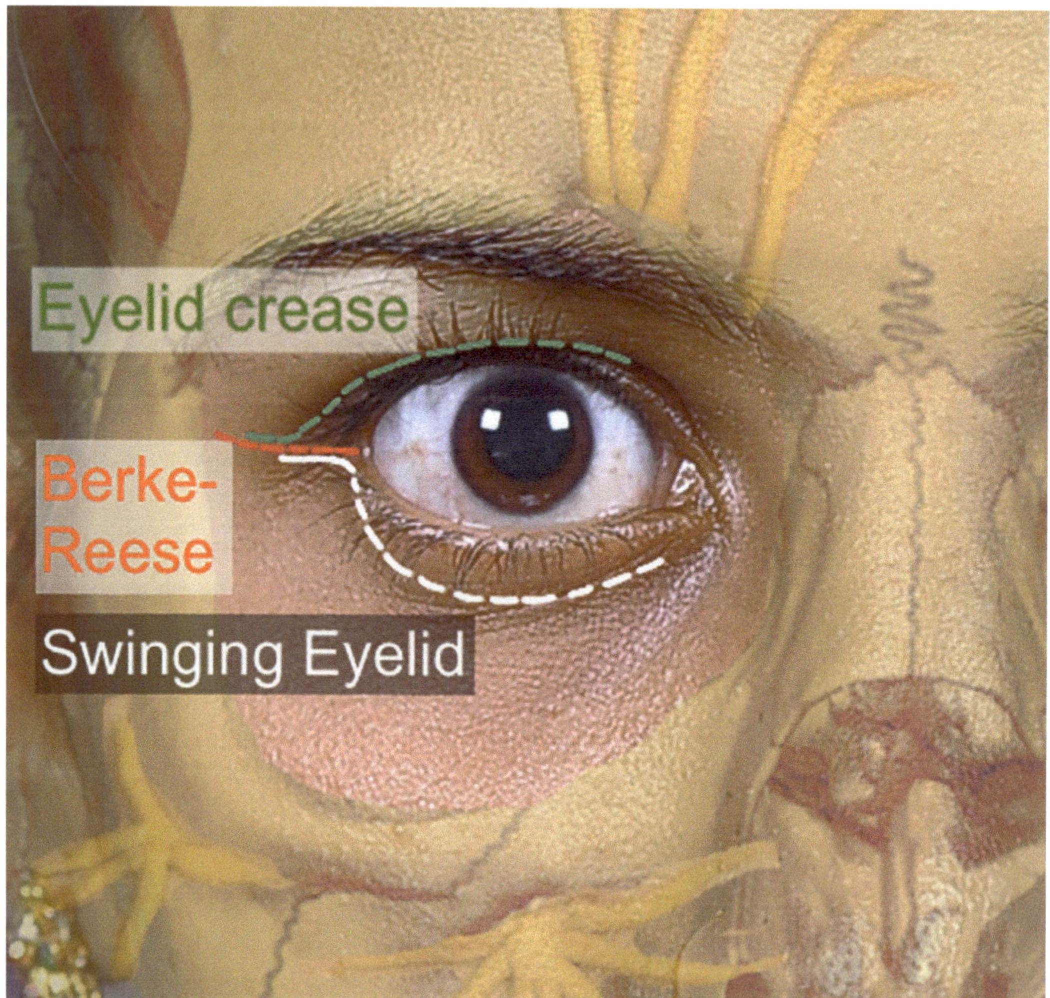

Fig. 10.1 The incisions used to reach the lateral orbital wall

[10]. The coronal approach provides unimpeded access to the deep lateral orbit, which is superior to a direct lateral orbitotomy. It leaves no visible scar (assuming an adequate hairline) and allows the performance of a simultaneous upper facelift when desired. Through a coronal approach, the lateral rim can be left in place and thinned. After elevating the medial canthal tendon and lacrimal sac from their periosteal attachment, excellent exposure is obtained through a coronal incision for medial and inferior orbital decompression.

The eyelid crease incision is considerably less time consuming than the coronal approach (Fig. 10.2). The eyelid crease incision is well hidden cosmetically and offers excellent exposure to the three areas of thick bone in the lateral wall, as discussed above.

10.3.3 Exposure of Lateral Wall

The periosteum is incised 4–5 mm outside the superolateral orbital rim, extending from the supraorbital notch medially, to the junction of the floor and lateral wall inferolaterally (Fig. 10.3). Periorbital dissection over the zygomatic prominence and superiorly over the frontal bone is necessary to achieve maximal deep orbital exposure.

The orbit is then entered extra-periosteally and exposure is taken back to the superior orbital fissure (Fig. 10.4). Separation of the periosteum here is easily done with a suction tip and malleable retractor. The zygomaticotemporal and zygomaticofacial neurovascular bundles are encountered along the lateral wall during the separation of the periosteum. Inferior dissection exposes the inferior orbital fissure, which is degloved, exposing the orbital floor.

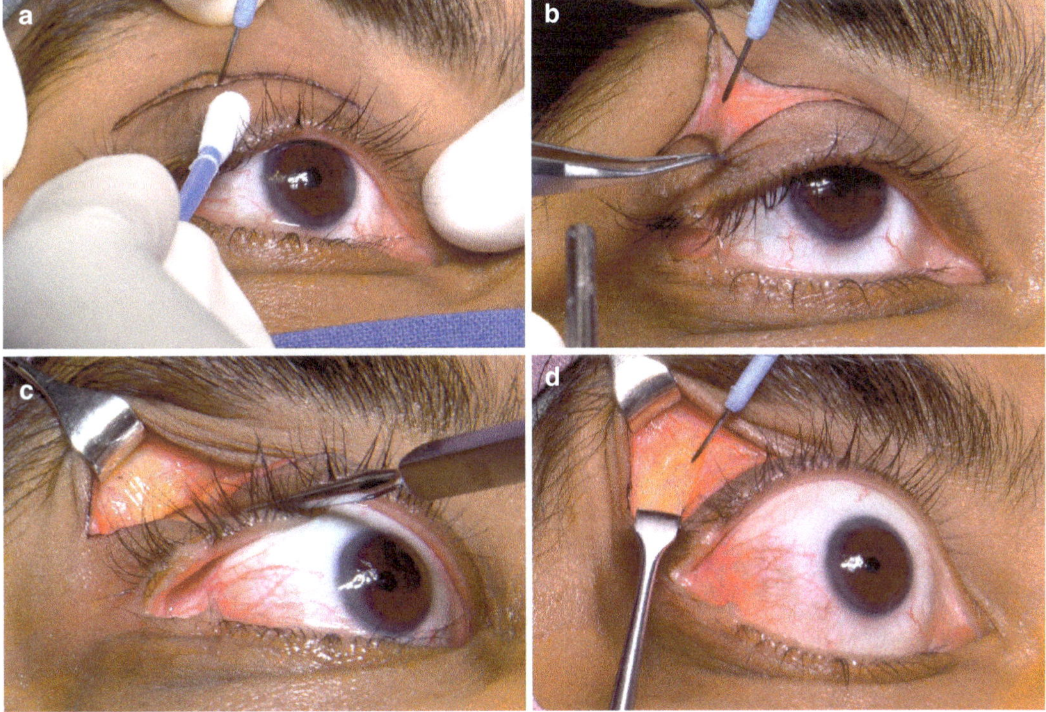

Fig 10.2 Eyelid crease incision design for lateral wall decompression. Skin incision (**a**), separation of orbicularis (**b**). Ascend towards the orbital rim in the sub-orbicularis plane to palpate the rim with a lens spatula (**c**). Periosteal incision is placed 4–5 mm away from bony orbital rim (**d**)

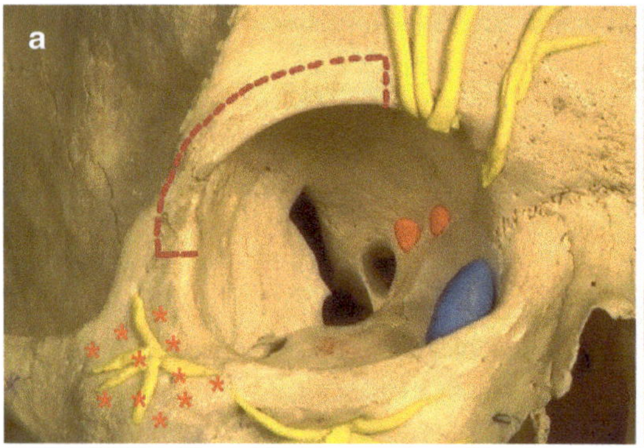

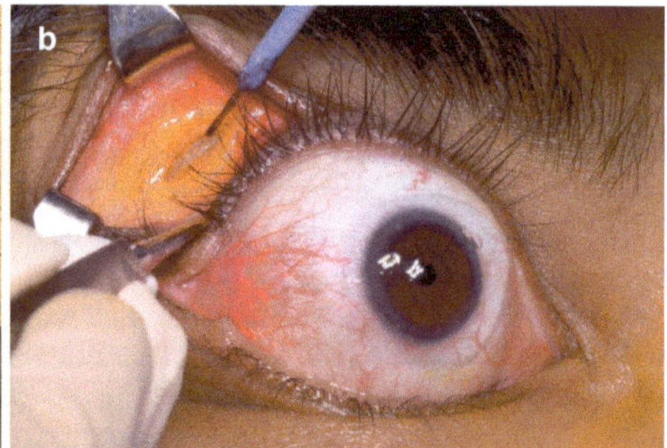

Fig. 10.3 Periosteal incision: Skull schematic showing the extent of periosteal incision after the eyelid crease incision is made. The periosteal incision is placed 4–5 mm outside the orbital rim. Inferolaterally, it extends just beyond the lateral canthus, and superomedially it stops short of the supraorbital notch, extending approximately 4 clock hours. (**a**). Note the periorbital area of dissection (asterisks) that is required for better exposure and access. Intraoperative photograph of the same step, showing periosteal incision being made through a thin layer of sub-brow fat (**b**)

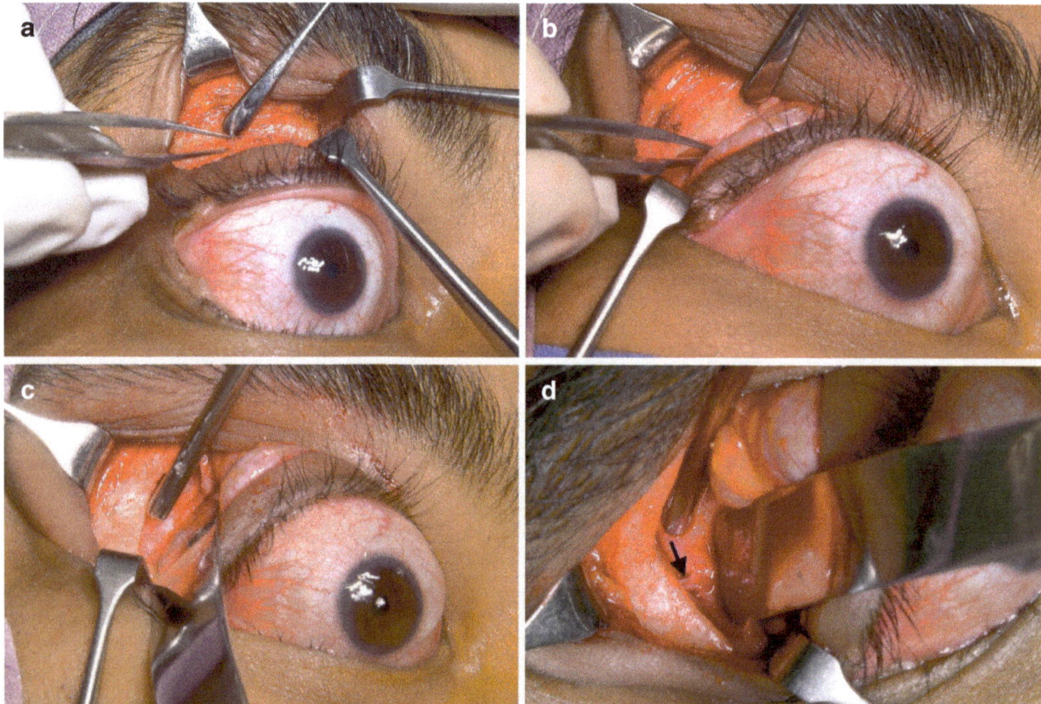

Fig. 10.4 After the periosteal incision, the periosteum is raised with a periosteal elevator (**a**) to reach the orbital rim along the entire length of the incision (**b**) and enter the orbit extraperiosteally (**c**). The orbital separation of periosteum can extend up to the superior orbital fissure posteriorly, lateral half of the roof supero-medially, and inferior orbital fissure infero-laterally. Superolaterally, the zygomaticotemporal neurovascular bundle is seen exiting the orbit (arrow), and requires cauterization (**d**). Similarly, the zygomaticofacial neurovascular bundle is encountered inferolaterally

10.3.4 Bony Sculpting

The anatomy of deep lateral orbital decompression can be intimidating, as the surgeon navigates around the dura of the anterior and middle cranial fossa. It is during this step, that navigation-guided surgery can be predictable and safe, although it is not mandatory to have navigation guidance (Fig. 10.5).

Focussing on the river of diploe that runs through the sphenoid bone, provides a reliable landmark that helps safely achieve maximal bone removal from the deep lateral orbit.

There are three areas of bone within the deep lateral orbit, which are available for removal in deep lateral orbital decompression surgery: *the doorjamb* of the greater wing of the sphenoid, the *lacrimal keyhole* in the frontal and zygomatic bone, and *the basin of the inferior orbital fissure* within the lateral maxilla (Figs. 10.6–10.8) [1].

The average total bone volume available for removal from the combined three areas is 5.6 cc. Averages for the door jamb, lacrimal keyhole, and basin are 2.9 cc, 1.2 cc, and 1.5 cc, respectively. The deep lateral orbital wall can provide significant room for volume expansion, and we have observed that up to 6 mm of proptosis reduction can be obtained utilizing the lateral wall alone.

The first bone removed is the *lacrimal keyhole*, in the fossa of the lacrimal gland (Fig. 10.6). The sculpting can begin by creating a notch at the orbital rim that helps stabilize the drill handpiece by providing a fulcrum. A groove is then drilled, starting from the superolateral notch in the direction of the superior orbital fissure. Then, internal sculpting is done from the superolateral orbital rim inwards (conceptually called lacrimal keyhole). It achieves proptosis reduction, allows the lacrimal gland to relax back within the orbital rim, and also gives a better view of the superior orbital fissure. This dissection is performed with a side cutting aggressive mechanized burr.

By aiming for the fissure, the surgeon naturally encounters the beginning of the diploic space within the greater wing of the sphenoid. Superiorly, this dissection is limited by the thin bone of the orbital roof, and particularly in a

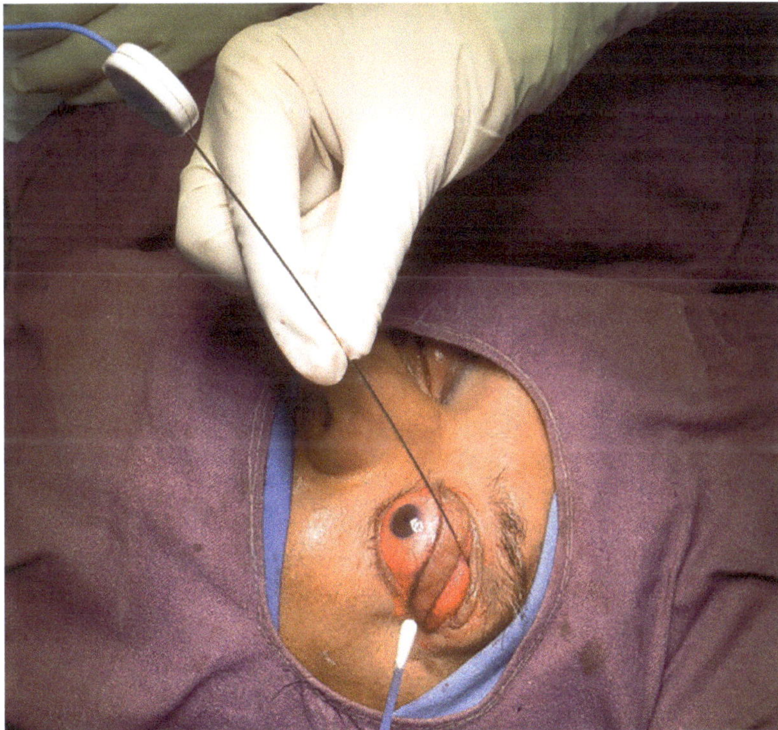

Fig. 10.5 Intraoperative use of navigation guidance during deep lateral wall decompression

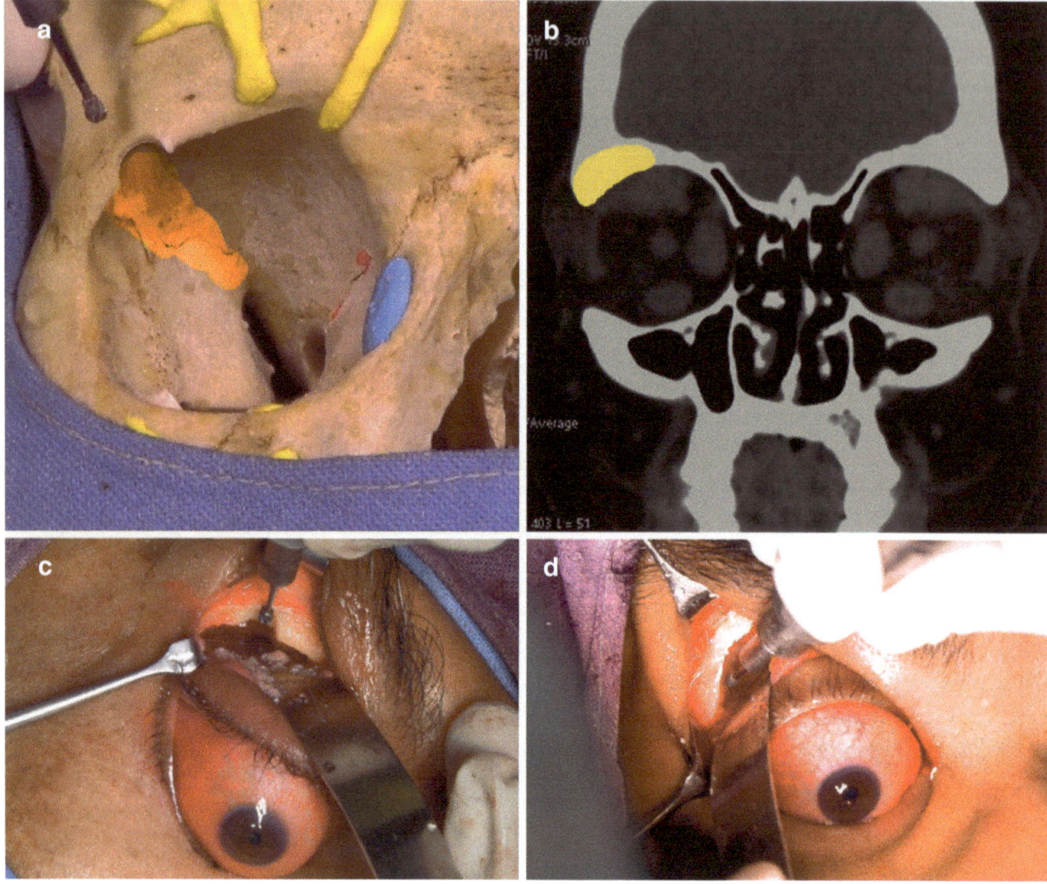

Fig. 10.6 Sculpting the Lacrimal keyhole. A superotemporal notch is first made in the orbital rim (**a**, **c**). Starting from the notch, a groove is made extending up to the superior orbital fissure (**a**, marked in red color). The frontal and zygomatic bones are drilled supero-temporally, which conceptually represents the lacrimal keyhole (**b**, **d**). Coronal CT scan of the orbit showing the anterior part of the lacrimal keyhole that is being drilled (**b**)

young patient, I have no hesitation to expose some of the frontal dura as I delineate the superior most edge of the thick bone of the deep lesser wing. The surgeon may switch to a 3-mm diamond burr for increased control as the deepest bone is removed.

The next bone removed is the sphenoid *doorjamb* (Fig. 10.7). The diploic space within the greater wing is hollowed out using burrs and curettes. This leaves a "cliff" of the orbital table of the diploe, which can be removed using the diamond burr, working back toward the superior orbital fissure. We then follow the diploe as it branches off inferiorly toward the inferior orbital fissure. Again, a combination of rough diamond burr and curettes can be used. Above the inferior orbital fissure, the diploic space typically widens to form a large lake of diploe that can be hollowed out along the edge of the inferior orbital fissure, creating a large cavity. The diploe in the greater wing of the sphenoid also leaves a cliff of bone in the deepest part of the greater wing, and this cliff of the orbital table can be removed using the diamond burr.

Once the diploe has been removed, and the inner table and "cliff" thinned, the remainder of the decompression is straightforward. The anterior lateral wall can be thinned over the tempora-

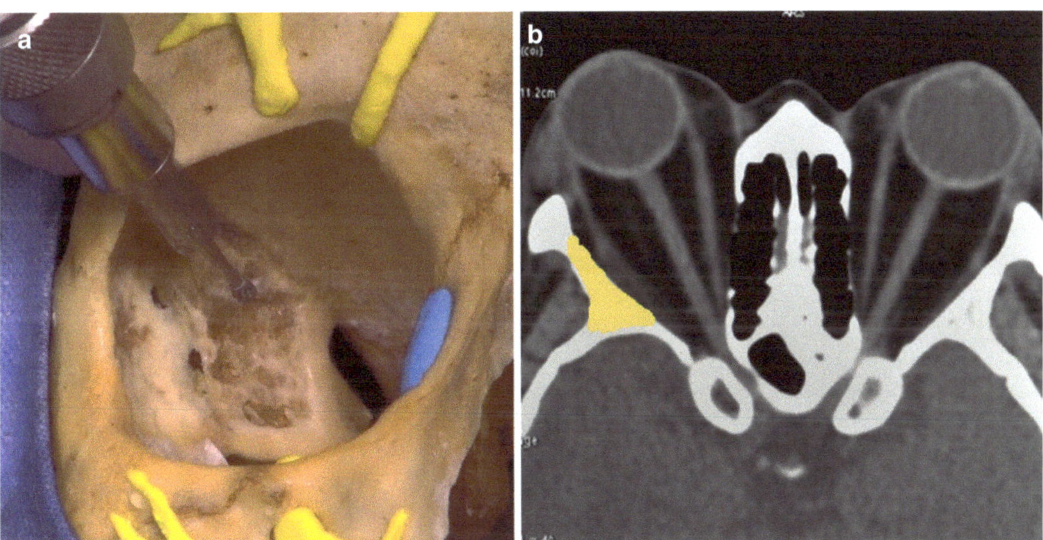

Fig. 10.7 Sculpting the sphenoid doorjamb. The sphenoid diploe is drilled to obtain maximum posterior displacement of the eyeball (**a**). Axial CT scan of the orbit showing the area of diploe that is removed in this step (**b**)

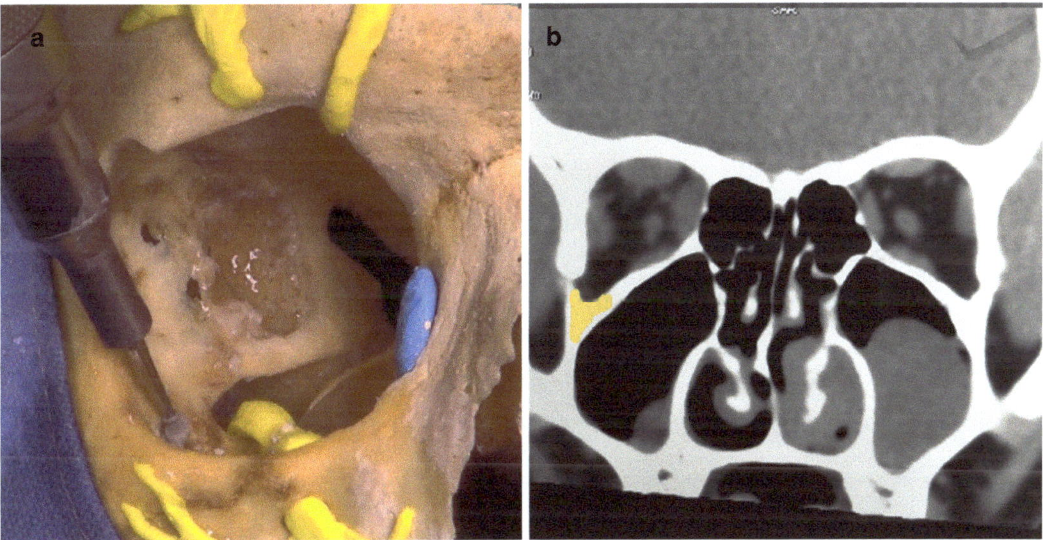

Fig. 10.8 Sculpting the basin of inferior orbital fissure. The bone in front of the anterior edge of inferior orbital fissure is drilled full thickness (**a**). Coronal CT scan of the orbit showing the area of the basin (**b**)

lis muscle. I try to leave an eggshell bone over the muscle, for the fear that extensive removal of bone over the muscle may result in oscillopsia with chewing. No bone should be removed directly lateral to the globe; otherwise lateral shift of the globe with increased inter-pupillary distance may result.

Finally, the *basin of the inferior orbital fissure* is addressed for more space (Fig. 10.8). This is the bone between the anterior end of inferior orbital fissure and the orbital rim. The bone here can be drilled out to expose the buccal fat and maxillary sinus mucosa. For more decompression, the cranial fossa of the diploe can be burred or ronguered to expose the dura of the middle cranial fossa.

10.3.5 Periosteal Release

The periosteum is then opened widely over all of the areas of bone removal, and intraconal fat can be accessed for graded removal as the assistant retracts the lateral rectus muscle superiorly using a curved malleable retractor (Fig. 10.9).

10.4 Outcome

The risk of post-operative strabismus is lessened compared to medial approaches, and good cosmetic outcomes can be achieved (Fig. 10.10). With experience, the lateral wall decompression can be performed in 45 minutes per side. Bone is removed directly behind the globe, allowing proptosis reduction even in "woody" orbits that have little ability to expand their shape horizontally. Bone is removed from the deep orbital apex, so it

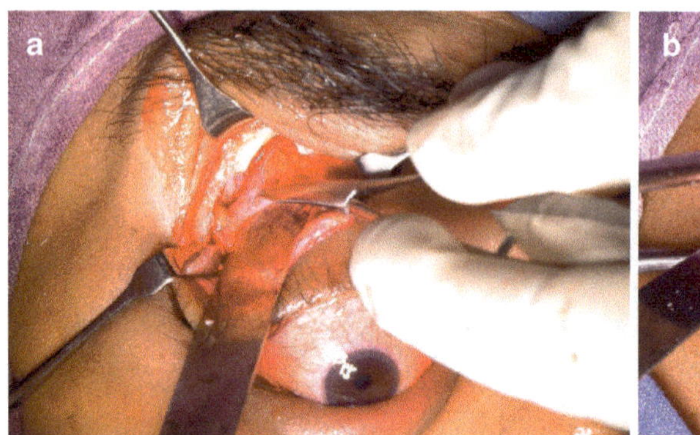

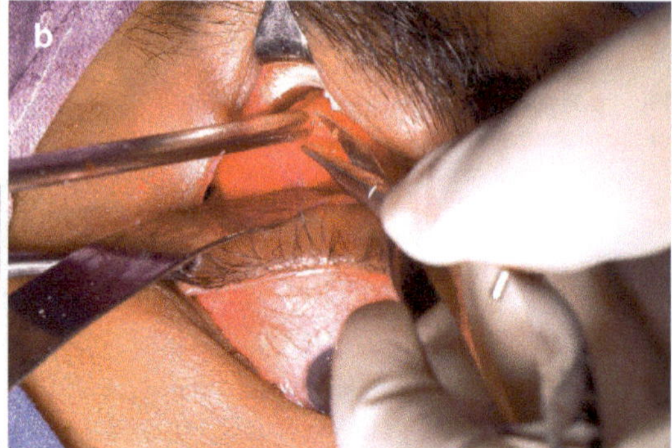

Fig. 10.9 Release of the superolateral periorbita using a Wescott scissors to allow fat prolapse (**a**). Conservative fat decompression superolaterally using a suction tip and Wescott scissors (**b**)

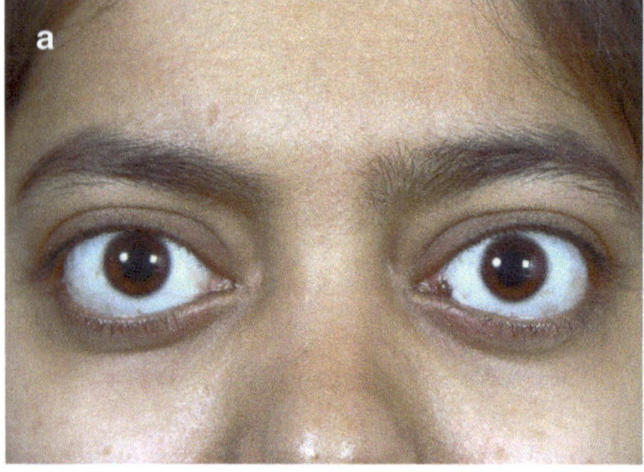

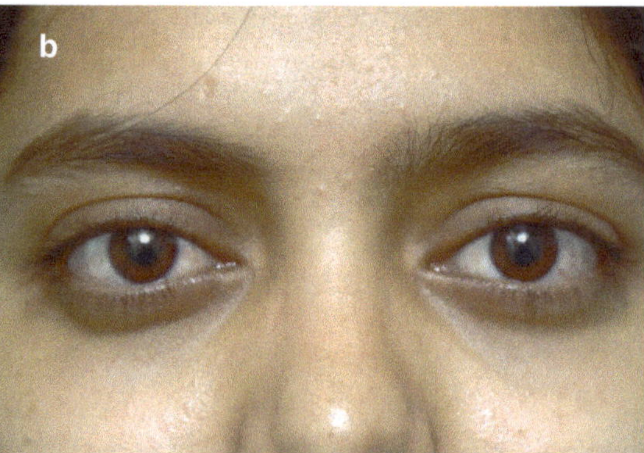

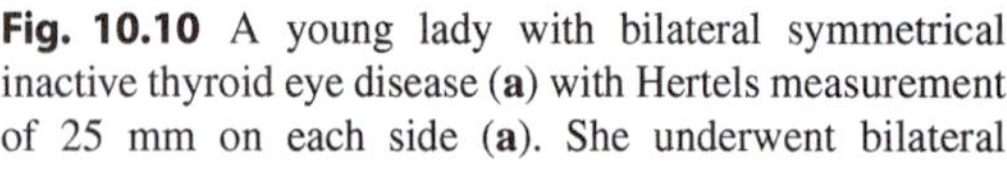

Fig. 10.10 A young lady with bilateral symmetrical inactive thyroid eye disease (**a**) with Hertels measurement of 25 mm on each side (**a**). She underwent bilateral sequential deep lateral wall decompression through an eyelid crease incision to achieve good correction of the proptosis without muscle disturbance (**b**)

should be equally efficacious for treating compressive optic neuropathy compared to the medial approach.

Ab interno decompression without marginotomy, irrespective of the incision or approach has been reported to achieve on an average between 2.7 mm and 4.0 mm of proptosis reduction [8, 11–16]. Addition of fat removal to this technique can give 4.5 mm of proptosis reduction [8, 16]. The ab-externo technique via the temporal fossa reports similar results with 4–4.5 mm proptosis reduction [17, 18]. One study comparing the two approaches found similar proptosis reduction close to 4.0 mm in each group [19].

With pure lateral decompression, without other walls, the rate of new-onset diplopia in primary position is typically in the range of 0–6% [11, 12]. Motility has been reported to be unchanged after ab interno decompression of the deep orbital bone [11].

10.4.1 Risks and Complications

Removal of deep bone in the lateral orbit requires sculpting away layers of cortical and marrow bone in an anatomically complex area. Knowledge of anatomy and experience in the cadaver lab are prerequisites for safe surgery. Good illumination and retraction are paramount.

Post-operative hypoaesthesia in the zygomaticotemporal and zygomaticofacial neurovascular distribution is a common complication, but self-limited. Supraorbital nerve anesthesia is reported for coronal approaches due to dissection around the supraorbital nerve.

Cerebrospinal fluid leaks occur in approximately 3–7% of cases [16]. These are typically self-limited and can be managed with bone wax, tissue glue, or by packing orbital fat into the tissues. The leak has no long-term egress route and is self-limited. Meningitis and vision loss are rare.

Other rare complications include motor nerve injury associated with coronal or pre-trichial dissections, alacrimia, temporalis muscle wasting, oscillopsia, and infection.

10.5 Conclusion

Removing bone from the deep lateral wall has several benefits over other walls. It causes less consecutive strabismus, eliminates the risk of sinusitis (as with floor or medial wall decompression), affects faster resolution of post-operative strabismus and is especially useful for woody/fibrotic orbits. Deep lateral wall decompression can be carried superiorly to include fossa for lacrimal gland and inferiorly up to the inferior orbital fissure.

References

1. Goldberg RA, Kim A, Kerivan KM. The lacrimal keyhole, orbital door jamb, and basin of the inferior orbital fissure. Three areas of deep bone in the lateral orbit. Arch Ophthalmol. 2000;116:1618–24.
2. McCord CD Jr. Current trends in orbital decompression. Ophthalmology. 1985;92:21–33.
3. Ramesh S, Nobori A, Wang Y, Rootman D, Goldberg RA. Orbital expansion in cranial vault after minimally invasive extradural transorbital decompression for thyroid orbitopathy. Ophthalmic Plast Reconstr Surg. 2018;35(1):17–21.
4. Garrity JA, Fatourechi V, Bergstralh EJ, et al. Results of transantral orbital decompression in 428 patients with severe Graves' ophthalmopathy. Am J Ophthalmol. 1993;116:533–47.
5. Walsh TE, Ogura JH. Transantral orbital decompression for malignant exophthalmos. Laryngoscope. 1957;67:544–68.
6. Leone CR Jr, Piest KL, Newman RJ. Medial and lateral wall decompression for thyroid ophthalmopathy. Am J Ophthalmol. 1989;108:160–6.
7. Goldberg RA, Shorr N, Cohen MS. The medial orbital strut in the prevention of postdecompression dystopia in dysthyroid ophthalmopathy. Ophthalmic Plast Reconstr Surg. 1992;8:32–4.
8. Goldberg RA, Perry JD, Hortaleza V, Tong JT. Strabismus after balanced medial plus lateral wall versus lateral wall only orbital decompression for dysthyroid orbitopathy. Ophthalmic Plast Reconstr Surg. 2000;16:271–7.
9. Sasim IV, de Graaf ME, Berendschot TT, Kalmann R, van Isterdael C, Mourits MP. Coronal or swinging eyelid decompression for patients with disfiguring proptosis in graves' orbitopathy? Comparison of results in one center. Ophthalmology. 2005;112:1310–5.
10. Goldberg RA, Weinberg DA, Shorr N, Wirta D. Maximal 3 wall orbital decompression through a coronal approach. Ophthalmic Surg. 1997;28:832–43.
11. Ben Simon GJ, Syed HM, Syed AM, Lee S, Wang DY, Schwarcz RM, et al. Strabismus after deep lateral wall

orbital decompression in thyroid-related orbitopathy patients using automated hess screen. Ophthalmology. 2006;113:1050–5.

12. Ben Simon GJ, Wang LL, McCann JD, Goldberg RA. Primary-gaze diplopia in patients with thyroid-related orbitopathy undergoing deep lateral orbital decompression with intraconal fat debulking: a retrospective analysis of treatment outcome. Thyroid. 2004;14(5):379–83.
13. Liao SL, Shih MJ, Chang TC, Lin LL. Transforniceal lateral deep bone decompression-a modified technique to prevent postoperative diplopia in patients with disfiguring exophthalmos due to dysthyroid orbitopathy. J Formos Med Assoc. 2006;105:611–6.
14. Nguyen J, Fay A, Yadav P, MacIntosh PW, Metson R. Stereotactic microdebrider in deep lateral orbital decompression for patients with thyroid eye disease. Ophthalmic Plast Reconstr Surg. 2014;30(3):262–6.
15. Rocchi R, Lenzi R, Marinò M, Latrofa F, Nardi M, Piaggi P, et al. Rehabilitative orbital decompression for graves' orbitopathy: risk factors influencing the new onset of diplopia in primary gaze, outcome, and patients' satisfaction. Thyroid. 2012;22:1170–5.
16. Sellari-Franceschini S, Lenzi R, Santoro A, Muscatello L, Rocchi R, Altea MA, et al. Lateral wall orbital decompression in graves' orbitopathy. Int J Oral Maxillofac Surg. 2010;39(1):16–20.
17. Chang EL, Piva AP. Temporal fossa orbital decompression for treatment of disfiguring thyroid-related orbitopathy. Ophthalmology. 2008;115(9):1613–9.
18. Korinth MC, Ince A, Banghard W, Gilsbach JM. Follow-up of extended pterional orbital decompression in severe graves' ophthalmopathy. Acta Neurochir. 2002;144(2):113–20.
19. Cho RI, Choe CH, Elner VM. Ultrasonic bone removal versus high-speed burring for lateral orbital decompression: comparison of surgical outcomes for the treatment of thyroid eye disease. Ophthalmic Plast Reconstr Surg. 2010;26(2):83–7.

11 Orbital Floor Decompression for Thyroid Eye Disease

Peter J. Dolman

11.1 Introduction

Decompression of the orbital floor is typically performed as an adjunct to medial and/or lateral bony wall decompression, often in combination with orbital fat resection [1]. In the active phase of the disease, it may be combined with a posterior medial wall decompression to relieve dysthyroid compressive optic neuropathy, as described in Chap. 7.

In the quiescent phase, the primary indications are for disfiguring or symptomatic proptosis (to prevent or treat corneal exposure or globe prolapse) (Fig. 11.1a, b), or for chronic periorbital soft tissue congestion from extraocular muscles that remain engorged despite immunomodulators or radiotherapy (Fig. 11.2a, b) [2].

P. J. Dolman (✉)
Department of Ophthalmology and Visual Sciences, University of British Columbia, Vancouver General Hospital, Vancouver, Canada

S. Rath, M. N. Naik (eds.), *Surgery in Thyroid Eye Disease*, https://doi.org/10.1007/978-981-32-9220-8_11

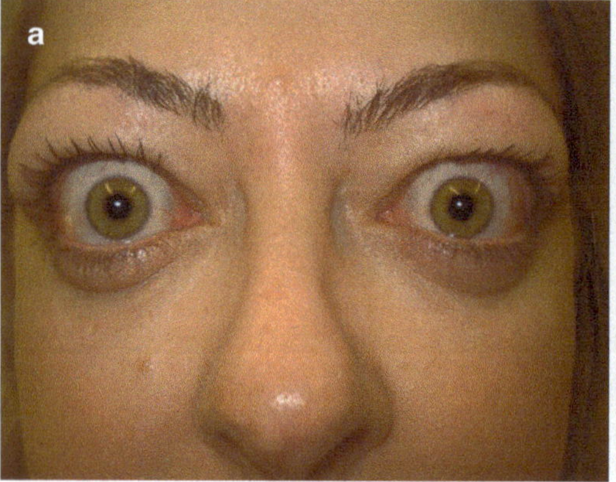

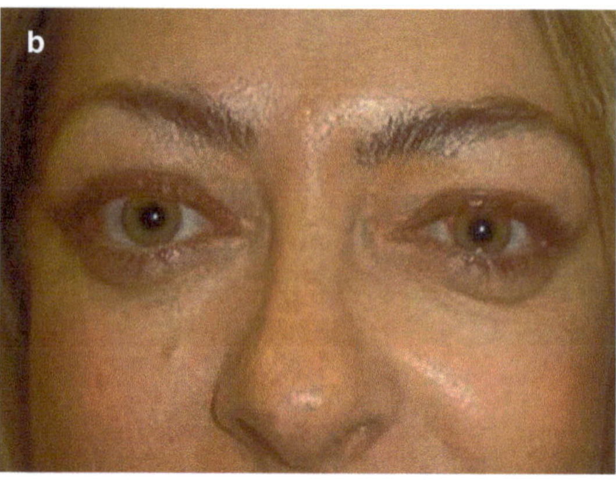

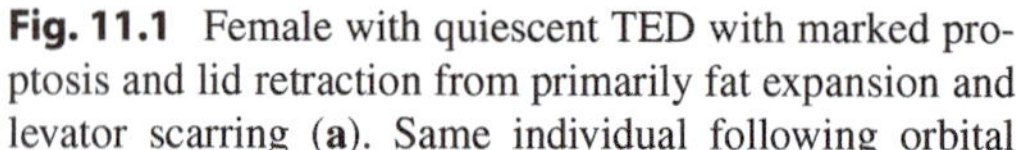

Fig. 11.1 Female with quiescent TED with marked proptosis and lid retraction from primarily fat expansion and levator scarring (**a**). Same individual following orbital floor and medial wall decompression along with levator recession (**b**)

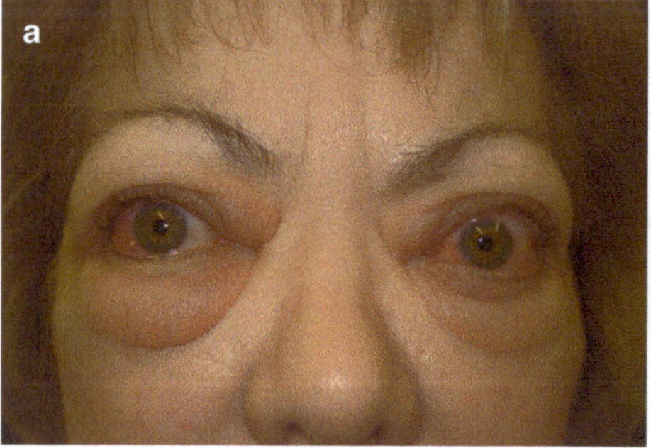

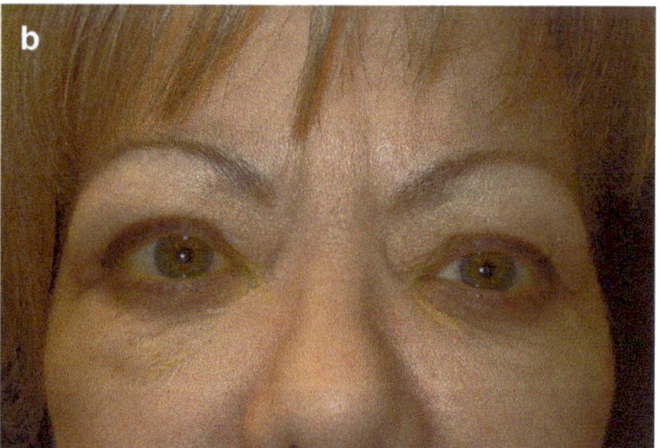

Fig. 11.2 Congestive TED from longstanding quiescent disease with enlarged muscles limiting orbital venous drainage (**a**). Same individual demonstrating resolution of congestive soft tissue features following orbital floor and medial wall decompression (**b**)

11.2 Surgical Anatomy of the Orbital Floor

The orbital anatomy is covered in detail in Chap. 2. However, elements of the orbital anatomy relevant to orbital floor decompression are reiterated below.

The orbital floor is a thin triangular structure that is bounded anteriorly by the orbital rim, posterolaterally by the inferior orbital fissure which separates it from the apex and the lateral wall, and nasally by the ethmoid and lacrimal bones which define the medial wall [3]. The back wall of the maxillary sinus defines the posterior limit of the floor and the anterior limit of the pterygopalatine fossa.

The floor is composed mainly of the maxillary bone with a small posterior segment of palatine bone and a larger anterolateral contribution from the zygoma. Extending forward from the inferior orbital fissure is the infraorbital groove or tunnel that is variably covered by a thin plate of bone at the level of the mid-orbit: this houses the maxillary division of the trigeminal nerve which erupts as the infraorbital nerve through the infraorbital foramen, 4–5 mm below the central orbital rim [3].

The lacrimal sac and duct lie at the anteromedial corner of the floor near its junction with the medial wall, while the inferior oblique muscle takes its origin from the bony floor immediately lateral to the sac. Care should be taken to identify and protect these structures during surgery.

11.3 Preoperative Assessment

The surgeon should determine how the condition affects the patient and what they hope to gain from the procedure. (Cosmetic concerns may involve eyelid retraction, fat prolapse, and soft tissue thickening in the eyelids, in addition to exophthalmos. Functional concerns may be related to exposure complaints with ocular surface irritation, tearing, and visual disruption, or to orbital discomfort from a tight orbital compartment or from recurrent globe prolapse.)

Both disease severity and activity should be clinically assessed to plan the type and timing of surgery. The VISA Classification scheme confirms the disease is quiescent by lack of progression in any of the four VISA parameters: V (optic neuropathy), I (periocular soft tissue congestion), S (strabismus and motility restriction), and A (appearance/exposure changes) [4]. Severity measures for appearance and exposure changes include exophthalmometry, lid position and fullness, and corneal exposure changes [5]. Asymmetric involvement is noted so that surgery may be titrated for each eye accordingly.

Old photographs help to identify the orbital changes resulting from the disease.

Laboratory studies include thyroid function to ensure the patient is euthyroid, and thyroid immune tests including thyrotropin-receptor (TSH-R) antibodies to ensure the immune process is relatively controlled.

Radiologic studies primarily include axial and coronal CT scans with or without contrast to document which tissues are involved including specific muscles, any evidence for non-thyroid-orbitopathy causes of the proptosis especially in unilateral cases, and the presence of any sinusitis, specifically in the maxillary sinus. A more detailed assessment of radiology is described in Chap. 3.

The surgical plan is reviewed with the patient, explaining with CT images what tissues are enlarged, and what surgery is planned for each eye. The normal post-operative course and management are described along with a printed list of instructions and a letter for sick leave. Possible complications (described below) and the need for subsequent procedures including possible ocular alignment or lid surgery are discussed.

11.4 Perioperative Considerations

Orbital floor decompressions are typically performed under general anesthesia, although a unilateral procedure can be performed with regional blocks using monitored sedation [6].

Anticoagulants and antiplatelet agents are generally discontinued several days prior to the surgery with permission from the treating cardiologist, family physician, or neurologist. Bridging low-molecular-weight subcutaneous heparin may be administered while warfarin is held for three days prior to the surgery [7].

Perioperative antibiotics (intravenous cefazolin) and corticosteroids (intravenous dexamethasone) are administered at the start of surgery.

Most surgeons favor lateral wall or fat decompressions for mild proptosis (2–3 mm) and 3-wall combined floor, medial wall, and lateral wall decompressions for severe proptosis (>5 mm) [1]. For moderate proptosis (3–5 mm), some surgeons advocate a "balanced" medial and lateral wall decompression, arguing that this might reduce the risk of new-onset strabismus [8]. Others, such as this author, prefer a combined medial and floor decompression, obtaining an excellent reduction in proptosis with a low incidence of strabismus for those patients with inactive disease, the majority of whom have minimal preoperative extraocular muscle enlargement or restriction [9].

11.5 Surgical Technique

The "swinging eyelid flap" provides access to the floor, medial, and lateral walls allowing any combination of bony wall and orbital fat removal (Fig. 11.3a). This involves a lateral canthotomy and inferior cantholysis, dissection to the inferior rim via an inferior fornix transconjunctival approach, incision, and reflection of the periorbita at the arcus marginalis, and exposure of the medial wall, floor, and lateral wall. Care is taken to avoid disruption of the inferior oblique muscle and the lacrimal sac nasally, while laterally the floor is exposed to the level of the anterior limit of the inferior orbital fissure, 1.5 cm behind the inferior rim [3]. A Desmarres retractor displaces the lower lid structures inferiorly while a malleable ribbon retractor contains the orbital soft tissue (Fig. 11.3b). A Cottle elevator is used to strip the periorbita posteriorly to expose the orbital floor (Fig. 11.3c).

The infraorbital canal or tunnel travels anteromedially from the leading edge of the inferior fissure; a small feeding arteriole may extend from the orbital soft tissue to the nerve within the canal

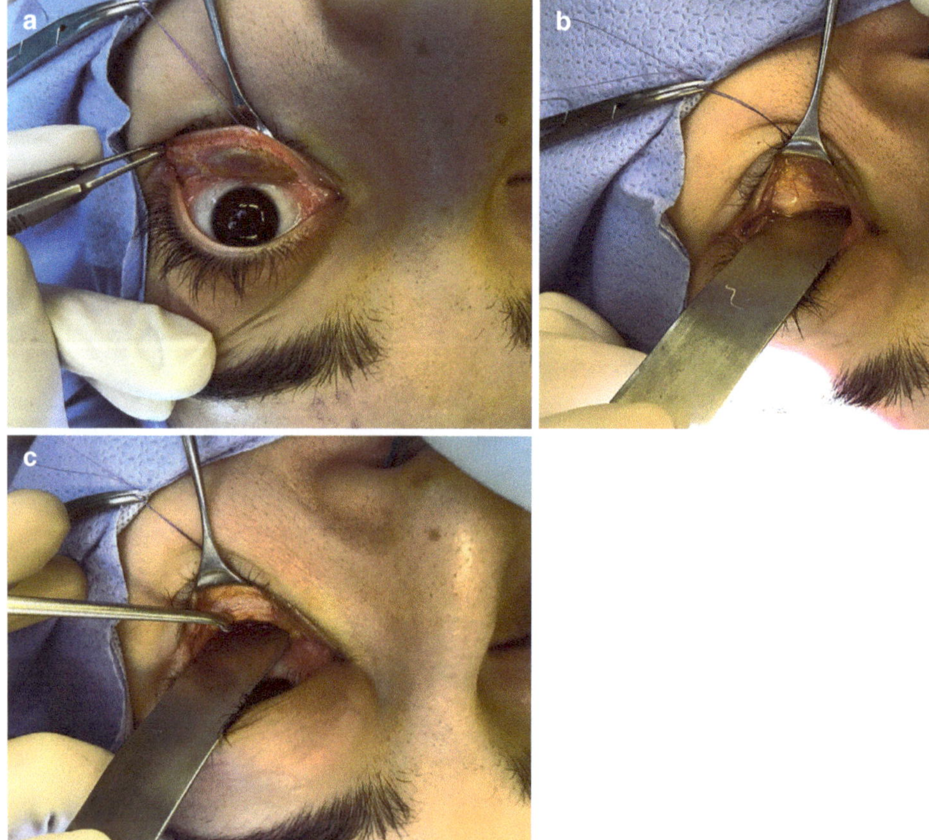

Fig. 11.3 Swinging eyelid approach to left orbital floor (**a**). A lateral canthotomy and inferior cantholysis are performed, the lower lid is everted over a Desmarres retractor, and a hot wire cautery is used to open infratarsal palpebral conjunctiva and lower lid retractors down to the inferior rim. The inferior rim and arcus marginalis are exposed using the Desmarres retractor and a broad malleable ribbon retractor (**b**). A monopolar cautery may be used to open the periosteum to bone. A Cottle elevator is used to strip the periorbita posteriorly to expose the orbital floor (**c**)

and maybe cauterized and divided, occasionally causing transient cheek numbness.

The thin bone medial to the canal is entered with a chisel a few millimeters posterior to the inferior orbital rim (Fig. 11.4a). Weil-Blakesley or Takahashi forceps can be used to remove bone fragments to the posterior wall of the maxillary sinus, with a Fraser suction used to identify the posterior wall by sounding through the opening in the floor (Fig. 11.4b). Bone is removed lateral to the orbital strut separating the medial wall and floor.

Bone may be removed anteriorly using a Kerrison rongeur: in unilateral decompressions, care must be taken to leave adequate bone to support the globe up to the equator to limit inferior displacement of the eyeball relative to the opposite side.

Medially, the bony strut may be removed behind the lacrimal drainage apparatus and origin of the inferior oblique muscle, avoiding disruption of the maxillary sinus drainage. If medial wall decompression is performed, bone and ethmoid sinus may be rongeured superiorly to the level of the ethmoidal vessels and nerves, located approximately at the level of the medial canthal ligament [3].

Temporally, the lateral wall of the maxillary sinus may be sounded underneath the infraorbital canal using the suction tip through the opening in

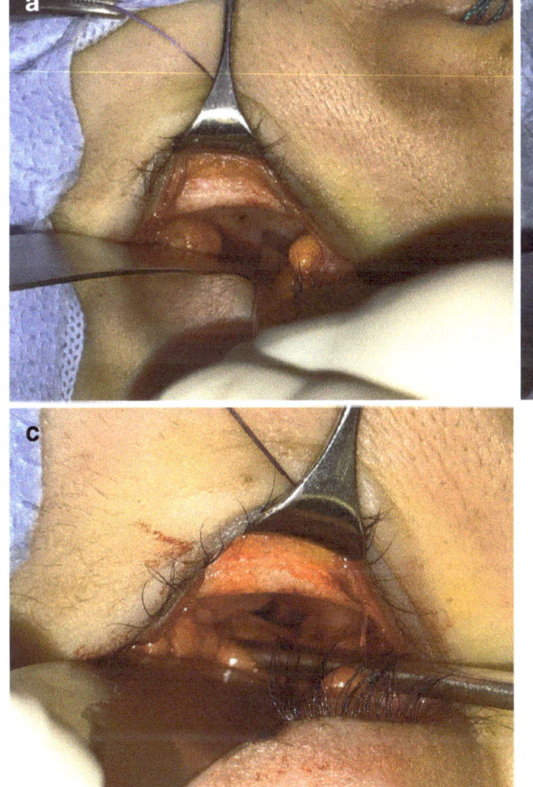

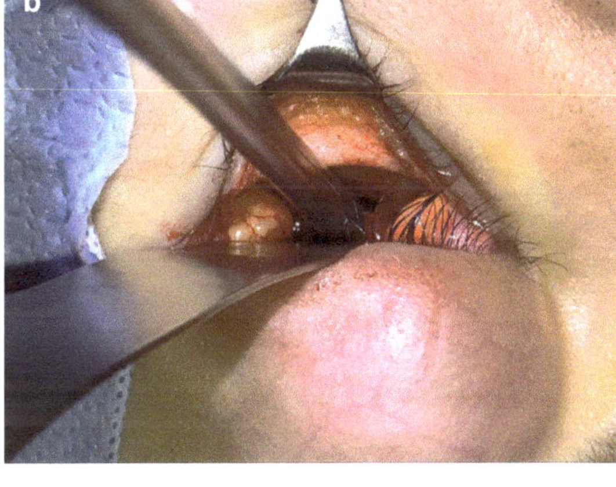

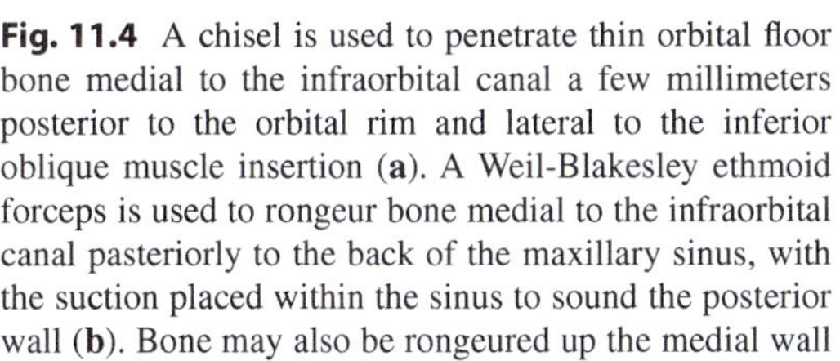

Fig. 11.4 A chisel is used to penetrate thin orbital floor bone medial to the infraorbital canal a few millimeters posterior to the orbital rim and lateral to the inferior oblique muscle insertion (**a**). A Weil-Blakesley ethmoid forceps is used to rongeur bone medial to the infraorbital canal pasteriorly to the back of the maxillary sinus, with the suction placed within the sinus to sound the posterior wall (**b**). Bone may also be rongeured up the medial wall to the level of the ethmoidal vessels, but care is taken to stay well posterior to the lacrimal sac apparatus, origin of the inferior oblique muscle, and the maxillary sinus drain. The suction may also be used to sound the lateral wall underneath the infraorbital nerve to determine if the bony floor lateral to the nerve may be chiselled and rongeured (**c**). Often there is little gain in removing this portion of the bony floor

the floor (Fig. 11.4c). The steps in floor decompression are depicted on the skull model in Fig. 11.5. Additional bone may be rongeured lateral to the groove if space can be identified. Although bone surrounding the infraorbital nerve may be carefully freed and removed, it is often left intact to avoid temporary post-operative cheek or upper lip anesthesia or paresthesia.

The lateral wall may be adjunctively drilled both anteriorly to the temporalis muscle or posteriorly through the marrow of the greater wing of the sphenoid bone up to the superior fissure [10].

The periorbita is then opened from its posterior aspect anteriorly parallel to the inferior rectus with caution to avoid trauma to either the inferior rectus or the oblique muscles (Fig. 11.6a). Orbital fat herniates through the periorbital windows and both the inferolateral and the inferomedial pockets may be resected, with each cubic centimeter of fat removed corresponding to a millimeter of reduced proptosis (Fig. 11.6b). The inferior oblique muscle must be identified to prevent trauma during fat resection (Fig. 11.6c). Remaining fat can be gently

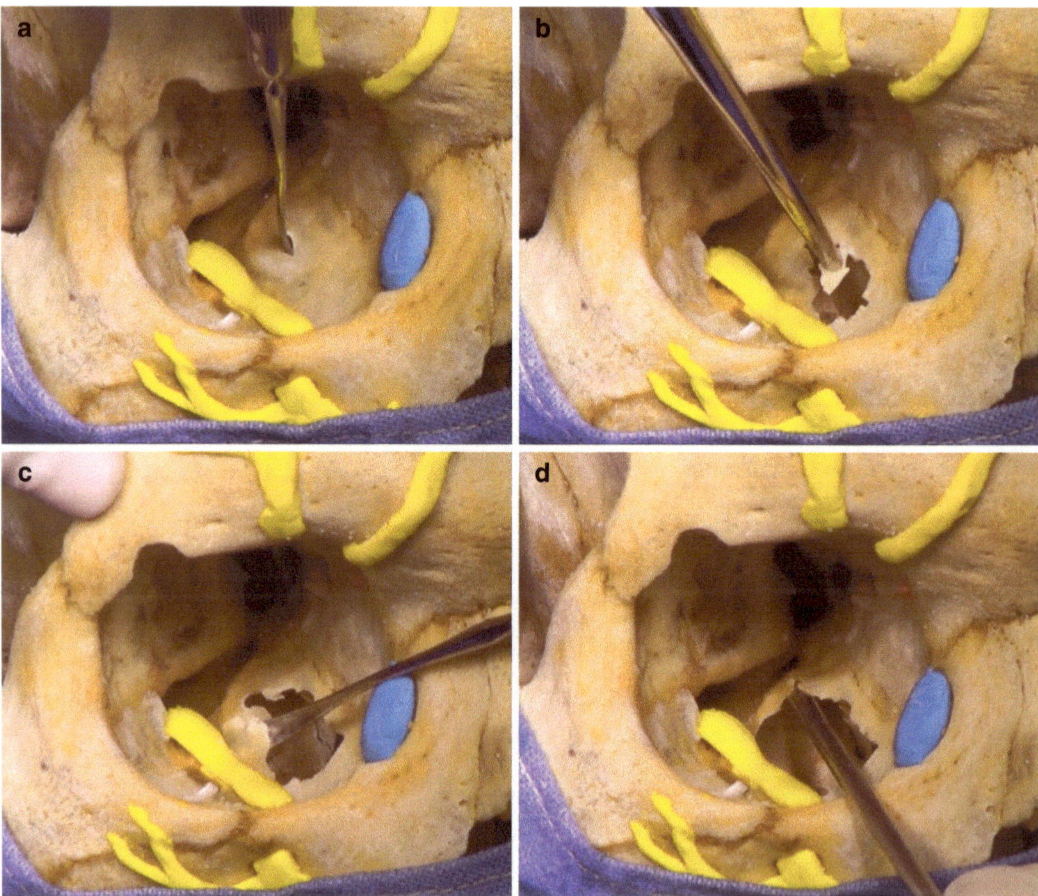

Fig. 11.5 Representation of Orbital floor decompression on a skull model. Penetration of the thin orbital floor (**a**), removal of floor medial to the infraorbital canal (**b**), careful elevation and removal of the bone adjoining the infraorbital canal (**c**), and removal of posterior floor using a suction tip (**d**)

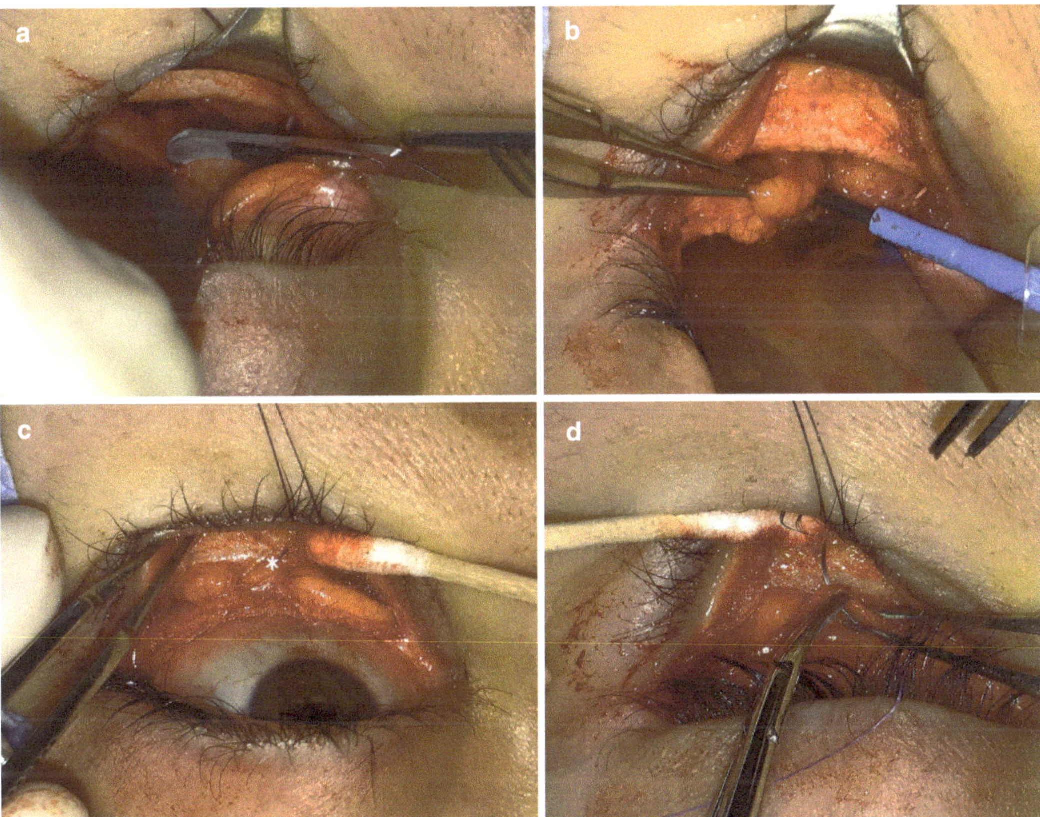

Fig. 11.6 With a #12 blade, myringotomy blade, or arthrotec Beaver blade may be used to penetrate the periorbita of the floor, starting posteriorly and advancing anteriorly, avoiding the inferior rectus and oblique muscles (**a**). Flaps are joined so that orbital flat is completely released. In cases of medial wall decompression, the periorbita is opened along the medial orbit. The inferotemporal and inferomedial fat pockets may be teased forward and portions excised (**b**). This is particularly helpful in cases of fat expansion in those cases with indolent onset disease and can also be used to reduce fat prolapse from the lower lids, although be cautious not to induce hollowing from excessive sculpting. The remaining orbital fat may be gently prolapsed into the sinus cavities. Care is taken not to damage the inferior oblique muscle (asterisk) as it courses obliquely between the medial and temporal inferior fat pockets (**c**). The inferior lid retractors and conjunctiva are closed with a running 6-0 absorbable suture (**d**)

prolapsed into the exposed sinus spaces by gentle retropulsion on the globe. Inferior orbital fat may also be removed to reduce lower lid fat pockets, with care to avoid hollowing of the lids.

The inferior retractors and conjunctiva are closed with a running 6-0 polyglactin 910 suture and the lateral canthus re-sutured to the rim (Fig. 11.6d). Horizontal tightening of orbicularis and skin may be performed to improve lower lid cosmesis, but horizontal shortening of the lower lid should be performed cautiously, as it may induce further lower lid retraction. I do not place any surgical drains, but the patient should be monitored for retrobulbar hematoma, compartment syndrome, or vision loss. Post-operative medications may include 3 days of oral corticosteroids and 5 days of oral broad-spectrum antibiotic (such as cefazolin) (Fig. 11.6d).

11.6 Surgical Tips and Outcomes

Orbital floor decompression reduces proptosis by an average of 2 mm. Additional medial or lateral wall decompression may add a further 2 mm of reduction for each wall [1]. Orbital roof decompression is seldom performed. Adjunctive orbital fat resection may reduce proptosis by a further 1 mm for every 1.5 cubic centimeter of fat excised [11].

Both floor decompression and inferior orbital fat resection may cause inferior globe displacement. This may reduce lower lid retraction, which will also be improved by reduced proptosis. However, in unilateral cases, one should consider avoiding floor surgery or restricting removal to the posterior floor to avoid unilateral globe dystopia and obvious asymmetry (Fig. 11.7). In cases of lower lid retraction greater than 2 mm, additional lid elevation may be achieved through a posterior lamellar graft at the time of closure of the inferior fornix [12].

Inferior displacement of the globe from floor decompression may also exaggerate upper lid retraction, and patients should be warned about this. Although reduction in proptosis improves lower lid retraction, it seldom improves upper lid retraction which is caused by enlargement and scarring of the levator complex [13].

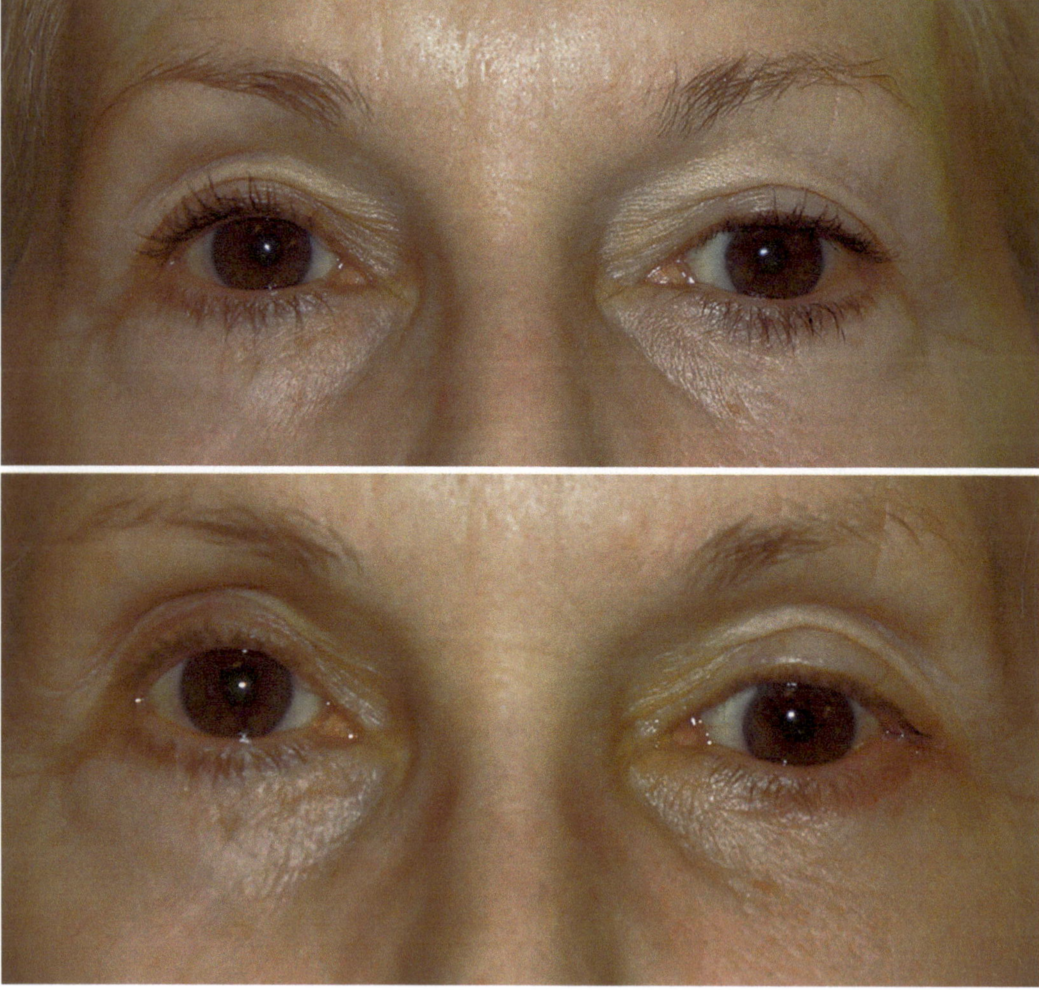

Fig. 11.7 This lady with 4-mm left proptosis and hypotropia (top) underwent unilateral left orbital floor and medial wall decompression with good resolution in proptosis and congestion, but developed some inferior dystopia from excessive anterior floor removal (bottom)

11.7 Complications

Temporary anesthesia or paresthesia may involve various regions of the V2 dermatome (lateral nostril, cheek, and upper lid/teeth) as a result of vascular or mechanical injury to the infraorbital nerve as the bony floor is exposed or removed. Complete exposure of the nerve by removing all the bone around its length increases the risk of secondary nerve injury and so should be avoided unless maximum decompression is needed. Bothersome infraorbital anesthesia usually resolves over weeks to months.

Various studies have reviewed the incidence of new-onset or worsening diplopia following different orbital decompression approaches. Lateral wall decompressions have been reported to have an incidence of new-onset strabismus of 7%, but maybe compromised by transient oscillopsia in 35% [14]. Balanced medial and lateral wall decompressions have a reported incidence of new-onset strabismus of 33% [15]. Another review by the same institution found balanced decompression had a significantly lower incidence of diplopia compared with combined floor and medial wall decompressions: however, it was not clear whether the indications for performing each type of surgery differed. At our institution, we recently compared combined medial wall and floor decompressions performed by the author over a one-year period for different indications, and identified that the incidence of worsening diplopia was greater than 50% when performed for compressive optic neuropathy (active phase, muscles enlarged), approximately 20% when performed for congestive orbitopathy (inactive phase, muscles enlarged), and less than 10% when performed for quiescent proptosis (inactive phase, fat expansion) [9]. In other words, in cases without diplopia nor muscle enlargement, the risk of new-onset strabismus is no worse than any other approaches for combined orbital floor and medial wall decompression.

Disruption of the insertion of the inferior oblique should be avoided to reduce the risk of developing torsional vertical diplopia [16]. Treatment for this is weakening of the ipsilateral superior oblique muscle.

Epiphora or dacryocystitis results from inadvertent trauma to the lacrimal outflow apparatus during dissection or retraction of the periosteum during medial wall exposure and decompression. This should be avoided by identifying and protecting these structures.

Maxillary sinus opacification with hematoma may occur following floor decompression but the blood usually clears spontaneously. Rarely disruption of the maxillary sinus drainage apparatus may lead to chronic congestion or sinusitis (Fig. 11.8) [17].

Compartment syndrome and loss of vision may rarely occur in the week following surgery from a post-operative orbital hemorrhage or less likely from air emphysema from a contained sneeze forcing air through a bony defect between the orbit and the nasal cavity. Patients should monitor the vision, position, and movement of each eye, and to proceed immediately to their local emergency facility to release the lateral canthus should signs of compartment syndrome development. This is an unlikely event, but could have a devastating outcome if ignored by an uninformed patient.

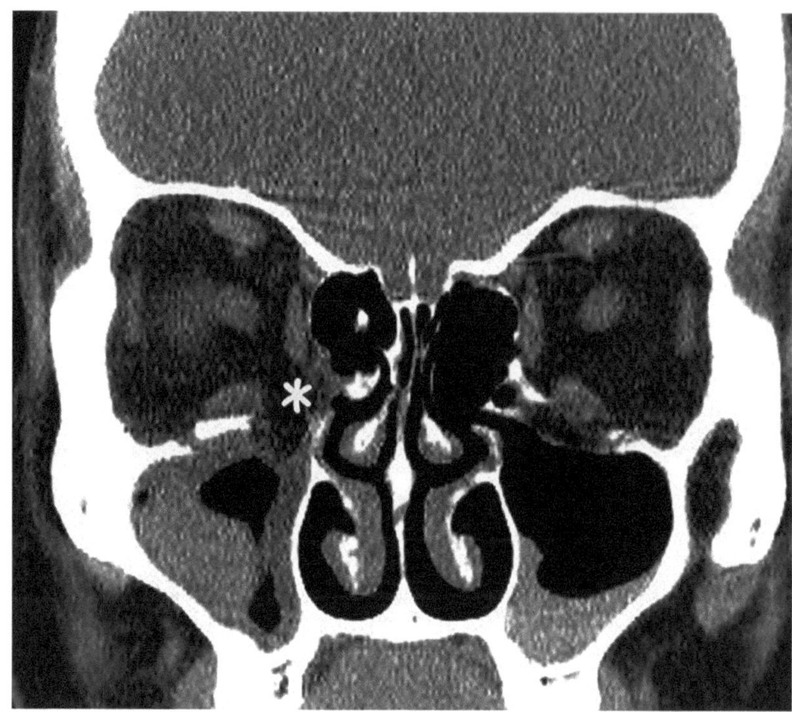

Fig. 11.8 Right sinus congestion developed following bilateral orbital floor and medial wall decompressions from disruption in the right maxillary sinus drainage (asterisk)

11.8 Conclusion

Orbital floor decompression yields gratifying and predictable results in reducing proptosis in inactive thyroid eye disease. Careful selection of patients, knowledge of the regional anatomy, and proper surgical maneuvres are critical for avoiding complications and yielding positive outcomes.

References

1. Kikkawa DO, Pornpanich K, Cruz RC Jr, Levi L, Granet DB. Graded orbital decompression based on severity of proptosis. Ophthalmology. 2002;109(7):1219–24.
2. Dolman PJ. Evaluating Graves orbitopathy. Best Pract Res Clin Endocrinol Metab. 2012;26(3):229–48.
3. Dutton JJ. Applied anatomy of the orbit and ocular adnexa. In: Fay, Dolman, editors. Diseases and disorders of the orbit and ocular adnexa. London: Elsevier; 2017.
4. Dolman PJ, Rootman J. VISA classification for Graves orbitopathy. Ophthal Plast Reconstr Surg. 2006;22:319–24.
5. Dolman PJ. Assessment and management plan for Graves' orbitopathy. In: Bahn RS, editor. Graves' disease: a comprehensive guide for clinicians. New York: Springer; 2015.
6. Ben Simon GJ, Schwarcz RM, Mansury AM, Wang L, McCann JD, Goldberg RA. Minimally invasive orbital decompression: local anesthesia and hand-carved bone. Arch Ophthalmol. 2005;123(12):1671–5.
7. Ing E, Douketis J. New oral anticoagulants and oculoplastic surgery. Can J Ophthalmol. 2014;49(2):123–7. Review
8. Shepard KG, Levin PS, Terris DJ. Balanced orbital decompression for Graves' ophthalmopathy. Laryngoscope. 1998;108(11):1648–53.
9. Dolman PJ. Orbital decompression and its effect on strabismus. Presentation at Oculoplastics SUBDAY. Chicago: American Academy of Ophthalmology Fall Meeting; 2014.
10. Sagiv O, Satchi K, Kinori M, et al. Comparison of lateral orbital wall decompression with and without rim repositioning in thyroid eye disease. Graefes Arch Clin Exp Ophthalmol. 2016;254(4):791–6.
11. Adenis JP, Robert PY, Lasudry JG, Dalloul Z. Treatment of proptosis with fat removal orbital decompression in Graves' ophthalmopathy. Eur J Ophthalmol. 1998;8(4):246–52.
12. Norris JH, Ross JJ, O'Reilly P, Malhotra R. A review of combined orbital decompression and lower eyelid recession surgery for lower eyelid retraction in thyroid orbitopathy. Br J Ophthalmol. 2011;95(12):1664–9.
13. Davies MJ, Dolman PJ. Levator muscle enlargement in thyroid eye disease-related upper eyelid retraction. Ophthalmic Plast Reconstr Surg. 2017;33(1):35–9.

14. Fayers T, Barker LE, Verity DH, et al. Oscillopsia after lateral wall orbital decompression. Ophthalmology. 2013;120(9):1920–3.
15. Goldberg RA, Perry JD, Hortaleza V, Tong JT. Strabismus after balanced medial plus lateral wall versus lateral wall only orbital decompression for dysthyroid orbitopathy. Ophthal Plast Reconstr Surg. 2000;16(4):271–7.
16. Serafino M, Fogagnolo P, Trivedi RH, et al. Torsional diplopia after orbital decompression and strabismus surgery. Eur J Ophthalmol. 2010;20(2):437–41.
17. Antisdel JL, Gumber D, Holmes J, Sindwani R. Management of sinonasal complications after endoscopic orbital decompression for Graves' orbitopathy. Laryngoscope. 2013;123(9):2094–8.

Medial Wall Decompression for Thyroid Eye Disease

12

Suryasnata Rath

12.1 Introduction

The medial wall is often preferred for decompressing the orbit in thyroid eye disease (TED) because of the ease of access and short duration of surgery. Decompression of the medial wall is typically performed as an adjunct to the lateral bony wall decompression (balanced orbital decompression), or as a part of 3-wall decompression for severe TED.

S. Rath (✉)
Ophthalmic Plastic and Reconstructive Surgery Service, Director and Taraprasad Das Chair of Ophthalmology, Mithu Tulsi Chanrai Campus, LV Prasad Eye Institute, Bhubaneswar, India
e-mail: suryasnata@lvpei.org

S. Rath, M. N. Naik (eds.), *Surgery in Thyroid Eye Disease*,
https://doi.org/10.1007/978-981-32-9220-8_12

12.2 Anatomy

The medial wall of the orbit is formed by four skull bones—maxillary, lacrimal, ethmoid, and sphenoid. The medial walls of both the orbits are arranged parallel to each other and to the mid-sagittal plane. The orbital anatomy is covered in detail in Chap. 2. However, elements of the orbital anatomy relevant to medial orbital decompression are reiterated below.

The *Lamina papyracea* forms most of the lateral wall of the ethmoid labyrinth. It is thin and fragile, making it vulnerable to fractures and an easy option for medial decompression.

Fronto-ethmoid suture marks the roof of the ethmoid labyrinth and floor of anterior cranial fossa. In most individuals, the cribriform plate lies medial to the ethmoid labyrinth. However, sometimes the cribriform plate may extend below the fronto-ethmoid suture line thus increasing the risk of a breach and CSF leak.

Anterior (Fig. 12.1; white arrow) and posterior *ethmoid foramina* (Fig. 12.1; yellow arrow) typically lie within the fronto-ethmoid suture line and transmit neurovascular bundles. In a small minority (10–20%), they may lie above or below the suture. Anterior and posterior ethmoid foramina lie within a range of 20–25 mm and 25–41 mm from the anterior lacrimal crest, respectively, and about 4–15 mm from the optic canal. Body of sphenoid bone (Fig. 12.1; red arrow) is posterior-most part of the medial wall.

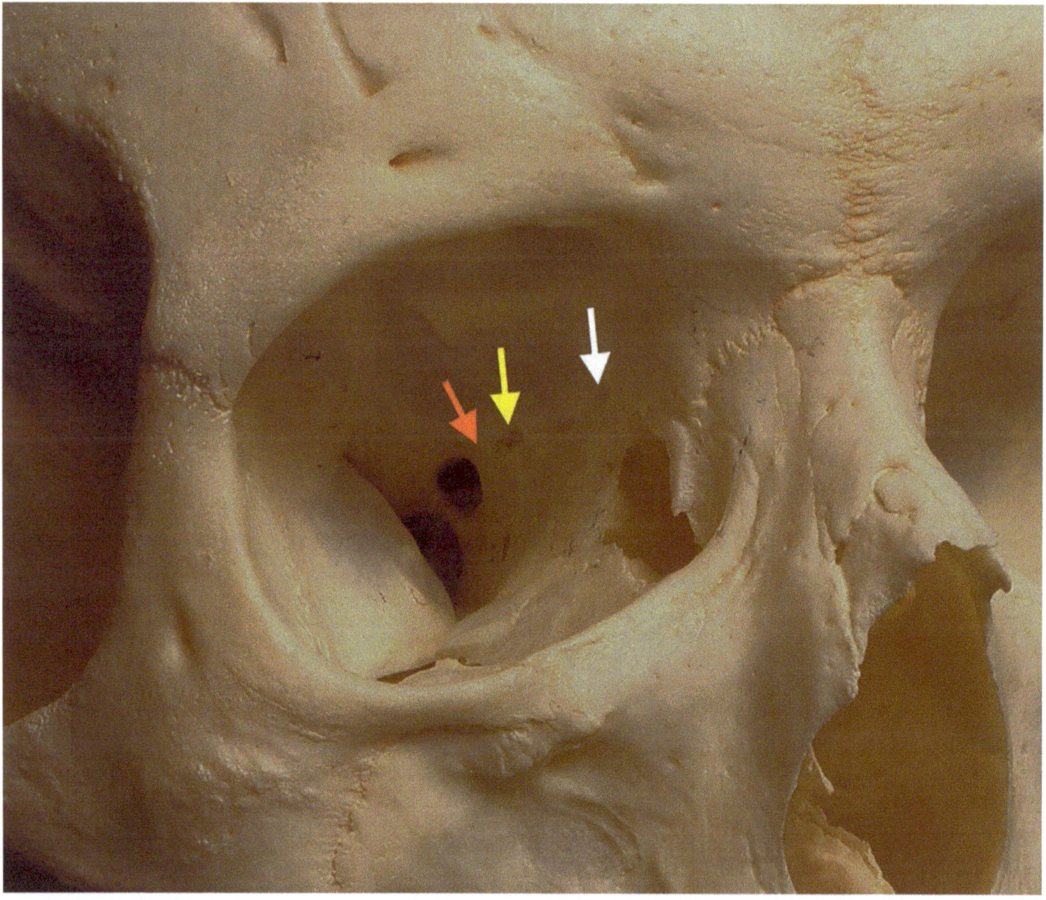

Fig. 12.1 Photograph showing the medial wall of the skull. The anterior (white arrow) and posterior (yellow arrow) ethmoidal foramina transmit the corresponding neurovascular bundles and lie on the fronto-ethmoid suture line. The optic canal is bounded by the body of sphenoid medially (red arrow) lesser wing of sphenoid superiorly and the optic strut inferolaterally

12.3 Indications

In the active phase, with optic nerve compromise, the medial wall offers a unique opportunity to decompress the apical orbit as described in Chap. 7 [1]. In the inactive phase, the medial orbital wall is rarely decompressed in isolation. Most often, the medial wall decompression is combined with other walls. When combined with floor, it achieves an inferomedial decompression, and when combined with the lateral wall, a balanced decompression [1]. Indications for medial orbital decompression are outlined in (Fig. 12.2) [1].

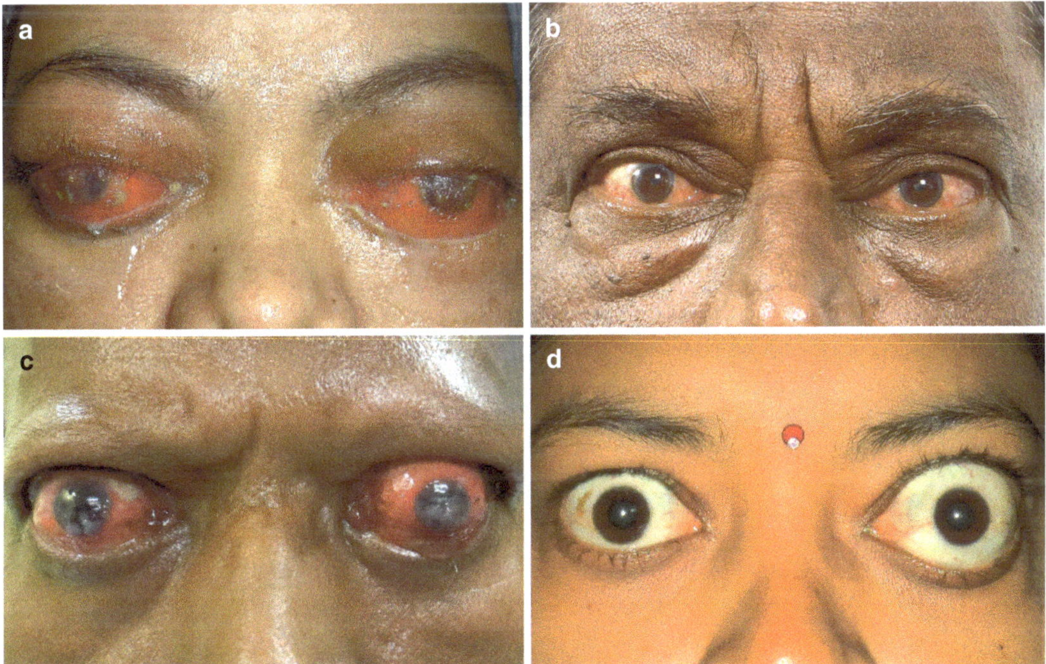

Fig. 12.2 Indications for medial wall decompression. (**a**) A 23-year-old lady presented with burnt-out TED showing long-standing exposure changes of the ocular surface. A 60-year-old man shown in (**b**) with coexisting diabetes mellitus presented with bilateral progressive TED with refractory dysthyroid optic neuropathy. Figure (**c**) shows a 50-year-old man who presented with active TED associated with Hansen's disease. The severity of exposure marked by the corneal breakdown in both eyes was compounded by the neurotrophic keratopathy of Hansen's disease necessitating an urgent inferomedial decompression with full-thickness skin grafts for the eyelids to salvage the eye and vision. Figure (**d**) shows a 35-year-old lady with inactive TED who needed a rehabilitative orbital decompression

12.4 Incision

Various approaches (and incisions) to medial orbital decompression (transorbital, transantral, and endonasal) are covered in Chap. 9 [1]. While preference of these approaches depends upon the training and background of the operating surgeon, we shall restrict to the transorbital approaches in this chapter. A medial orbital decompression is usually done through a Lynch, coronal, and transcaruncular incision (Fig. 12.3) [1]. When the medial wall and floor are decompressed together, the incision preferred is the swinging eyelid incision and/or transconjunctival approach.

The caruncle is split, and the incision is extended above and below for 4–6 clock hours in the conjunctival fornix (Fig. 12.4a). The plane of dissection lies between the Horners muscle overlying the posterior lacrimal crest, and the medial rectus (with extraconal fat) to expose the posterior lacrimal crest just behind the lacrimal sac (Fig. 12.4b).

12.5 Exposure of the Medial Orbital Wall

Exposure of the medial wall of the orbit is facilitated by blunt dissection using a blunt-tipped Steven's scissor over the posterior lacrimal crest (Fig. 12.5). The periorbital incision is placed beyond the posterior lacrimal crest and extends for 4–5 clock hours (Fig. 12.6a), for a good exposure of bony anatomy. Dissection is then carried along the subperiosteal space to expose the length of the bony medial wall (Fig. 12.6b, c) taking care not to breach the periosteum during the surgery and avoid fat prolapse. The anterior and posterior ethmoid vessels are identified and may be cauterized (Fig. 12.6d, e).

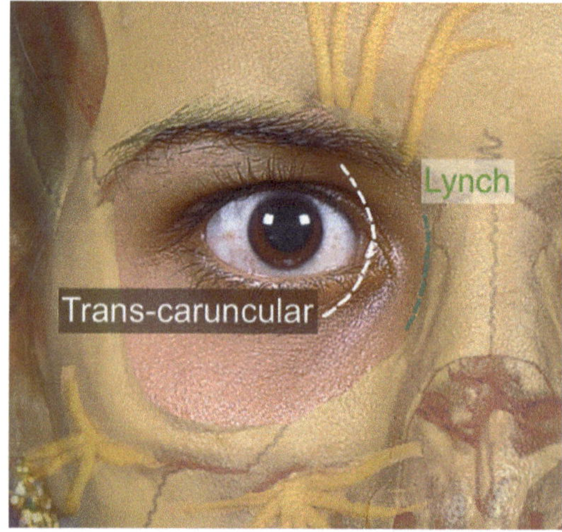

Fig. 12.3 Schematic representation of incisions to reach the medial wall. Transcaruncular incision is the most popular as compared to the transcutaneous Lynch incision

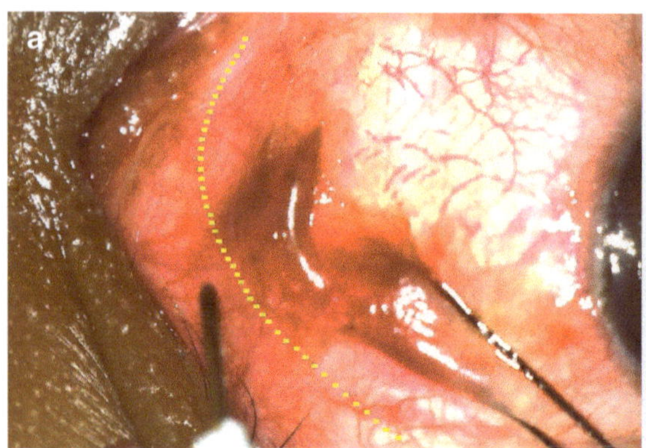

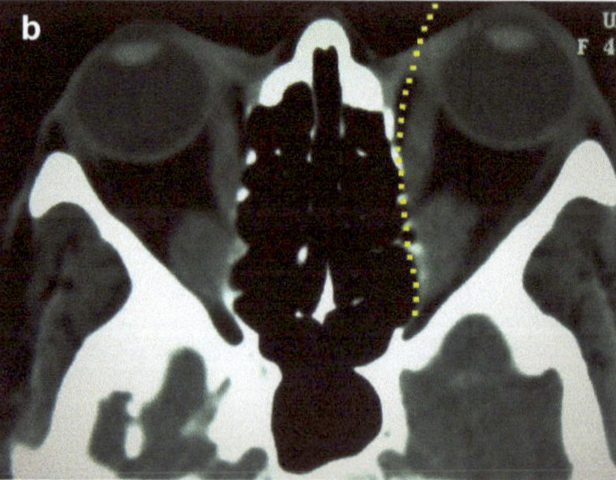

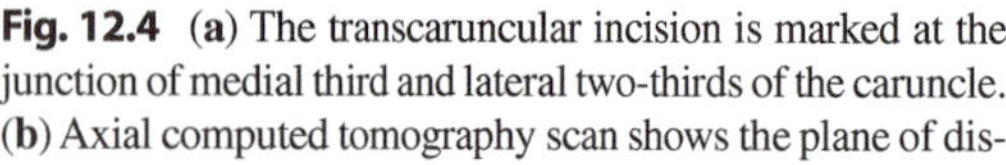

Fig. 12.4 (**a**) The transcaruncular incision is marked at the junction of medial third and lateral two-thirds of the caruncle. (**b**) Axial computed tomography scan shows the plane of dissection between Horner's muscle and medial rectus muscle to expose the medial orbital wall beyond the posterior lacrimal crest. This avoids damage to the lacrimal apparatus

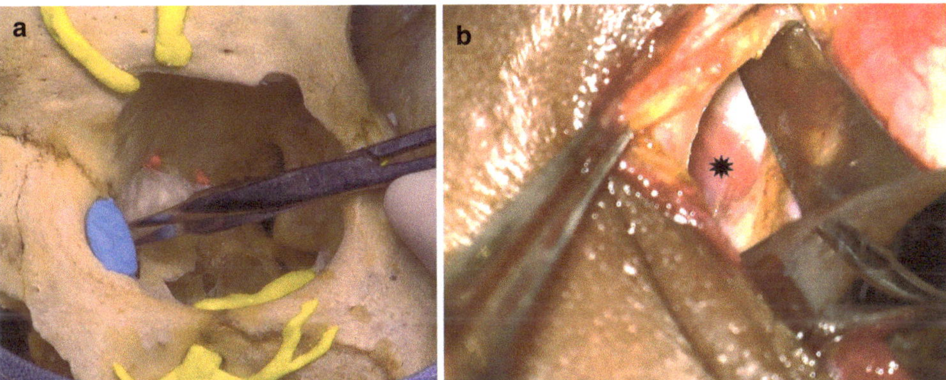

Fig. 12.5 Steven's scissor with its curve pointing posteriorly beyond the posterior lacrimal crest is used for blunt dissection. Figure 12.5a demonstrates the approach with Steven's scissor behind the lacrimal sac. The fronto-ethmoid suture with the foramina of anterior and posterior ethmoid neurovascular bundles (red dots) are also seen. Figure 12.5b shows the medial rectus muscle (black star) behind Steven's scissor

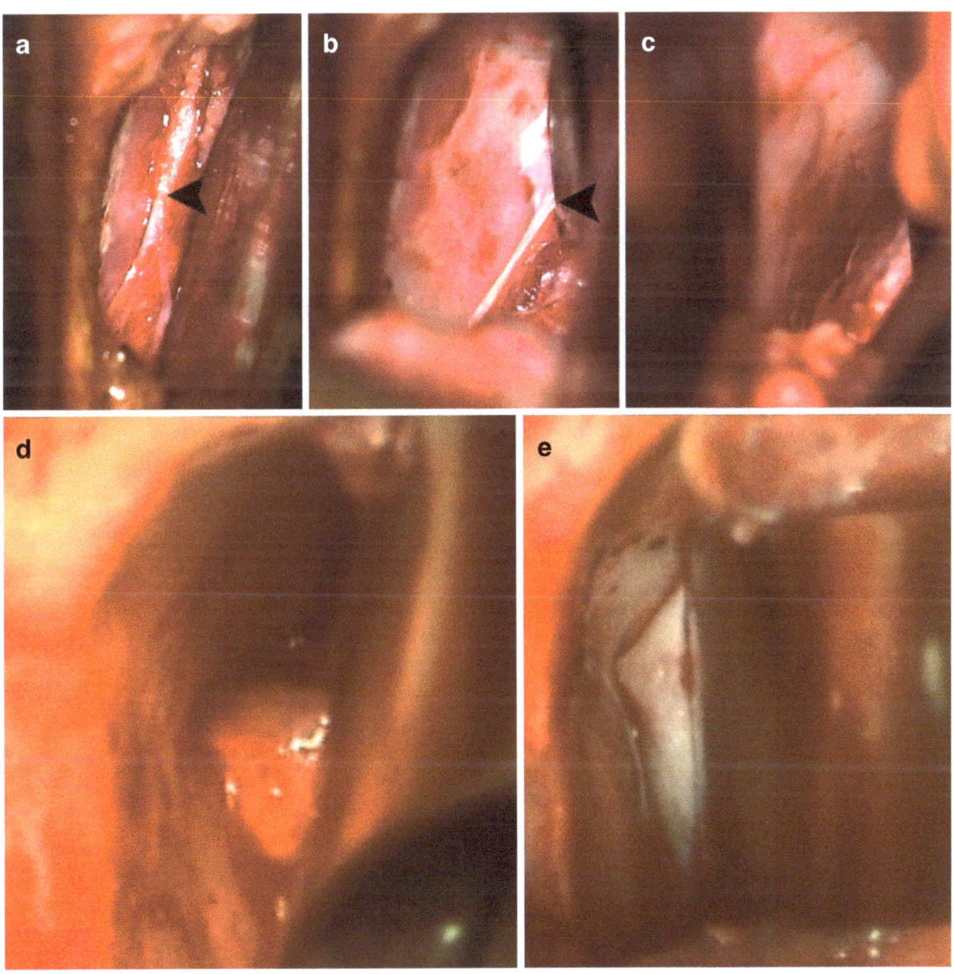

Fig. 12.6 (**a**) Clinical photograph showing the edge of the periorbita (black arrowhead) after incision. The periorbita is carefully dissected with the blunt end of the periosteal elevator to progressively expose the thin medial bony wall of the orbit (**b**, **c**). Care is taken to keep the periorbita intact to avoid premature prolapse of orbital fat making exposure of the deep orbit difficult. The anterior ethmoidal (**d**) and posterior ethmoidal (**e**) vessels are encountered along the fronto-ethmoid suture and can be carefully avoided or cauterized

12.6 Bony Decompression

The bony decompression is usually commenced with a Freer elevator, and can be completed with a bone rongeur or with the suction tip. The lamina papyracea (Fig. 12.7a) is removed from the sphenoid–ethmoid junction posteriorly to fall short of the posterior lacrimal crest anteriorly, and from the fronto-ethmoid suture superiorly to the maxilloethmoidal strut inferiorly. The exposed ethmoid air cells can be seen (Fig. 12.7b) Anterior and posterior bony landmarks to be respected include the posterior lacrimal crest (Fig. 12.8a) and anterior wall of sphenoid sinus respectively. Skeletonized ethmoidal air cells (Fig. 12.8b) are seen posteriorly.

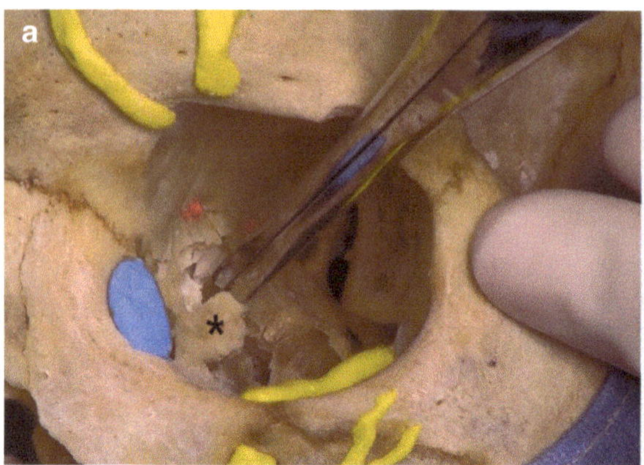

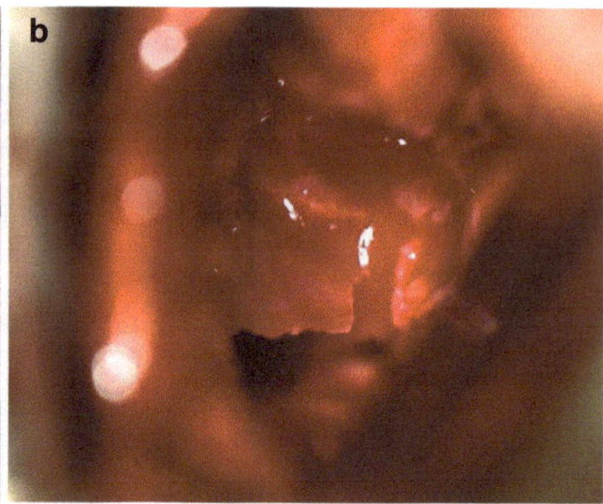

Fig. 12.7 (**a**) Bony decompression of the medial wall is achieved by removal of the lamina papyracea black asterisk to expose the anterior and posterior ethmoidal air cells. The fronto-ethmoid suture line (red dots) defines the superior limit of the bony decompression. The junction of the medial wall and the floor marks the inferior extent of decompression. Removal of the orbital process of the palatine bone joins decompression of the floor with medial wall and is especially useful in relieving dysthyroid optic neuropathy. (**b**) Ethmoid air cells are exposed which need to be removed with their lining mucosa

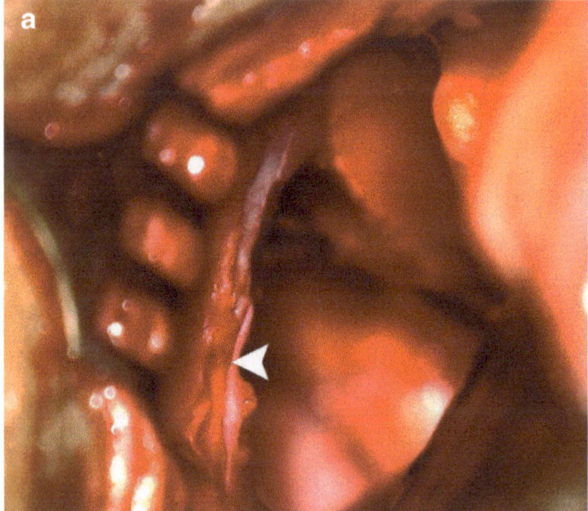

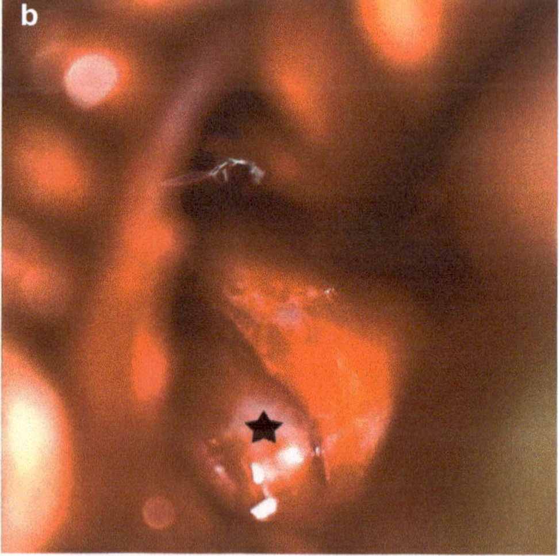

Fig. 12.8 (**a**) Medial wall bony decompression can maximally extend anteriorly to spare the posterior lacrimal crest (white arrowhead) to avoid damage to the lacrimal apparatus. (**b**) Skeletonized ethmoid air cells (black star) are seen posteriorly. The anterior wall of the sphenoid sinus marks the posterior extent of the bony decompression

12.7 Management of the Periorbita

The periorbita is released in a linear fashion, longitudinally above and below the medial rectus muscle to allow effective fat prolapse (Fig. 12.9a). Following bony decompression and release of the periorbita, the extraconal and intraconal fat from around the medial rectus muscle can be debulked. Coronal sections on CT scan done after an optimal medical decompression shows prolapse of the orbital structures (Fig. 12.9b) in the mid orbit.

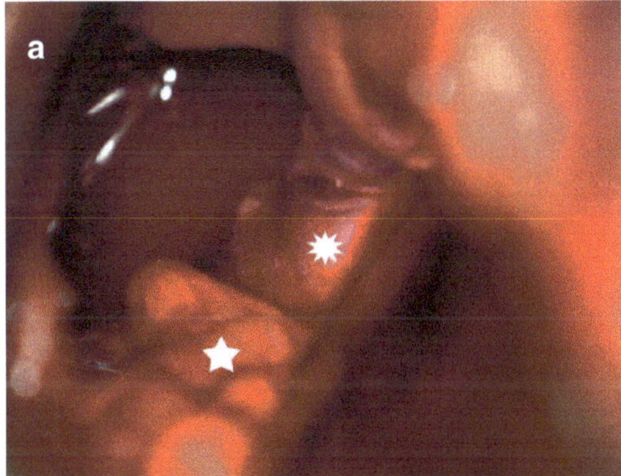

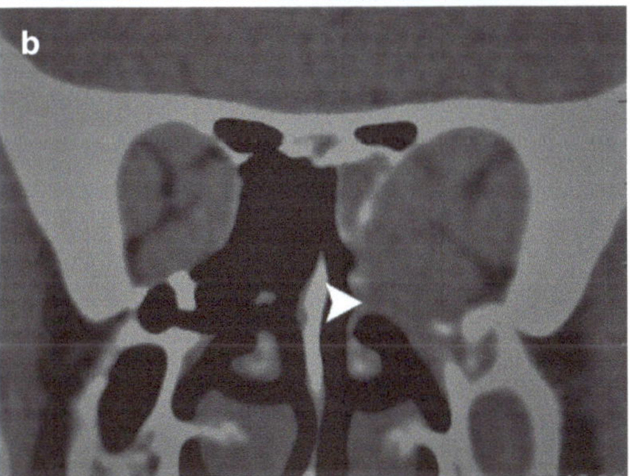

Fig. 12.9 (**a**) Effective decompression of the orbit can be achieved by opening the periorbital lining. Intact periorbita (white 10-point star) prevents the prolapse of orbital structures while adjacent area shows prolapse of orbital fat (white 5-point star) after the periorbita has been opened. Periorbita may be opened in a linear or cross-hatched pattern. (**b**) Coronal section in CT scan of orbit shows the decompressed medial wall and floor (white arrowhead) in contrast to the contralateral orbit

12.8 Outcomes

For dysthyroid optic neuropathy, good apical decompression can be achieved (Fig. 12.10). In the inactive phase, medial wall decompression whether balanced or un-balanced gives good outcome (Figs. 12.11a, b and 12.12a–d). Meta-analyses data of combined inferomedial decompression show reduction of proptosis to range between 4 and 5 mm with a transorbital or trans-antral approach [2, 3]. This may be augmented by adding fat decompression. Endoscopic medial wall decompressions tend to achieve about 3.5 mm of proptosis reduction [3].

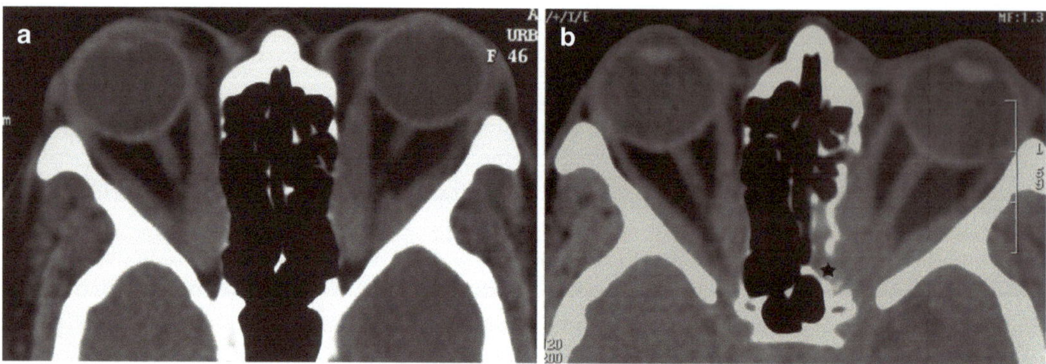

Fig. 12.10 Axial section of CT scan of orbit in a 46-year-old lady with TED and dysthyroid optic neuropathy of the left side before (**a**) and after surgery (**b**) clearly shows the decompression of the medial wall extending to the anterior wall of the sphenoid sinus (black 5-point star)

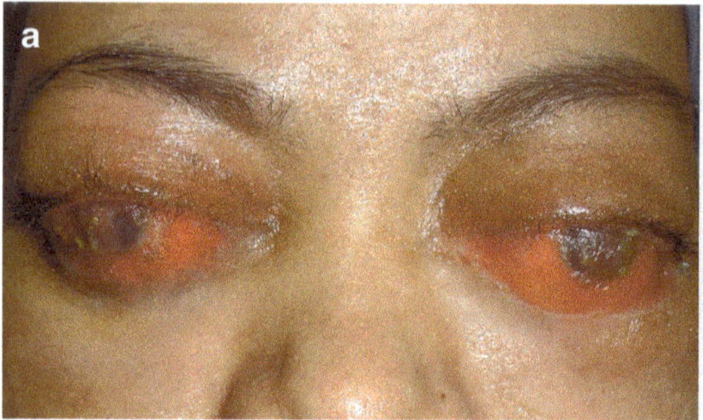

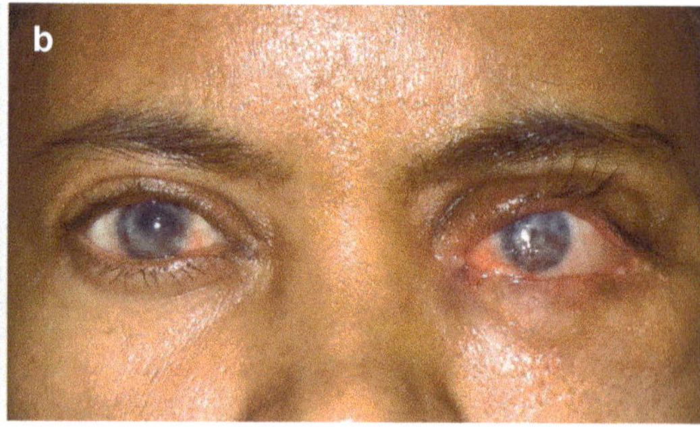

Fig. 12.11 (**a**) A 23-year-old lady presented with long-standing exposure changes of the ocular surface including the cornea. The marked ocular surface exposure in both eyes was predominantly a result of passive congestion with the thyroid eye disease having burnt-out over time. (**b**) The same lady after bilateral 2 wall-inferomedial decompression followed by eyelid surgery and right penetrating keratoplasty. Her best-corrected visual acuity in the right eye measured 20/50

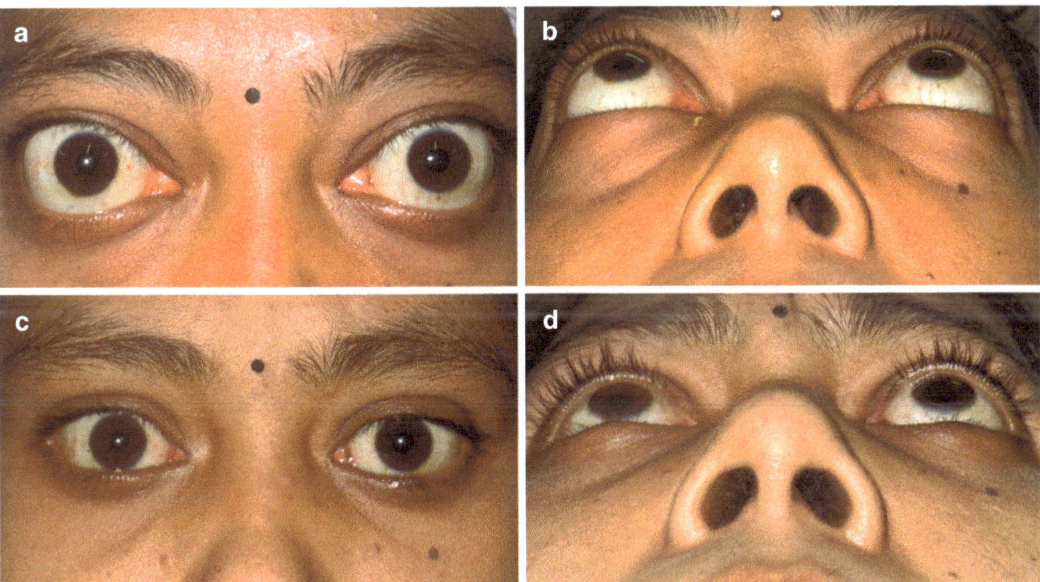

Fig. 12.12 (**a**–**b**) Preoperative clinical photographs of a 26-year-old lady who presented with inactive TED, VISA type A. (**c**–**d**) The same lady after simultaneous single-stage bilateral 2 wall-inferomedial decompression. Eyelid surgery to correct retraction was done later

12.9 Complications

Transorbital inferomedial decompressions result in new-onset and worsening diplopia in the range 10–35% [2–4]. Leaving part or all of the inferomedial strut intact is reported to reduce the globe dystopia and diplopia after decompression (Fig. 12.13) [5, 6]. Other complications though rare include sensory hypoesthesia, sinusitis, and cerebrospinal fluid leak [7].

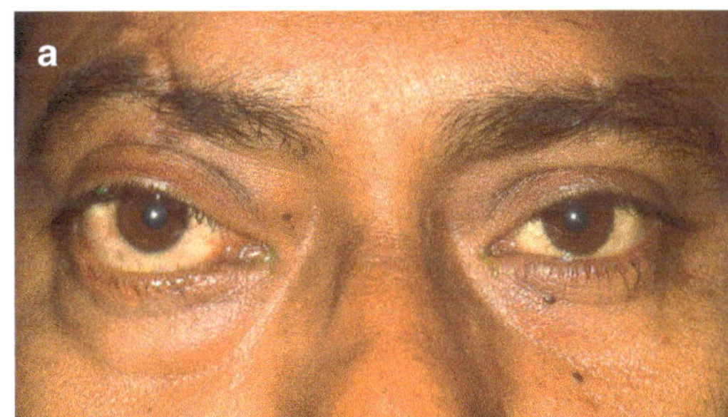

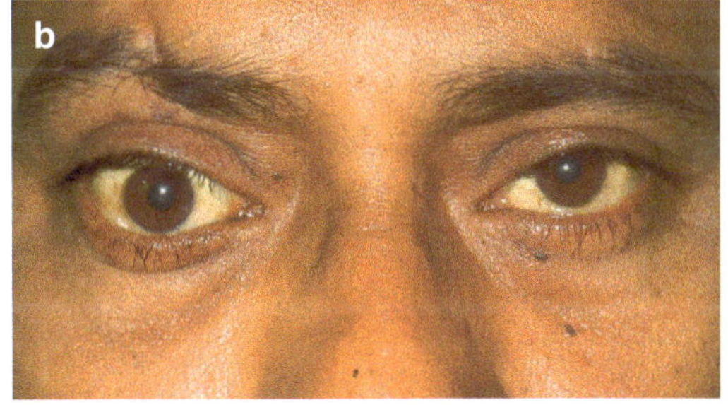

Fig. 12.13 Clinical photographs showing a 45-year-old male with TED and proptosis in his right eye. He was orthotropic before (**a**) and developed right hypotropia after inferomedial orbital decompression (**b**) of the right side. He was rehabilitated by prisms

12.10 Conclusion

Transorbital approaches to medial orbital decompression provide optimum exposure of the medial wall and give good outcomes. The medial wall is preferred when decompression is needed for refractory dysthyroid optic neuropathy. In orbital decompression for moderate and severe inactive disease, the medial wall is usually combined with floor and/or lateral wall in a 2–3 wall bony decompression.

References

1. Rootman DB. Orbital decompression for thyroid eye disease. Surv Ophthalmol. 2018;63:86–104.
2. Borumandi F, Hammer B, Kamer L, von Arx G. How predictable is exophthalmos reduction in graves' orbitopathy? A review of the literature. Br J Ophthalmol. 2011;95:1625–30.
3. Leong SC, Karkos PD, Macewen CJ, White PS. A systematic review of outcomes following surgical decompression for dysthyroid orbitopathy. Laryngoscope. 2009;119(6):1106–15.
4. Paridaens D, Lie A, Grootendorst RJ, van den Bosch WA. Efficacy and side effects of 'swinging eyelid' orbital decompression in Graves' orbitopathy: a proposal for standardized evaluation of diplopia. Eye (Lond). 2006;20:154–62.
5. Goldberg RA, Shorr N, Cohen MS. The medial orbital strut in the prevention of post decompression dystopia in dysthyroid ophthalmopathy. Ophthalmic Plast Reconstr Surg. 1992;8(1):32–4.
6. Wright ED, Davidson J, Codere F, Desrosiers M. Endoscopic orbital decompression with preservation of an inferomedial bony strut: minimization of postoperative diplopia. J Otolaryngol. 1999;28(5):252–6.
7. Woo KI, Kim YD. Isolated caruncular approach for orbital decompression. Jpn J Ophthalmol. 2004;48(4):397–403.

13 Transantral Orbital Decompression

Michael Burnstine and Mica Y. Bergman

13.1 Introduction

When thyroid-associated ophthalmopathy results in vision-threatening compressive optic neuropathy, orbital ache, or significant aesthetic deformity, orbital decompression may be indicated. Several operative techniques exist, and the choice of which to employ is a function of the patient's orbital disease, the patient's systemic condition, and the surgeon's preference.

Transantral orbital decompression offers several advantages over other techniques, including decreased procedure time, providing more posterior orbital decompression, and avoiding an orbital approach in active orbits [1–4]. Additionally, the procedure often results in greater improvement of eyelid retraction and scleral show than do the other choices. The possible drawbacks of this technique include dysesthesia in the V2 distribution and worsening strabismus. In this chapter, we provide a detailed guide for performing transantral orbital decompression, paying particular attention to relevant anatomy and surgical pearls to avoid potential pitfalls.

M. Burnstine (✉)
Ophthalmology, USC Roski Eye Institute,
Keck medicine of USC, Eyesthetica Oculofacial and Cosmetic Surgery Associates, Los Angeles, CA, USA
e-mail: burnstin@usc.edu

M. Y. Bergman
Ophthalmology, Sansum Clinic, Santa Barbara, USA
e-mail: mbergman@sansvmclinic.org

S. Rath, M. N. Naik (eds.), *Surgery in Thyroid Eye Disease*,
https://doi.org/10.1007/978-981-32-9220-8_13

13.2 Instrumentation

The instrumentation used in transantral orbital decompression procedure is depicted in Fig. 13.1. Proper instrumentation will aid in the safety, ease, and success of this operation.

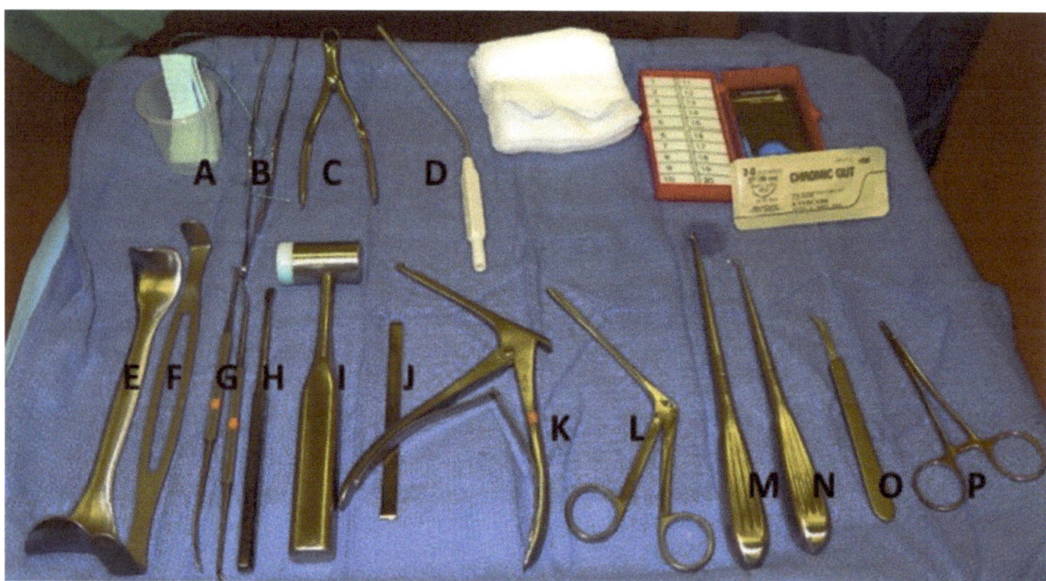

Fig. 13.1 Instrumentation for transantral orbital decompression. Preoperative packing of the naris with cottonoids soaked in 4% cocaine (**a**) is accomplished using the nasal speculum (**b**) and bayonet forceps (**c**). Frazier suction tip (**d**) is critical for visualization throughout the procedure. Retractors to retract the upper lip are Goelet (**e**) and Army-Navy (**f**). Freer elevators (**g**) are used to initiate the reflection of mucoperiosteum in the mouth at the start of the procedure, and later in the procedure to infracture the medial orbital wall. Key elevator (**h**) is used to complete the reflection of mucoperiosteum off the anterior wall of the maxillary sinus to the inferior aspect of the infraorbital nerve. Mallet (**i**) and osteotome (**j**) are used to create the antrostomy. Kerrison rongeur (**k**) is used to expand the antrostomy. Takahashi forceps (**l**) are used to remove ethmoid sinus mucosa. Curettes (**m**, **n**) are used to remove maxillary sinus mucosa. Sichel (#12) blade (**o**) is used to incise the periosteum of the orbital floor and medial wall (if needed) to prolapse orbital contents. Curved hemostat (**p**) is used to assist with maxillary sinus mucosa removal and placement of packing between the maxillary sinus and the nose at the conclusion of the procedure (*Not pictured is the nasal antral rasp, used to make an opening between the nasal cavity and the maxillary sinus it is pictured in Fig. 13.8a*)

13.3 Anesthesia

This operation is typically done under general anesthesia with local infiltrative anesthesia. Prior to the procedure, the buccogingival mucosa is infiltrated with local anesthetic. Given that the operation is performed through an incision in this tissue, adequate hemostasis with local anesthesia containing epinephrine for its vasoconstrictive properties is crucial. The addition of hyaluronidase (7.5 U/cc) will promote distribution of the anesthetic agent. Lidocaine alone is typically sufficiently long-acting, though many surgeons will choose to employ a 1:1 mixture of lidocaine and bupivacaine (Fig. 13.2a). Approximately 5 cc of local anesthetic agent per side is sufficient. Infiltration of the buccogingival mucosa with local anesthetic is by two to three deep injections into the fornix of the upper lip (Fig. 13.2b). Care should be taken to avoid injecting the centrally located frenulum.

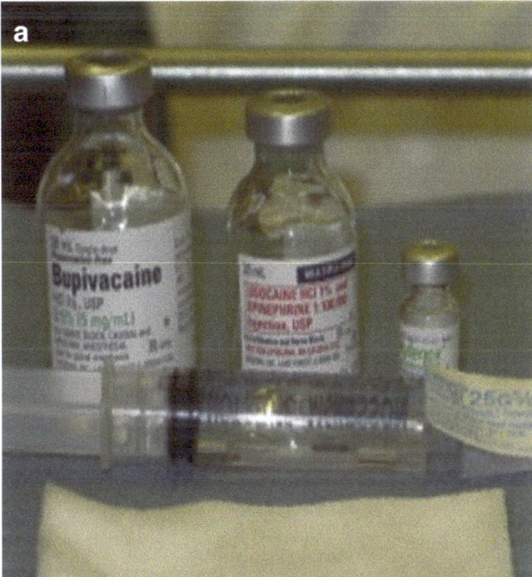

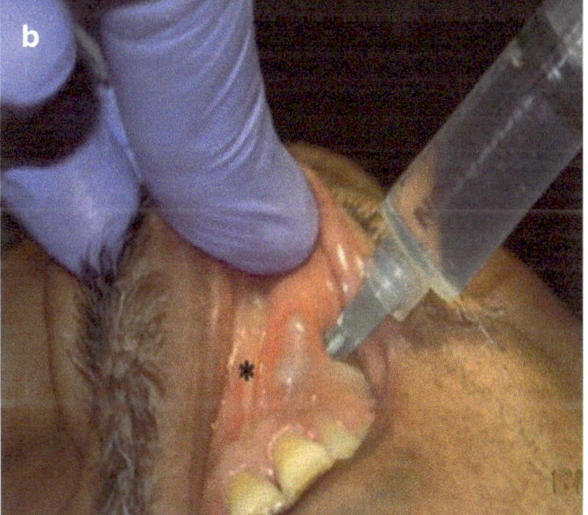

Fig. 13.2 Local anesthesia used in transantral orbital decompression procedure. (**a**) Components of anesthetic solution. (**b**) Injection of local anesthetic into the buccogingival mucosa. The asterisk marks the frenulum, which should be avoided

13.4 Preoperative Steps

Prior to beginning the operation, the nares are packed with cocaine-soaked cottonoids, and proptosis is quantified. Using a nasal speculum for visualization, bayonet forceps are used to pack the nose with cottonoids soaked in 4% cocaine (Fig. 13.3a) to promote mucosal vasoconstriction and reduce bleeding during the operation. The cottonoids should be placed along the lateral nasal wall. Two cottonoids per side are usually sufficient. If cocaine is not available, oxymetazoline may be used.

It is critical to measure proptosis at the start of the operation. This will allow appropriate titration of the decompression intraoperatively, and a means of quantifying the reduction in proptosis at the conclusion of the operation. Measurement should be taken from the lateral orbital rim at the lateral canthus to the anterior central cornea (Fig. 13.3b).

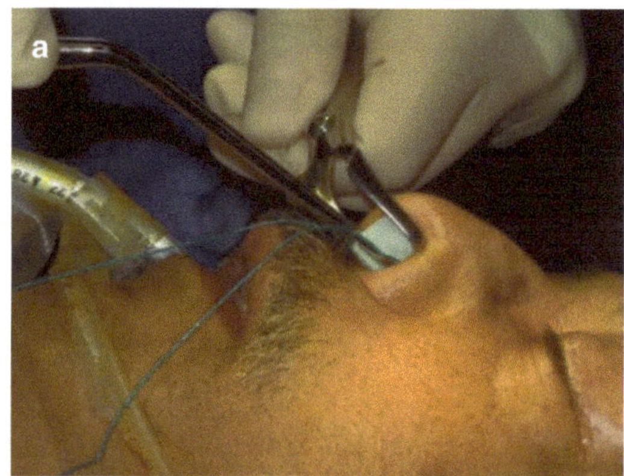

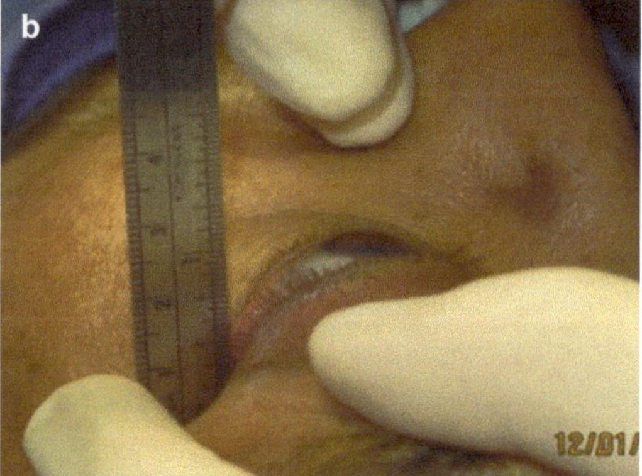

Fig. 13.3 Preoperative steps. (**a**) The nose is packed with cottonoids soaked in 4% cocaine. (**b**) Preoperative proptosis is measured

13.5 Buccogingival Sulcus Incision and Mucoperiosteal Reflection

Access to the maxillary sinus is achieved by incision into the buccogingival sulcus followed by upward reflection of the mucoperiosteum to expose the anterior wall of the maxillary sinus (Fig. 13.4).

Care must be taken to avoid Stenson's duct, the exit point of the parotid gland, which enters the oral cavity at the parotid ampulla, next to the upper second molar. The mucoperiosteum is reflected upward using the Freer and then Key elevators. Initially, the Goelet retractor is used to hold the upper lip away from the surgical site (Fig. 13.4a). The Army-Navy retractor may then be used in its place for better visualization, holding both the superior cut edge of the mucosa and the lip (Fig. 13.4b). The Frazier suction tip is used both to clear blood and to assist in the distraction of tissue (Fig. 13.4c). It is important to identify the inferior aspect of the infraorbital nerve during dissection (Fig. 13.4d).

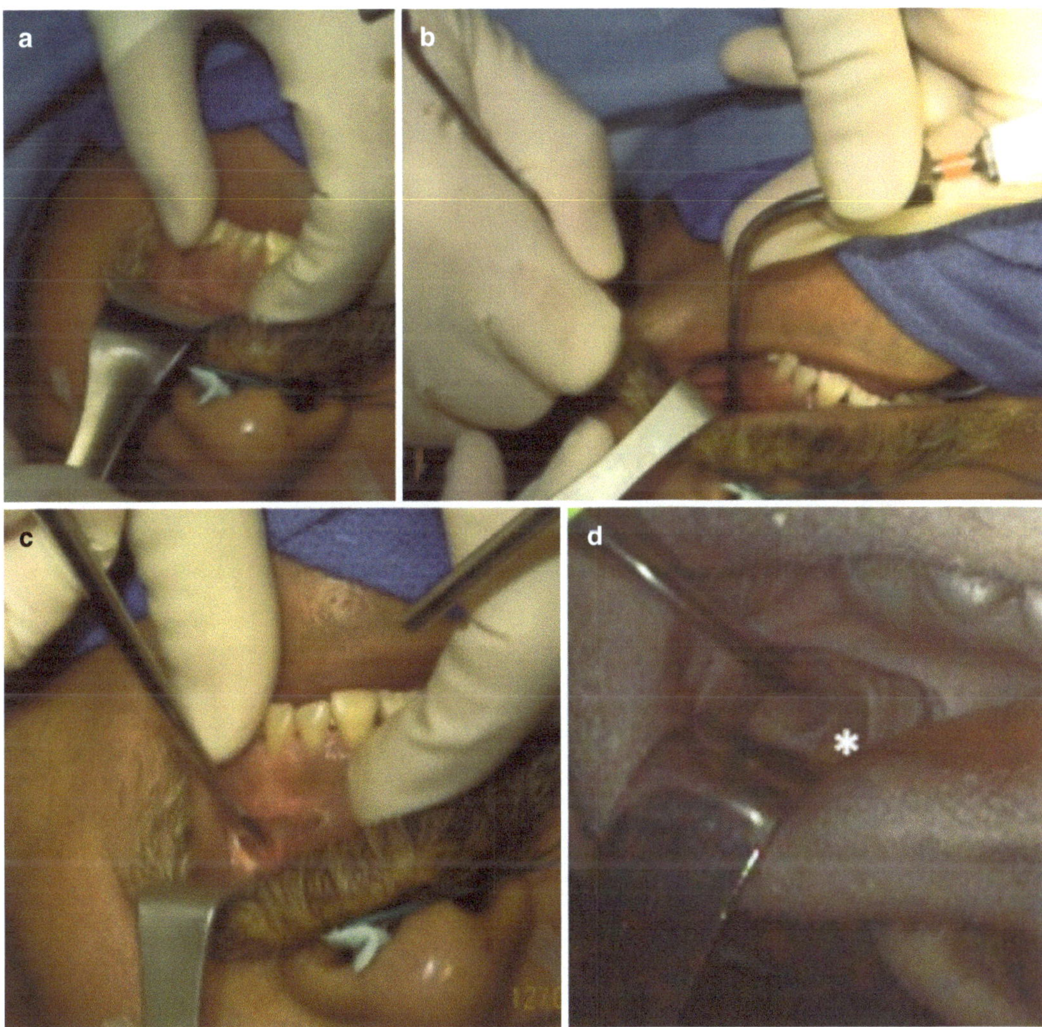

Fig. 13.4 Buccogingival sulcus incision and mucoperiosteal reflection. (**a**) Goelet retractor retracts upper lip to show completed buccogingival sulcus incision. (**b**) With Army-Navy retractor in place, Freer elevator is used to initiate periosteal reflection. (**c**) While elevating the periosteum, the Frazier suction tip may be used to clear blood and to distract tissue. (**d**) The Key elevator is used to complete the majority of the periosteal reflection. The infraorbital nerve (marked with an asterisk) exits the maxillary bone about 5-mm below the orbital rim at the level of the medial limbus, and must be avoided

13.6 Antrostomy

Entrance to the maxillary sinus is achieved with Caldwell-Luc antrostomy, wherein a large opening is created in the sinus' anterior wall (Fig. 13.5). Using an osteotome and mallet, the osteotomy is created in the canine fossa (Fig. 13.5a), which is a shallow depression on the anterior wall of the maxillary sinus, just lateral to the ridge associated with the canine tooth (third from center). Care must be taken to avoid damage to the infraorbital nerve (Fig. 13.4d), which exits the maxillary bone about 5-mm below the inferior orbital rim. The osteotomy is expanded using a Kerrison rongeur (Fig. 13.5b, c), and the superior and nasal maxillary mucosa is peeled away with a curette and hemostat (Fig. 13.5d).

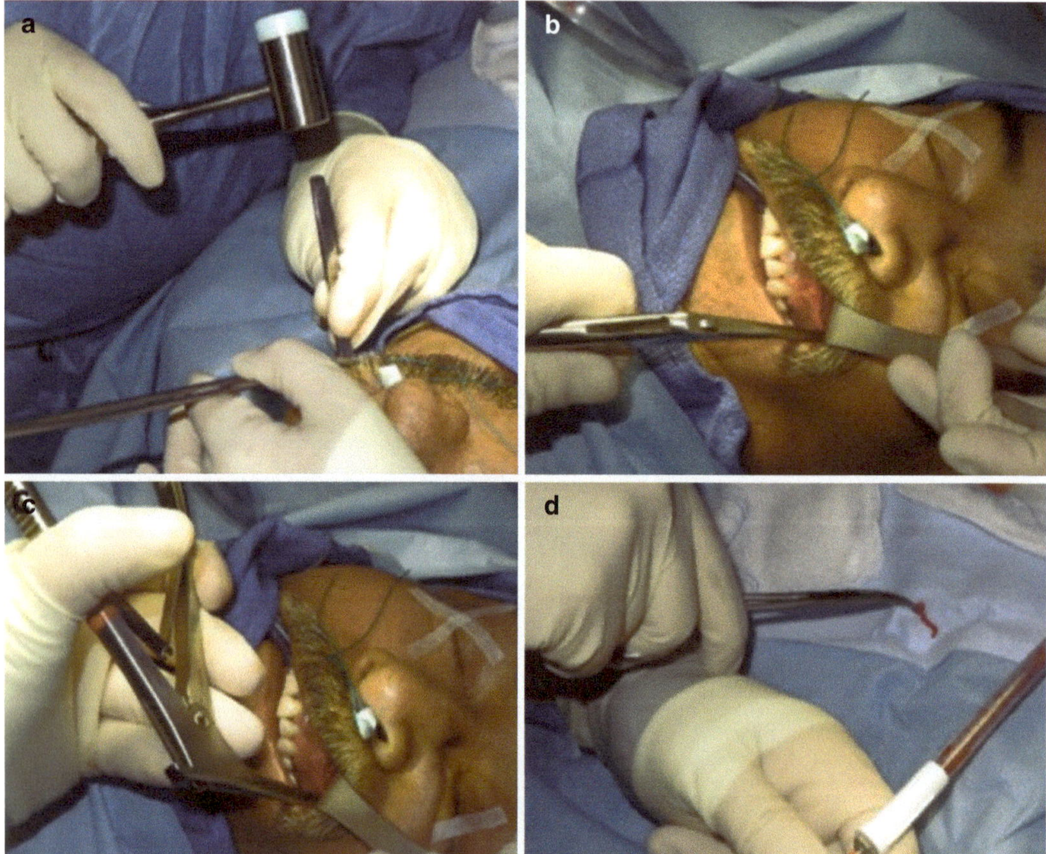

Fig. 13.5 Maxillary antrostomy. (**a**) An osteotome and mallet are used to create the osteotomy. (**b**) Kerrison rongeurs are used to expand the osteotomy. (**c**) The orientation of the Kerrison rongeurs is adjusted to facilitate bone removal. (**d**) Maxillary mucosa that has been stripped

13.7 Ethmoidectomy

Ethmoidectomy is required to gain access to the medial wall of the orbit (Fig. 13.6). This step is performed blindly, so an understanding of the anatomy is critical. The ethmoid air cells are positioned posterior to the nasolacrimal duct. Superiorly is the frontal bone, with the cribriform plate located superolaterally. They are bounded laterally by the medial orbit, inferiorly by the roof of the maxillary sinus, and medially by the lateral nasal wall. The ethmoid air cells are gently fractured using a Freer elevator or Frazier suction tip. The ethmoid air cells are then removed using Takahashi forceps (Fig. 13.6a). Although the procedure is not performed endoscopically, Fig. 13.6b, c demonstrate an endoscopic view of ethmoid air cell removal in a cadaver specimen. Removal of the ethmoid air cells will expose the medial orbital wall laterally, and the frontal bone superiorly.

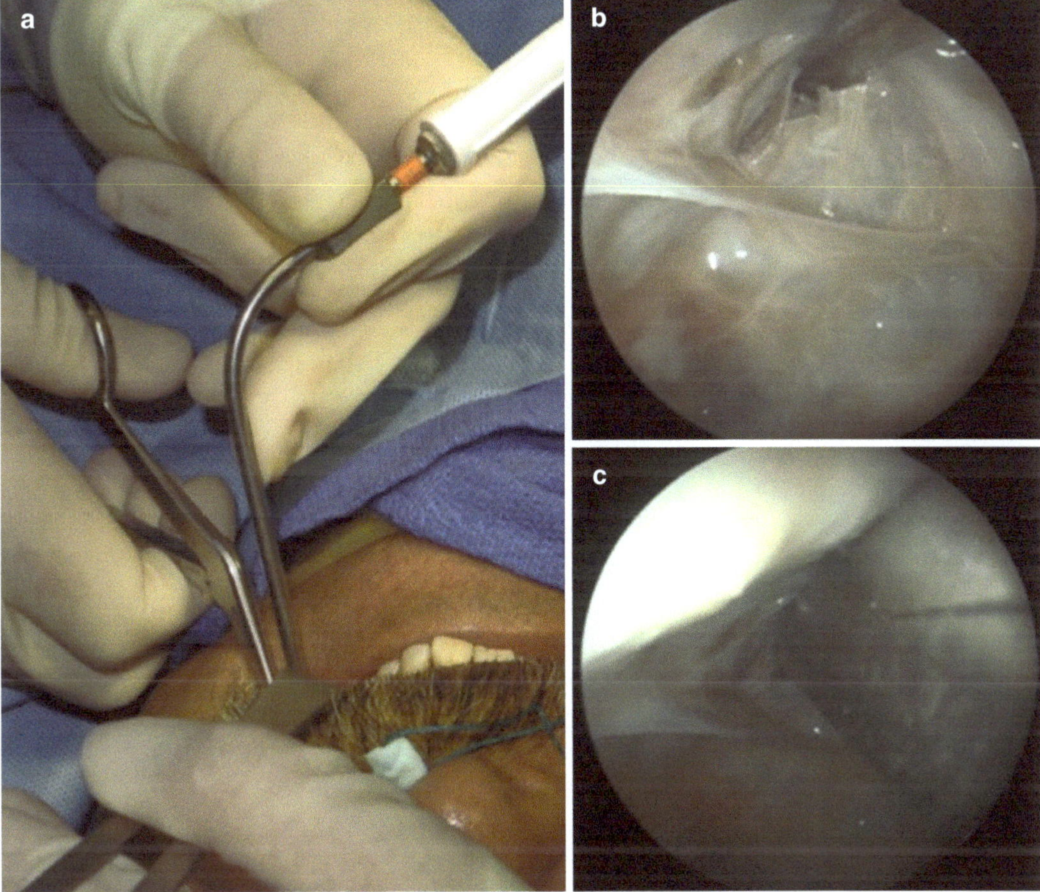

Fig. 13.6 Ethmoidectomy. (**a**) Takahashi forceps are used to remove the ethmoid air cells following their fracture with the Frazier suction tip. (**b**) Endoscopic view of ethmoid air cell removal in a cadaver specimen. (**c**) Magnified view of (**b**)

13.8 Removal of Floor and Medial Wall of Orbit

The orbital floor is fractured medial to the infraorbital bundle (visualized as a dark line running posterolateral to anteromedial along the orbital floor). The lateral portion of the floor may also be removed if decompression needs to be augmented. The floor is removed as far posteriorly as is necessary to achieve optimal decompression, reaching the posterior maxillary sinus as needed. The medial wall is infractured or removed with a Freer elevator depending on the extent of decompression required.

The periosteal incisions are initiated with a Sichel (#12) blade at the medial wall and floor windows (Fig. 13.7a, b). A hemostat or forceps is then used to grasp this periosteal reflection and release orbital fat. Manual pressure is applied gently to the globe to encourage fat prolapse into the maxillary sinus, thus decompressing the orbit (Fig. 13.7c, d—asterisk shows prolapsed orbital fat). The globe position is then checked. Fat decompression should be performed after the floor and medial wall removal.

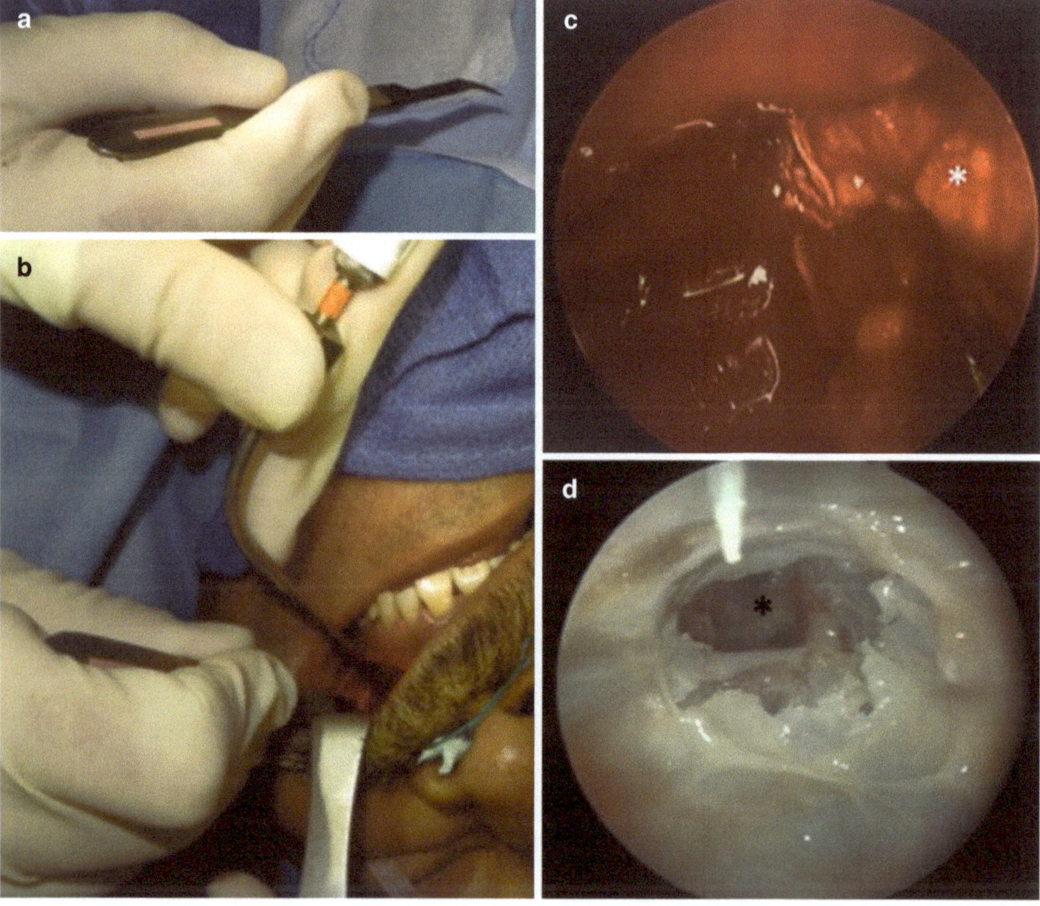

Fig. 13.7 Removal of the orbital floor and medial wall of the orbit and fatty decompression. (**a**) Sichel (#12 blade). (**b**) Sichel blade is used to incise periosteum on the orbital floor and medial wall windows, which allows fat prolapse. (**c**) Endoscopic view of fat (marked with an asterisk) prolapsing into the maxillary sinus. (**d**) In a cephalus specimen, endoscopic view of fat (marked with an asterisk) prolapsing into the maxillary sinus

13.9 Medial Antrostomy and Sinus Packing

At the conclusion of the decompression, an opening is created between the nasal cavity and the maxillary sinus by fracturing the lateral nasal wall/medial maxillary sinus wall. A nasal antral rasp (Fig. 13.8a) is used to create this antrostomy. The rasp is placed into the naris, and directed toward the maxillary sinus (Fig. 13.8b). It is then used to fracture the thin bone separating the nasal cavity from the maxillary sinus. This opening is located inferior to the middle turbinate. The maxillary sinus is then packed with bacitracin-soaked iodoform gauze, which is placed into the naris with a hemostat, and retrieved from the sinus with bayonet forceps (Fig. 13.8c). The packing is covered with a mustache dressing (Fig. 13.8d).

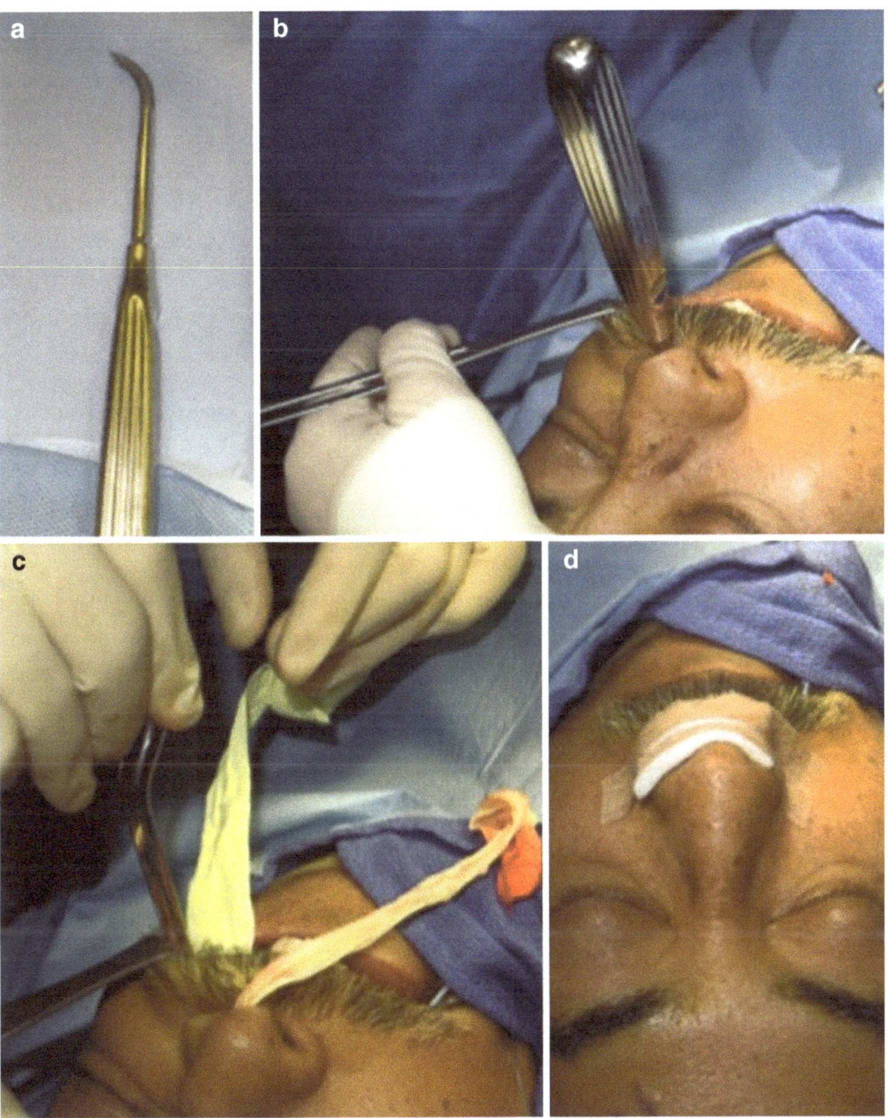

Fig. 13.8 Creation of medial antrostomy and sinus packing. (**a**) Nasal antral rasp used to create the antrostomy. (**b**) The rasp is inserted into the nare and directed laterally to create an opening in the medial wall of the maxillary sinus. (**c**) Iodoform gauze soaked in bacitracin is fed into the nare with a hemostat and retrieved from the maxillary sinus with a bayonet forceps. (**d**) A nasal mustache dressing secures the packing at the nares

13.10 Closing Wound

At the conclusion of the operation, the buccogingival incision is closed using a running 3-0 chromic gut suture (Fig. 13.9). Patients are not bothered by this suture in their mouth, though the ends should be cut short to minimize irritation.

13.11 Post-operative Care and Follow Up

Post-operative medications typically include:

1. Oral pain medication as needed
2. Oral antibiotic (Cephalexin or Ciprofloxacin) for 1 week
3. Methylprednisolone Oral (6-day course)
4. Viscous lidocaine to swish and spit four times a day for 1 week
5. Antibacterial mouthwash (e.g., Cepacol) to swish and spit four times a day for 1 week

On post-operative day zero, the patient should be seen prior to discharge to assess for optic nerve function (gross visual acuity and pupillary examination) and extraocular motility.

The patient is seen on post-operative day one for removal of the sinus packing from the nose. Assuming a routine course, the patient is seen again at post-operative week one.

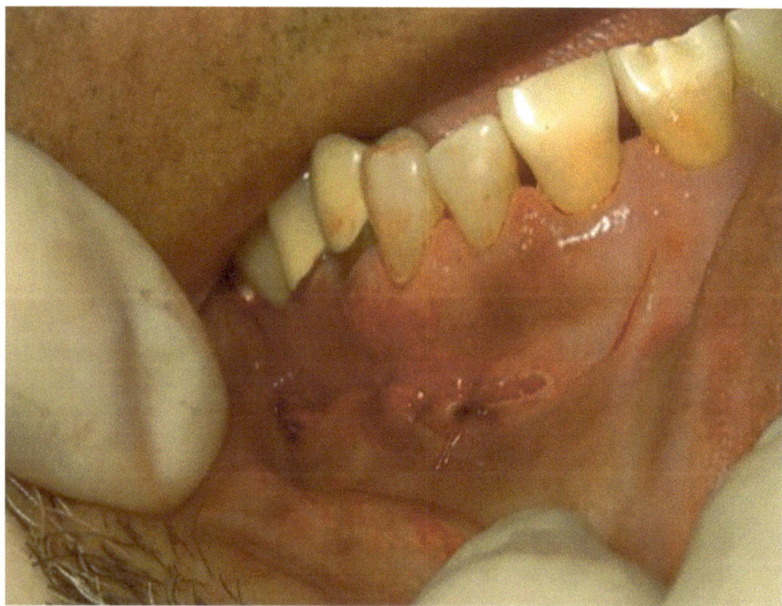

Fig. 13.9 Completed closure of the buccogingival incision with 3-0 chromic gut suture

13.12 Representative Case

DE is a 46-year-old male with thyroid-related immune orbitopathy resulting in bilateral proptosis, left greater than right (Fig. 13.10). He underwent left-sided transantral orbital decompression, with removal of the orbital floor medial to the infraorbital nerve and infracture of the medial orbital wall. Following decompression, his rim to cornea measurement on the left side decreased from 30 mm to 26 mm (right side remained stable at 27 mm). On post-operative day 1, symmetry in exophthalmos between the globes was noted.

Figure 13.10 shows the patient preoperatively (Fig. 13.10a), and on post-operative month 1 (Fig. 13.10c). In addition to the documented improvement in proptosis, note the marked improvement in eyelid position. The CT images show profound enlargement of the inferior rectus, medial rectus, and superior rectus muscles preoperatively (Fig. 13.10b) and at post-operative month 1 (Fig. 13.10d). In the post-operative image, note the expansion of the intraorbital space with removal of the orbital floor and infracture of the medial orbital wall with preservation of the orbital strut (Fig. 13.10d).

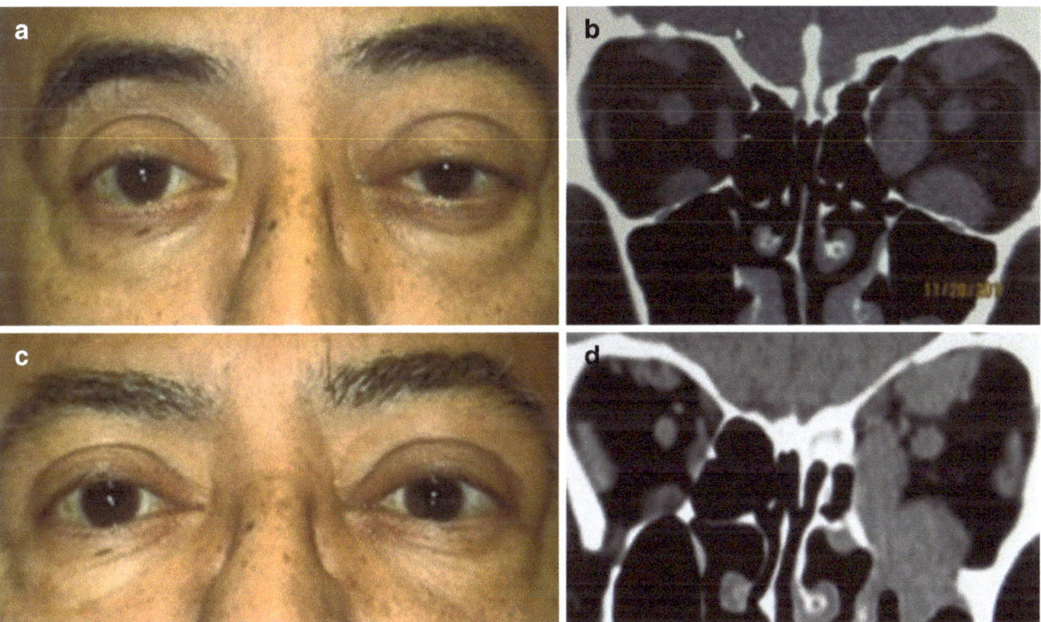

Fig. 13.10 Preoperative photographs and computed tomography images of a patient who underwent left-sided transantral orbital decompression (**a**, **b**). Post-operative clinical photograph and coronal section of CT scan one month after surgery (**c**, **d**)

13.13 Conclusion

Transantral approach avoids an going through the orbital approach in active orbits. It allows more posterior decompression and has a beneficial effect on eyelid retraction and inferior scleral show. It is a useful approach in the armamentarium of the orbital surgeon treating thyroid eye disease.

References

1. Walsh TE, Ogura JH. Transantral orbital decompression for malignant exophthalmos. Laryngoscopes. 1957;67(6):544–68.
2. Garritty JA, Fatourechu V, Bergstralh EJ, et al. Results of transantral orbital decompression in 428 patients with severe Graves ophthalmology. Am J Ophthalmol. 1993;116(5):533–47.
3. Tallstedt L, Papatziamos G, Lundblad L, Anggard A. Results of transantral orbital decompression in patients with thyroid-associated ophthalmopathy. Acts Ophthalmol Scand. 2000;78(2):206–10.
4. Lu JE, Pfeiffer ML, Burnstine MA. Graded transantral orbital decompression outcomes in stable thyroid eye disease: a series of 47 orbits. Orbit 2020; epub ahead of print.

Part IV

Strabismus and Eyelid Surgery in Inactive TED

14 Management of Strabismus in TED

Mithila Negalur and Ramesh Kekunnaya

14.1 Introduction

The relationship between thyroid gland dysfunction and the severity of induced orbitopathy still remains to be well established and can manifest itself in a myriad of ophthalmic symptoms and signs ranging from mild ocular irritation to severe proptosis, strabismus, and optic nerve compression [1]. Of these manifold presentations, strabismus due to thyroid induced myopathy has been reported in a huge number of patients (about 17–51%) whereas diplopia as the initial presentation may be seen in 15–20% of cases [2–5].

In the initial active phase of TED, there is inflammatory enlargement of extraocular muscles due to lymphocytic infiltration and deposition of glycosaminoglycans and hyaluronic acid accompanied by adipogenesis [6]. This involvement may be unilateral or bilateral or sometimes may involve only one muscle. The commonest muscle to be affected is the inferior rectus being a bulky and tonically active extraocular muscle, followed by the medial and superior rectus muscle (Fig. 14.1) [7]. Later, as the inflammation subsides, there are fibrotic changes in the orbit leading to tightness and restriction of movement of the extraocular muscles.

Management of this myopathy is challenging due to the constantly changing nature of this disease as well as the differences in the properties of inflamed and fibrosed muscles and hence surgery is generally avoided in the absence of functional disability [8, 9].

M. Negalur
LV Prasad Eye Institute, Hyderabad, India

R. Kekunnaya (✉)
Paediatric Ophthalmology and Strabismus Service,
Child Sight Institute, LV Prasad Eye Institute,
Hyderabad, India
e-mail: rameshak@lvpei.org

S. Rath, M. N. Naik (eds.), *Surgery in Thyroid Eye Disease*,
https://doi.org/10.1007/978-981-32-9220-8_14

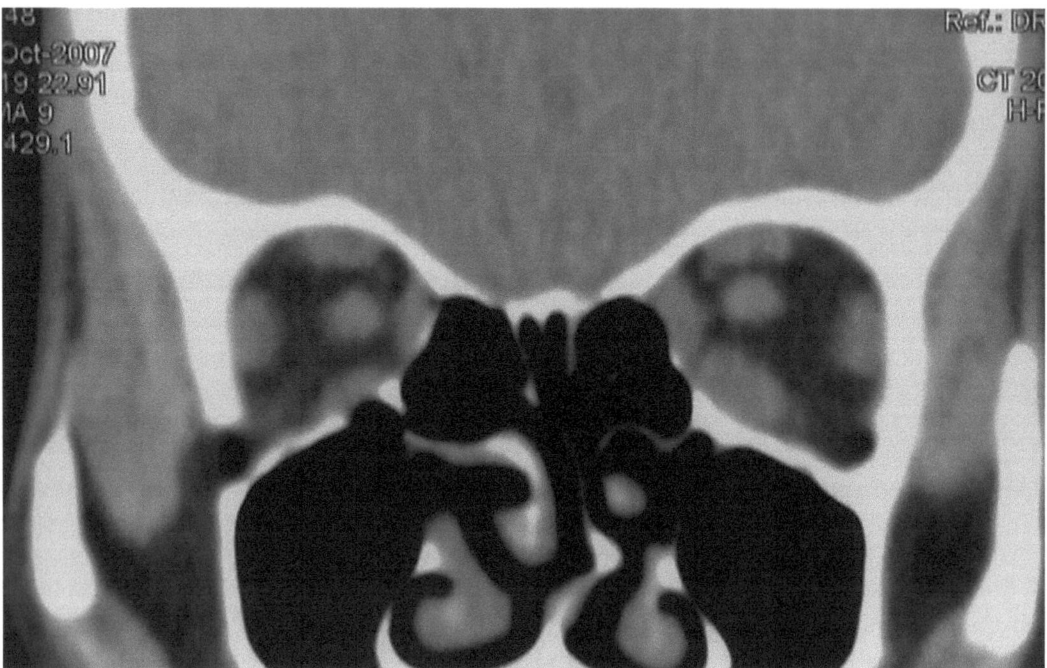

Fig. 14.1 Coronal CT scan image showing enlargement of the left inferior and medial rectus muscles in TED

14.2 Management of Diplopia During the Active Phase

Conservative measures, such as lowering the bifocal segment of glasses or separate glasses for distance and near can aid in near activities. The use of *Fresnel or ground-in prisms* for smaller deviations or monocular occlusion of the more hypotropic/strabismic eye can be used to relieve diplopia during the active phase [8]. Patients should also be advised to control thyroid hormone levels and cessation of smoking if any during this period. It has been studied that smokers with TED have twice the risk of requiring strabismus surgery compared to nonsmokers [8].

Other means of conservative management during the active phase includes intramuscular injection of *botulinum toxin type A* to treat thyroid myopathy [9, 10]. A study using Botulinum toxin in a dose of 5 units per muscle showed improvement in the alignment from a mean deviation of 19.5 Prism Dioptres (PD) to 2.25 PD [10]. Also, Akbari et al. found that the success following intramuscular Botulinum toxin injections in thyroid-induced myopathy was significantly higher in cases with esotropia, especially smaller deviations, small angles of vertical deviation, and lower degrees of excyclotorsion [9]. But, these studies have shown good outcomes in the active stage of the disease with limited benefit once the fibrotic stage had set in [10].

14.3 Management of Strabismus in the Inactive Phase

As discussed previously, any extraocular muscle may be affected in TED, though there is a predilection for the inferior and the medial recti. Usually, there is relative sparing of the antagonist muscle causing the eye to deviate in the direction of the affected muscle. If its yoke muscle is also spared these patients might have an overshoot on motility testing.

14.3.1 Indication and Timing

Traditionally surgical intervention for strabismus in TED is advisable in cases of disability in functional positions of gaze and should be avoided unless stable alignment has been noted for at least 6 months [11]. But, in spite of this the deviation may not be truly stable even after 6 months. Mills et al. reviewed strabismus surgery in adults, and noted an overall need for re-surgery in 21% of cases while in cases of strabismus with TED it increased to 50% [12]. So one can presume that longer the follow-up period of these patients, lower is the surgical success and more the need for re-surgery.

Hence, whenever surgery is indicated, the course of disease must be explained to the patients and realistic goals must be set, i.e., binocular single vision in primary and reading positions. More recently, newer surgical goals have included the expansion of a single binocular field and even the elimination of prism use [13]. Qahtani et al. in their study of 139 patients of TED operated for strabismus found that though vertical strabismus was more common due to inferior rectus involvement (Fig. 14.2), surgery for horizontal deviations had 84% success rate while that for vertical strabismus was only 66% [14]. Similarly, Volpe et al. in their series of 54 patients with vertical strabismus due to TED found that 65% of cases had a successful result after a single adjustable surgery [15].

As mentioned earlier, these muscles are fibrosed or inflamed and hence have highly variable and unpredictable outcomes with standard

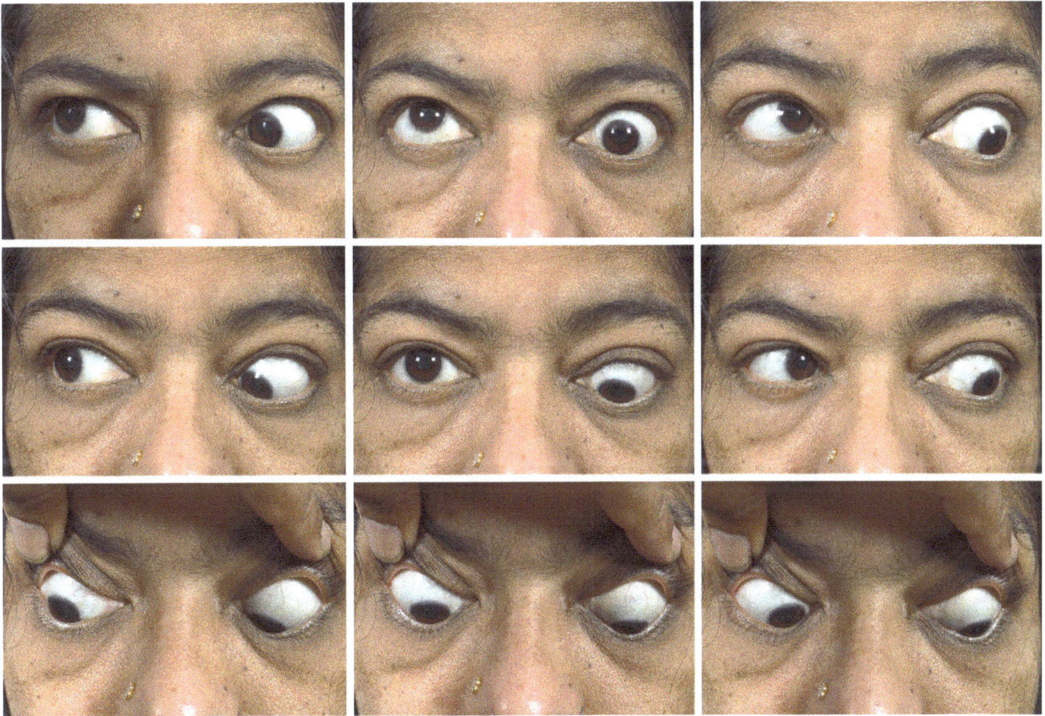

Fig. 14.2 Nine-gaze photograph showing left hypotropia with limitation of elevation (more in abduction than adduction) along with lid retraction due to tight left inferior rectus in TED

surgical nomograms [16]. The general dictum is larger than expected recessions for smaller deviations and smaller than expected recessions for larger deviations as described by Buckley and Von Noorden [17]—the "*a lot gets you a little and little gets you a lot*" dictum. However, it must be kept in mind that patients with vertical strabismus develop a large fusional range for their deviation mandating a small post-operative hypodeviation to allow easy fusion and prevent diplopia. Thus, a patient with right hypotropia will have developed the ability to remain binocular despite a large right hypophoric deviation and is best corrected with a small hypodeviation [18]. Before performing surgery, careful forced duction testing should be performed and repeated after each muscle is disinserted.

14.3.2 Vertical Muscle Surgery

Inferior rectus recession is the most commonly performed surgery in patients of TED with strabismus (Figs. 14.3 and 14.4) and is challenging due to the need for binocularity in the primary and reading positions and prisms may frequently

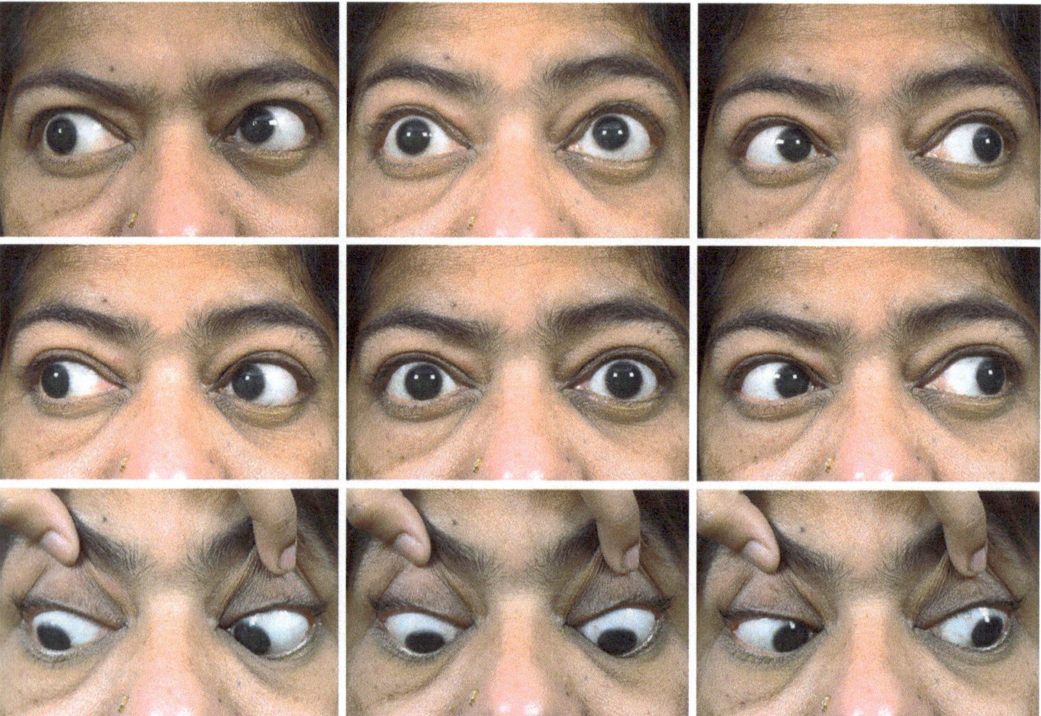

Fig. 14.3 Post-operative 9-gaze photograph of the same patient following left inferior rectus recession surgery

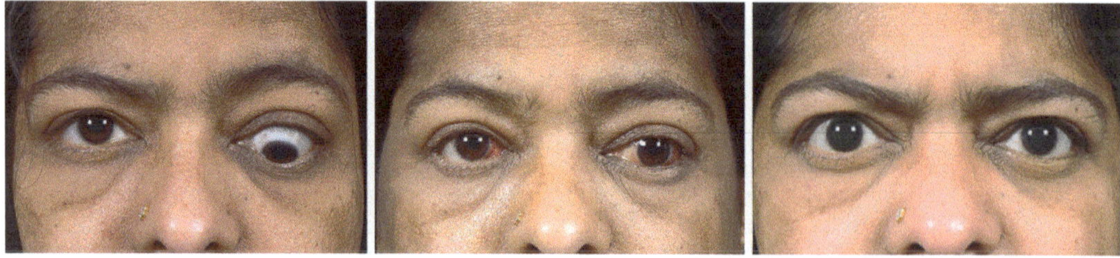

Fig. 14.4 Picture collage of the same patient showing pre-operative, immediate post-operative, and 3 months post-operative status

be needed [19]. Usually, these patients have hypotropia secondary to inferior rectus involvement and need careful evaluation including Hess charting, motility assessment, and passive ductions to rule out the involvement of contralateral inferior rectus. If found, it mandates bilateral (may be asymmetric) inferior rectus recession to improve the symmetry of ductions in both eyes. In large vertical deviations, inferior rectus recession may be combined with contralateral superior rectus recession as well. However, inferior rectus recession in TED has its own challenges [20].

Large inferior rectus recessions result in limitation of depression causing superior oblique, the other depressor to overact in downgaze. As superior oblique is an abductor the eye abducts in downgaze post-operatively, resulting in an A-pattern with incyclotorsion, and diplopia in downgaze [21]. Transposing the inferior rectus medially by a tendon width at the time of recession surgery can reduce this abduction effect, but increases the tendency for incyclotorsion. Posterior tenotomy (sparing torsion) of the superior oblique muscles can be considered though this may aggravate the limitation in downgaze [20].

Dagi et al. have also described bilateral transposition of the inferior oblique border to the superior border of the lateral rectus to correct torsional diplopia [8]. Each transposition can improve up to 10 degrees of incyclotorsion and the effect can be enhanced by resecting the muscle. Large recessions of the inferior rectus can also decrease innervation to the contralateral superior oblique muscle thereby causing apparent inferior oblique overaction contralaterally. For hypotropia persisting even after vertical rectus surgery, inferior oblique recession has been proposed by Salchow with good outcomes [22, 23]. This may be preferred to exploring the inferior rectus as it may be technically difficult and associated with complications [21].

Another concern with recession of the inferior rectus is the resulting lower lid retraction and the patient should be counselled preoperatively. This can be avoided to some extent by using a Desmarres retractor to enhance surgical exposure followed by meticulous dissection of the lower lid retractor fibers from the inferior surface of the inferior rectus muscle [20].

Also, recession of inferior rectus is frequently complicated by consecutive hypertropia, termed as progressive overcorrection as coined by Sharma and Reinecke, reported in 42–50% of patients post-operatively following inferior rectus recession. Various theories have been postulated to explain this phenomenon. Inferior rectus slippage was commonly proposed as the cause of overcorrection [21]. This muscle has been found to have a high risk of slippage, especially after large recession due to its short arc of contact and presence of thick Tenon capsule which may cause non-adhesion to the globe. Post-operative slippage of the inferior rectus has led to controversy about the use of hang-back or adjustable sutures in this situation. Hence, meticulous dissection of the Tenon capsule and use of nonabsorbable sutures has also been suggested.

But in the analysis by Qahtah et al. muscle slippage was found to be the reason in less than 10% of cases and more often than not the inferior rectus was seen at the correct position at the time of re-surgery [23]. In a study by Wright on the inferior rectus recession even without coexisting TED, 12% of patients developed consecutive hypertropia [19]. In those who underwent a second surgery, inferior rectus was found at normal position but very slack due to scarring of the lower lid retractors as a result of excessive dissection.

Thus, factors other than muscle slippage were also found to be contributory. As explained by Sharma and Reinecke, there is repeated contraction of the inferior rectus due to Bell's phenomenon, predisposing it to gradual overcorrection. Other reasons implicated include increased force from the ipsilateral superior rectus which is believed to be masked due to tight inferior rectus. Moreover, if the contralateral inferior rectus is also affected, there is increased innervation to its superior rectus. This produces a fixation duress and due to Hering's law, there is increased innervation of the contralateral superior rectus causing a hypertropia in the operated eye.

14.3.3 Horizontal Muscle Surgery

Large esotropias can require large recessions of both medial rectus muscles once again aiming for a small undercorrection. These patients are at a high risk of post-operative exotropia due to lateral rectus involvement [20]. Post-operatively, convergence may be limited, interfering with near activities and may be managed by incorporating base-in prisms into the patient's reading glasses [22].

14.3.4 Role of Resection Surgery

As in all forms of restrictive strabismus, it has been proposed that muscle resection should be avoided as it may be difficult to perform and may even worsen the restriction thereby impairing motility further. However, in some situations resection may be necessary as in cases of monocular patients or those who refuse binocular surgery, patients with undercorrection despite maximal recession and those with undercorrections and free ductions. A recent study by Yoo et al. on muscle resections in thyroid strabismus found good short-term post-operative results, with 87.5% of patients orthotropic in primary gaze and no cases with overcorrection or aggravated inflammation [24]. Few other studies on muscle resection in TED have found good post-operative alignment without any overcorrection [25, 26].

Hence, resections can be considered as a safe procedure, especially if it is limited to the tendon and there is minimal restriction [19].

Other challenges faced during surgery for thyroid-associated strabismus include limited exposure due to lid swelling accompanied by a friable conjunctiva, especially if radiation therapy has been administered and tight muscles. This mandates very careful handling of the muscles to avoid "pulled in two" syndrome or "PITS" as termed by Greenwald [27]. This is an infrequent complication involving rupture of the muscle, most commonly the medial rectus followed by the inferior rectus [28].

A guarded strabismus hook such as Wright, Wilson, Suh, Kowal, or Bishop grooved hook is useful when operating on very tight muscles to minimize risk of complications such as inadvertent globe perforation or inadequate capture of the muscle tendon [20, 23]. Also, instead of using tenotomy scissors to disinsert the muscle, it may be much easier and safer to cut the tendon over the hook using a no. 15 Bard-Parker blade.

When closing the conjunctiva one needs to keep in mind that large muscle recessions may need to be accompanied by conjunctival recession to avoid post-operative conjunctival tethering, which can worsen the restriction. To ensure this does not occur, the eye should be held in the position of fullest possible duction and the forced duction test should be repeated after conjunctival closure.

Post-operatively other than topical medication various regimes may be used keeping in mind the basic etiology of TED. The use of oral steroids, for even a short pulse, is recommended as it may lower the risk of reactivation due to surgery.

Another issue here is that most patients undergoing strabismus surgery for TED may have also undergone orbital decompression surgery, which in turn can cause deviation in muscle pathways resulting in new-onset strabismus [20]. Shorr et al. found a 30% incidence of diplopia in the primary position following decompression surgery. They also found that bony decompression surgery was associated with worsening of esotropia and hypotropia, specifically, in their cohort of 50 patients. They also found that patients more likely to develop diplopia in the primary position were those with preexisting limitations in ductions. More recently, it has been observed that different approaches to decompression are associated with differing rates of post-operative diplopia [29]. So, while some authors believe that prior decompression is a poor prognostic factor for post-operative alignment, some propose that it does not affect the final outcome and the poor results are possibly due to more severe disease in these eyes. Following decompression, the inflamed muscles get space to relax and may help convert an incomittant deviation into a comittant one with better surgical outcomes. It is, therefore, better to perform strabismus surgery after decompression.

14.4 Modifications of Strabismus Surgery in TED

In order to overcome these challenges in managing thyroid-associated strabismus, various modifications of standard strabismus surgery have been described.

Dal Canto et al. have described the "*intraoperative relaxed muscle positioning* technique" for thyroid strabismus [30]. This involves the positioning of disinserted muscle at its relaxed position with the globe in the primary position without taking into consideration the pre-operative deviations. Of the 24 patients in their series, 83.3% had excellent outcomes of no diplopia in primary or reading gaze after single surgery and the reoperation rate was 8% at an average follow-up of 5.4 months

Another approach described is the *correction of the deviation based on limitation of ductions* rather than preoperative deviations [23]. In this technique, the muscle to be recessed is disinserted and reattached at a point such that it matches the maximum duction of the contralateral eye. A 74% success rate has been reported with this procedure compared to 44% in the control group.

An additional significant introduction into the management of strabismus surgery is the use of *adjustable sutures*, which was found to have a higher success rate compared to traditional surgery. In the series by Volpe et al, adjustable suture recession of inferior rectus was found to have excellent post-operative alignment in primary and reading positions in 65% of patients while 31% of cases had post-operative alignment within 6 prism diopters [15]. However, concerns about adjustable suture surgery in TED include the possibility of muscle slippage, scar elongation, and progressive overcorrection and hence it's use remains controversial.

14.5 Conclusion

Thus, management of strabismus due to thyroid orbitopathy is complex and technically demanding as it is a dynamic entity. Treatment outcomes with both, nonsurgical and surgical modalities can be very unpredictable. Successful results often require a multidisciplinary approach to take care of the patient.

Some of the key points to consider for a good and consistent surgical outcome are as follows:

- Surgery should be planned only in cases with a functional or cosmetic disability and should not be performed before the alignment has been documented to be stable for 6 months.
- Surgical goals and expectations should be defined and clearly discussed with the patient.
- Assess disease activity, as it is not advisable to operate in the active stage of the disease.
- Cessation of smoking and thyroid hormone control is important in overall disease control and for better outcomes.
- Forced duction testing intraoperatively is crucial when deciding on or varying the surgical plan.
- Resection of muscles is generally avoided unless the deviation is very large or in patients where only monocular surgery can be done.
- Progressive overcorrection following inferior rectus recession is an important cause of recurrent diplopia in these patients; therefore, planned undercorrection of patients undergoing inferior rectus recession is advocated.
- The existence of unusual strabismus-like exotropia in TED, or presentation of ptosis in TED must alert one to look for associated myasthenia gravis.

References

1. Bartley GB, Fatourechi V, Kadrmas EF, et al. Long-term follow-up of Graves ophthalmopathy in an incidence cohort. Ophthalmology. 1996;103(6):958–62.
2. Lee HB, Rodgers IR, Woog JJ. Evaluation and management of Graves' orbitopathy. Otolaryngol Clin N Am. 2006;39(5):923–42.
3. De Waard R, Koorneef L, Verbatin B Jr. Motility disturbances in Graves' ophthalmopathy. Doc Ophthalmol. 1983;56(1-2):41–7.
4. Asman P. Opthalmological evaluation in thyroid-associated ophthalmopathy. Acta Ophthalmol Scan. 2003;81(15):437–48.
5. Kendler DL, Lippa J, Rootman J. The initial characteristics of Graves' orbitopathy vary with age and sex. Arch Ophthalmol. 1993;111(2):197–201.
6. Eckstein AK, Johnson KT, Thanos M, Esser J, Ludgate M. Current insights into the pathogenesis of Graves' orbitopathy. Horm Metab Res. 2009;41(6):456–64.
7. Dyer JA. The oculorotary muscles in Graves' disease. Trans Am Ophthalmol Soc. 1976;74:425–56.
8. Dagi LR, Elliott AT, Roper-Hall G, Cruz OA. Thyroid eye disease: honing your skills to improve outcomes. J AAPOS. 2010;14(5):425–31.
9. Akbari MR, Ameri A, Keshtkar Jaafari AR, Mirmohammadsadeghi A. Botulinum toxin injection for restrictive myopathy of thyroid-associated orbitopathy: success rate and predictive factors. J AAPOS. 2016;20(2):126–30.
10. Granet DB, Ventura RH, Kikkawa DO, Levi L. Management of restrictive endocrine myopathy with botulinum toxin. American academy for paediatric ophthalmology and strabismus, 26th annual conference, San Diego: 2000
11. Nardi M. Squint surgery in TED—hints and fints, or why Graves' patients are difficult patients. Orbit. 2009;28(4):245–50.
12. Mills MD, Coats DK, Donahue SP, Wheeler DT. American Academy of Ophthalmology. Strabismus surgery for adults, a report by the American Academy of Ophthalmology. Ophthalmology. 2004;111(6):1255–61.
13. Wallang BS, Kekunnaya R, Granet D. Curr Ophthalmol Rep. 2013;1:218.
14. Al Qahtani ES, Rootman J, Kersey J, Godoy F, Lyons CJ. Clinical pearls and management recommendations for strabismus due to thyroid orbitopathy. Middle East Afr J Ophthalmol. 2015;22(3):307–11.
15. Volpe NJ, Mirza-George N, Binenbaum G. Surgical management of vertical ocular misalignment in thyroid eye disease using an adjustable suture technique. J AAPOS. 2012;16(6):518–22.
16. Sharma P, Reinecke RD. Single-stage adjustable strabismus surgery for restrictive strabismus. J AAPOS. 2003;7(5):358–62.
17. Buckley EG. Restrictive strabismus. In: Plager DA, editor. Strabismus surgery: basic and advanced strategies. Oxford: Oxford University Press; 2004.
18. Fells P, Kousoulides L, Pappa A, Munro P, Lawson J. Extraocular muscle problems in thyroid eye disease. Eye (Lond). 1994;8(Pt 5):497–505.
19. Ellis FD. Strabismus surgery for endocrine ophthalmopathy. Ophthalmology. 1979;86(12):2059–63.
20. Shorr N, Neuhaus RW, Baylis HI. Ocular motility problems after orbital decompression for dysthyroid ophthalmopathy. Ophthalmology. 1982;89(4):323–8.
21. Flanders M, Hastings M. Diagnosis and surgical management of strabismus associated with thyroid-related orbitopathy. J Pediatr Ophthalmol Strabismus. 1997;34(6):333–40.
22. Salchow DJ. Inferior oblique recession in thyroid-related orbitopathy. JAAPOS. 2015;19(3):274–7.
23. Nguyen VT, Park DJJ, Levin L, Feldon SE. Correction of restricted extraocular muscle motility in surgical management of strabismus in Graves' ophthalmopathy. Ophthalmology. 2002;109(2):384–8.
24. Yoo SH, Pineles SL, Goldberg RA, Velez FG. Rectus muscle resection in Graves' ophthalmopathy. J AAPOS. 2013;17(1):9–15.
25. Yan J, Zhang H. The surgical management of strabismus with large angle in patients with Graves' ophthalmopathy. Int Ophthalmol. 2008;28(2):75–82.
26. Mourits MP, Koorneef L, van Mourik-Noordenbos AM, van der Meulen-Schot HM, Prummel MF, Wiersinga WM, Berghout A. Extraocular muscle surgery for Graves' ophthalmopathy: does prior treatment influence surgical outcome? Br J Ophthalmol. 1990;74(8):481–3.
27. Greenwald MJ. Intraoperative muscle loss due to muscle-tendon dehiscence. American Association for Pediatric Ophthalmology and Strabismus Sixteenth Annual Meeting, July 30, 1990
28. Ellis EM, Kinori M, Robbins SL, Granet DB. Pulled-in-two syndrome multicenter survey of risk factors, management and outcomes. J AAPOS. 2016;20(5):387–91.
29. Ruttum MS. Effect of prior orbital decompression on outcome of strabismus surgery in patients with thyroid ophthalmopathy. J AAPOS. 2000;4(2):102–5.
30. Dal Canto AJ, Crowe S, Perry JD, Traboulsi EI. Intraoperative relaxed muscle positioning technique for strabismus repair in thyroid eye disease. Ophthalmology. 2006;113(12):2324–30.

Surgical Management of Eyelid Retraction

15

Milind N. Naik

15.1 Introduction

The early attempts to alleviate GUER consisted of cervical sympathectomy, tarsorrhaphy, and blepharorrhaphy [1, 2]. Most surgical techniques till date have targeted either the Muller muscle or the levator for correction of upper eyelid retraction [3].

15.1.1 Indications for Surgery

The indications to undergo correction of eyelid retraction can be either cosmetic or functional. *Cosmetically*, the wide-eyed or staring look is disliked by the patients, and want it corrected. *Functionally*, the wide aperture due to eyelid retraction can lead to rapid tear evaporation leading to drying of the ocular surface.

Clinically, upper eyelid retraction is classified into mild (no superior scleral show), moderate (<2 mm scleral show), and severe (>2 mm scleral show) as shown in Fig. 15.1. At the milder end of the spectrum, patients may only complain of burning and watering, especially in windy and outdoor conditions. In moderate cases, nocturnal lagophthalmos may lead to exposure. In severe cases, infectious keratitis can be sight threatening.

15.1.2 Timing of the Surgery

Correction of eyelid retraction is usually performed in the inactive phase of the disease. Orbital decompression, and strabismus surgery if required, should be performed prior to the correction of eyelid retraction since it may influence the degree of retraction [4].

In the active phase of the disease, extreme cases of severe exposure keratopathy, or microbial keratitis may require urgent correction of eyelid retraction for corneal protection [5]. In such cases, reoperation may be required later for cosmetic correction of the palpebral fissure height.

M. N. Naik (✉)
Ophthalmic Plastic Surgery Service,
LV Prasad Eye Institute, Hyderabad, India
e-mail: milind@lvpei.org

S. Rath, M. N. Naik (eds.), *Surgery in Thyroid Eye Disease*,
https://doi.org/10.1007/978-981-32-9220-8_15

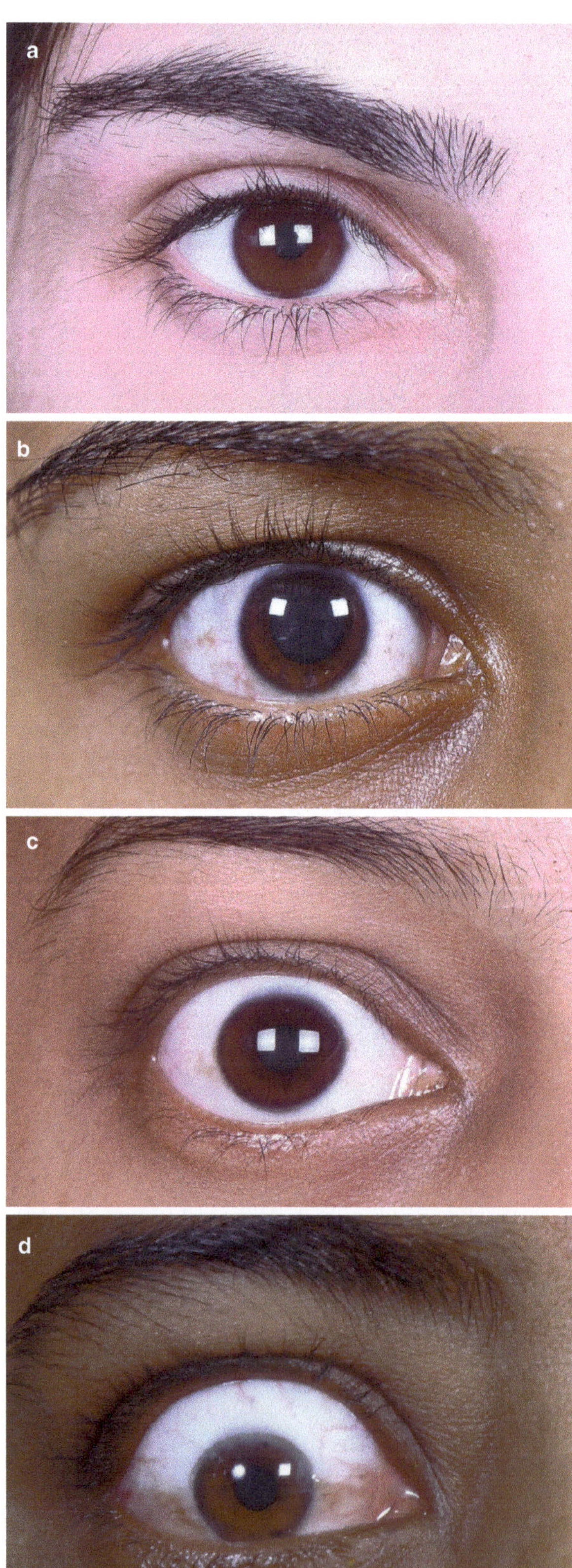

Fig. 15.1 Clinical grading of Upper Eyelid retraction. Normal position of upper and lower eyelid (**a**). Mild (**b**), moderate (**c**), and severe (**d**) upper eyelid retraction

15.2 Surgical Treatment

Surgery is recommended either for functional (persistent or symptomatic corneal exposure) or cosmetic reasons.

15.2.1 Tarsorrhaphy

Eyelid retraction has been identified as one of the risk factors for the development of microbial keratitis in patients with thyroid eye disease [5]. A lateral, paramedian or central tarsorrhaphy can help protect the ocular surface, and augment the healing of frank microbial keratitis (Fig. 15.2). Similarly, in mild cases, an extreme lateral tarsorrhaphy can give satisfactory results. An extreme lateral tarsorrhaphy can reduce the eyelid fissure where it is usually widest, i.e. it can cosmetically improve mild upper eyelid retraction (temporal flare) as well as lower eyelid retraction in a predictable manner (Fig. 15.2).

15.2.2 Surgeries of the Muller Muscle

In various procedures performed for the correction of upper eyelid retraction, three primary Muller muscle surgeries have been described. It can either be *recessed*, *recessed and re-sutured* or *excised* (Fig. 15.3) [1, 6–9]. Conjunctival division (Henderson, 1965) is one of the oldest surgery, where the conjunctiva is divided and recessed with the Muller muscle thereby lengthening the posterior lamella, and the defect is left to re-epithelize (Fig. 15.3a) [6]. The recessed conjunctiva and Muller can also be resutured to the levator in its new position, to hold it in place (Fig. 15.3b).

In mild cases (retraction up to superior limbus), excision of the Muller muscle (Mullerectomy) is sufficient (Fig. 15.3c). Mullerectomy surgery is described here.

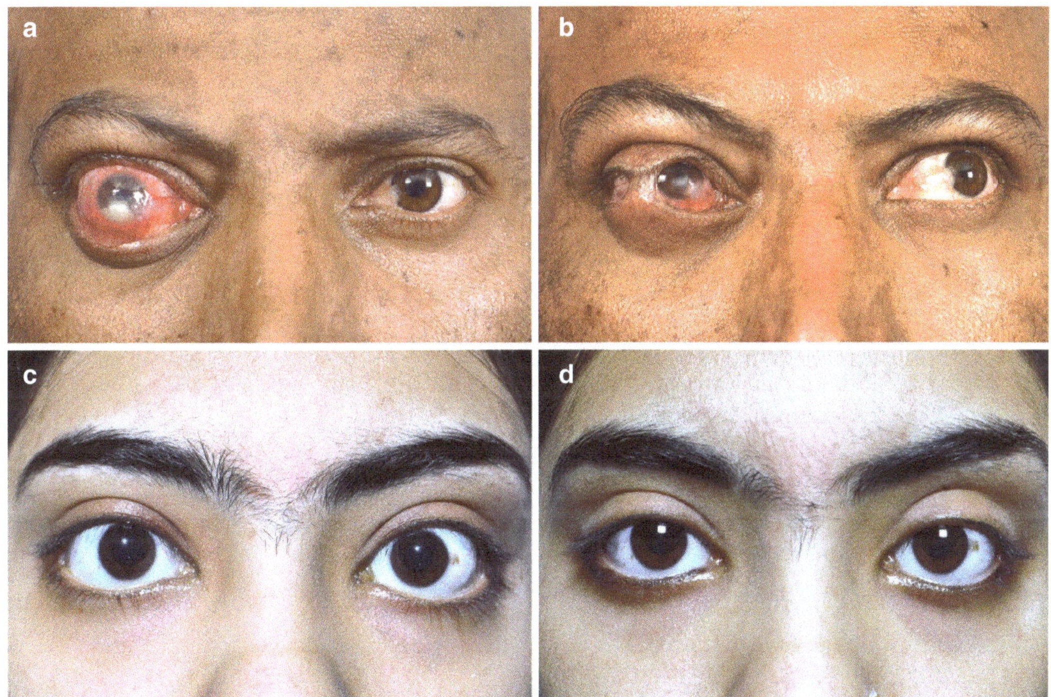

Fig. 15.2 Role of tarsorrhaphy in functional and cosmetic indications. A lateral paramedial tarsorrhaphy aids in early healing of microbial keratitis in a patient with thyroid eye disease (**a**, **b**). An extreme lateral tarsorrhaphy predictably corrects mild temporal flare and lower eyelid retraction at the same time (**c**, **d**)

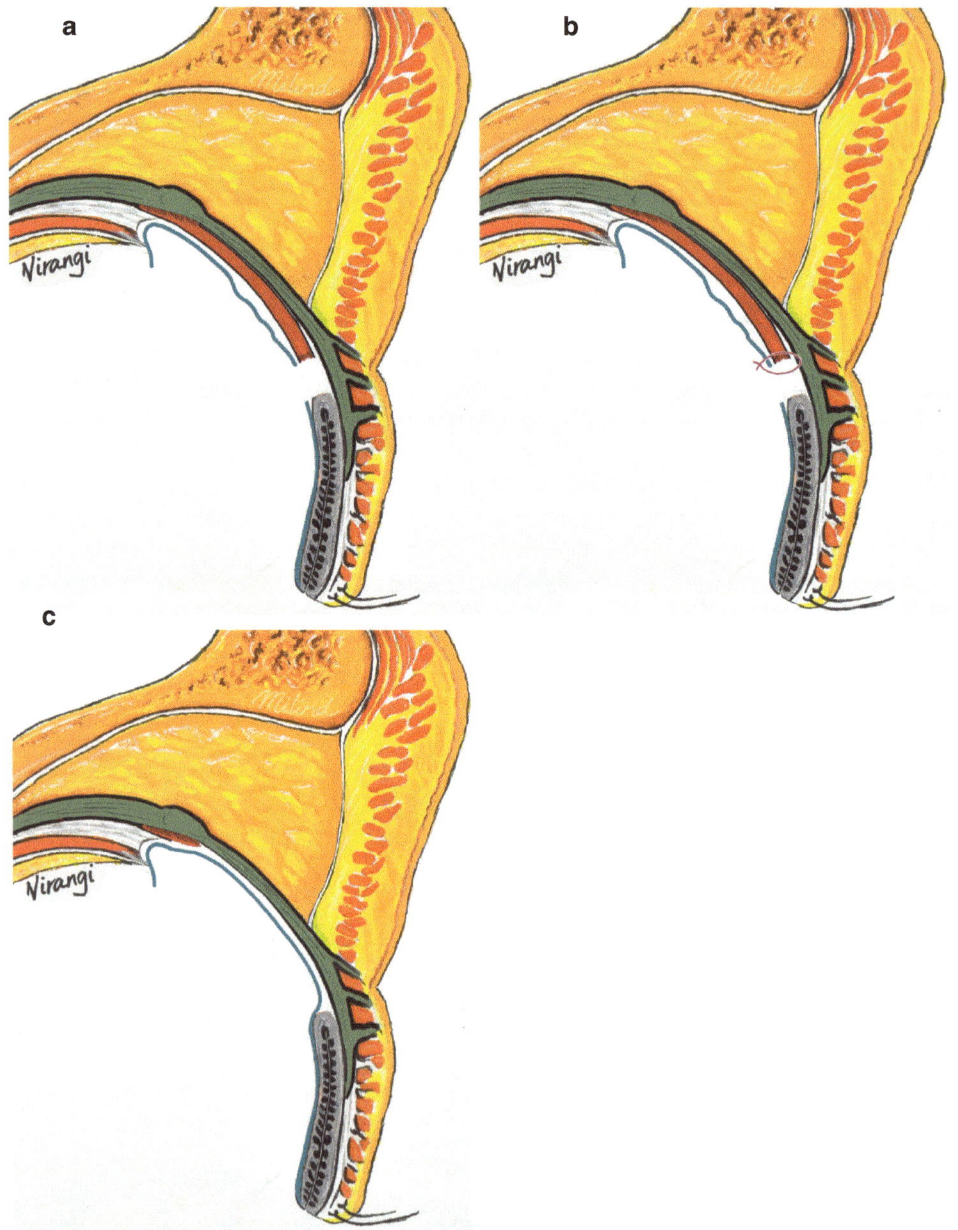

Fig. 15.3 Schematic diagram showing Muller muscle surgeries in the management of mild upper eyelid retraction. Muller and conjunctival recession (**a**), recession with suturing to the levator muscle (**b**), and Mullerectomy (**c**)

15.2.2.1 Mullerectomy

Excision of the Muller muscle can correct *mild* upper eyelid retraction. A trans-conjunctival approach is preferred, and the procedure involves separation of the Muller muscle from the levator anteriorly, and the conjunctiva posteriorly before it is excised (Fig. 15.4). The surgery can be performed under local anesthesia (Fig. 15.5). Infiltration of local anesthetic is performed subconjunctivally just above the upper edge of the tarsus after everting the eyelid over a Desmarre retractor. With a monopo-

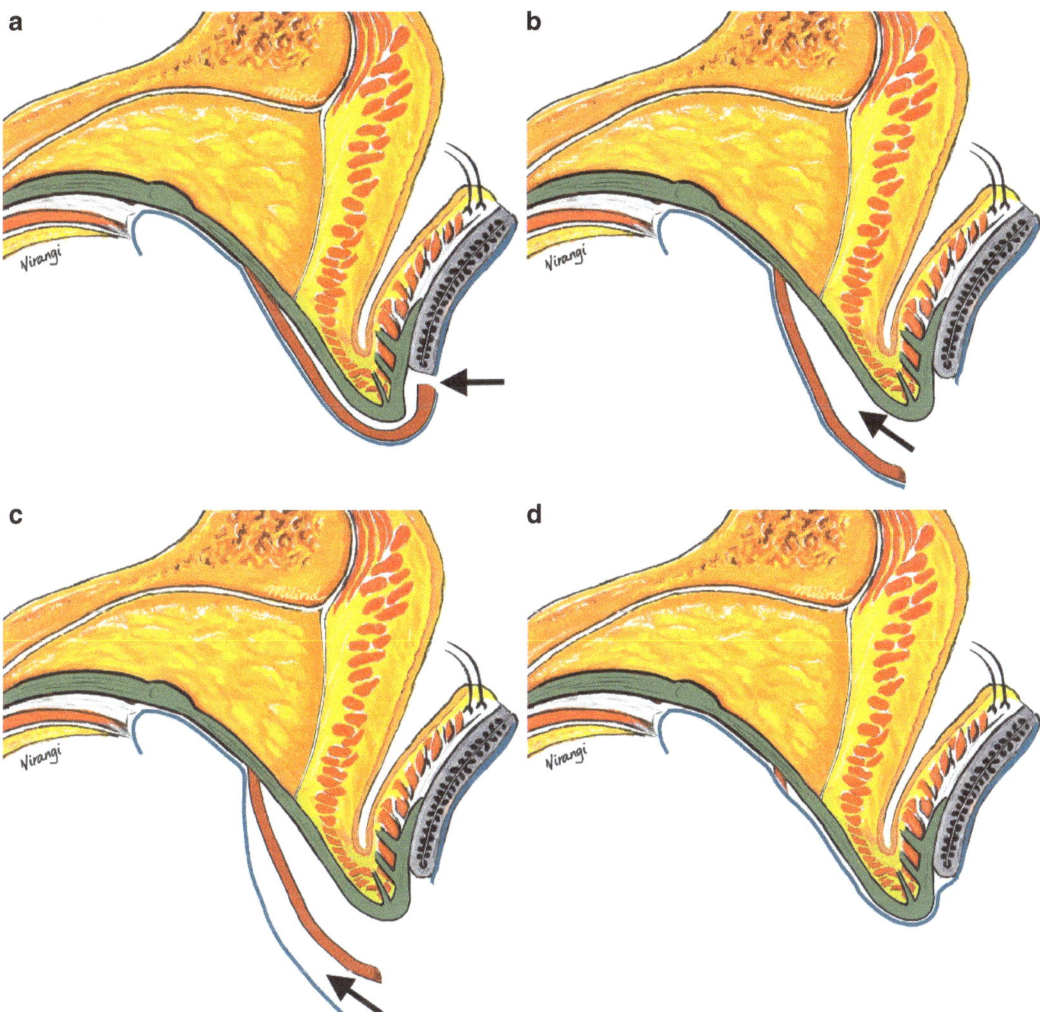

Fig. 15.4 Schematic diagram showing Mullerectomy surgery. Trans-conjunctival incision at the upper border of the tarsus (**a**). The plane between the Muller muscle (red) and levator (green) is dissected next (**b**). The conjunctiva (blue) is then separated from the Muller muscle (**c**). The muscle is separated from the levator and conjunctiva for its entire vertical distance and then excised. Conjunctiva is placed back with fibrin glue (**d**)

lar radiofrequency cautery, the conjunctiva is incised along the central 4/5th of the upper edge of tarsus. The incision is deepened until the levator (white line) is visible (Fig. 15.5). The Muller and levator are then separated along this plane until we reach the upper edge of Muller muscle close to the fornix. The plane between the Muller muscle and conjunctiva is then entered, to separate the muscle (Fig. 15.6a). Muller muscle is now separate from the levator anteriorly, and conjunctiva posteriorly (Fig. 15.6b). Then a 10–12 mm vertical height of Muller muscle is excised along the entire dissected length of the eyelid (Fig. 15.6c), and hemostasis is achieved. At the end of the procedure, only conjunctiva and levator are visible (Fig. 15.6d). The wound can be left as it is or can be sutured. We prefer fibrin glue to approximate the conjunctiva (Fig. 15.7). The surgery avoids an external scar and is predictable in providing up to 2 mm of drop in the eyelid position (Fig. 15.8).

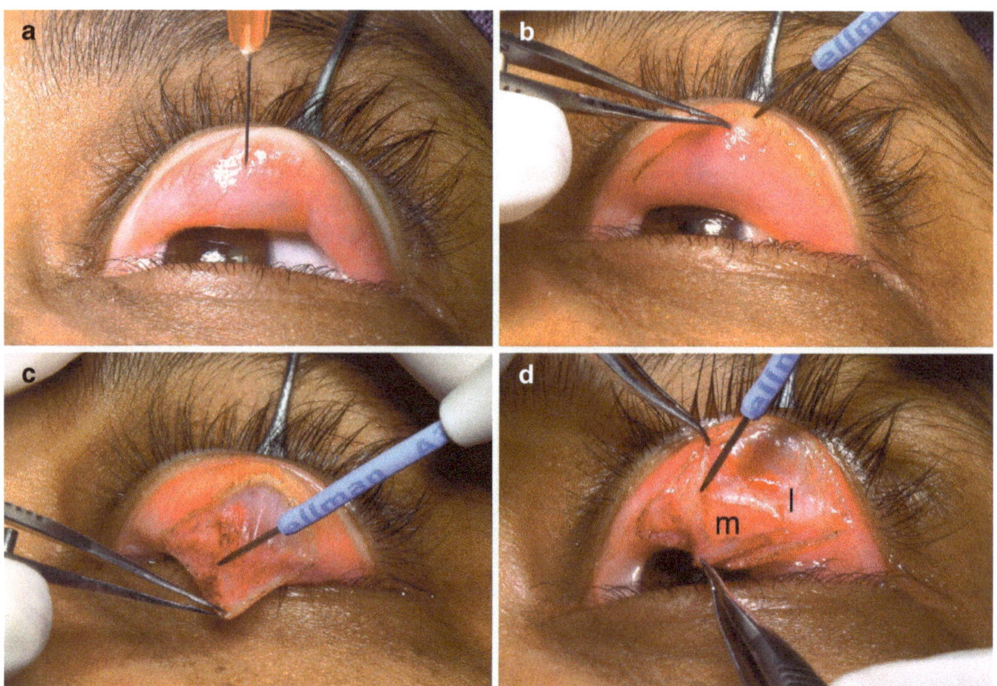

Fig. 15.5 Mullerectomy surgery for mild upper eyelid retraction. Subconjunctival infiltration anesthesia over an everted eyelid (**a**). Conjunctival incision at the upper border of the tarsus (**b**). Conjunctiva-Muller flap is raised (**c**). Levator muscle (l) is identified as a white line (**d**)

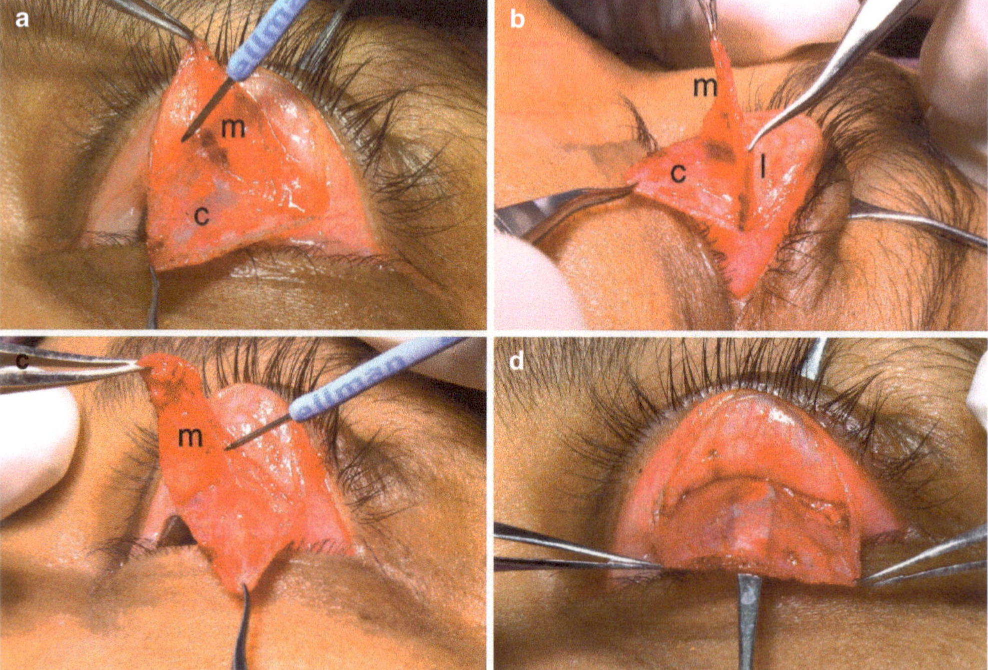

Fig. 15.6 Mullerectomy surgery for mild upper eyelid retraction *continued*. The Muller muscle (m) is now separated from the conjunctiva (c) in upward direction toward the fornix along the entire length of the eyelid (**a**). The Muller muscle is now separate from the levator, and the conjunctiva (**b**). The Muller muscle is excised (**c**). Note the conjunctiva and the levator at the conclusion of the procedure with no residual Muller muscle left (**d**)

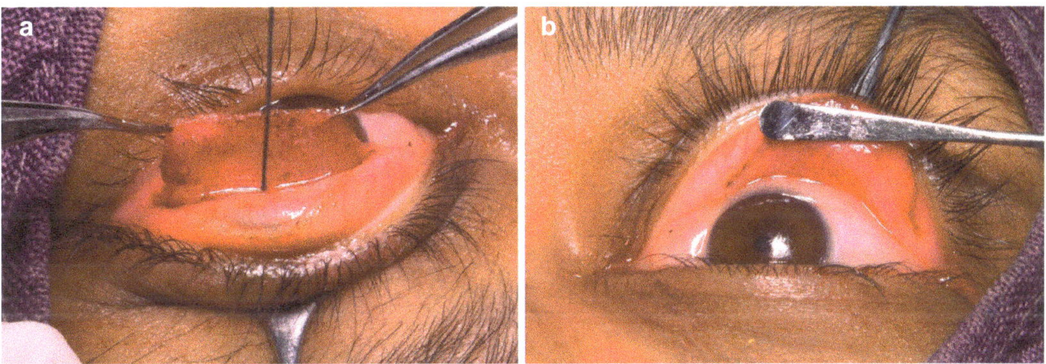

Fig. 15.7 Application of fibrin glue (**a**), and closure of the Mullerectomy surgery wound (**b**)

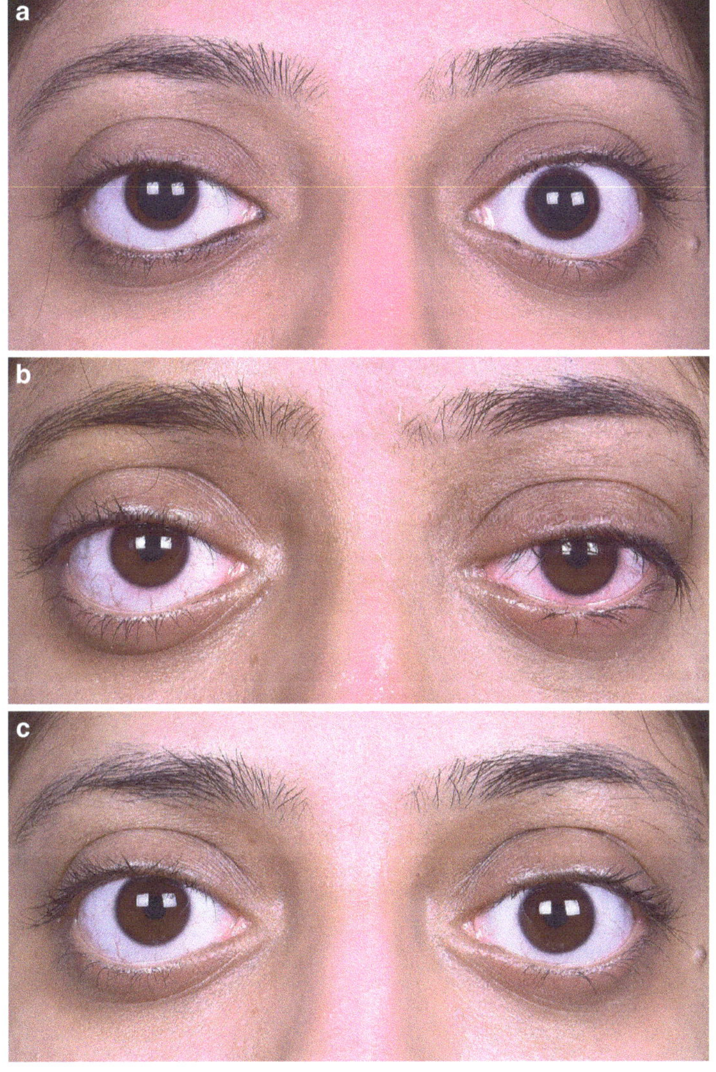

Fig. 15.8 Bilateral inactive thyroid eye disease with mild proptosis and left mild upper eyelid retraction (**a**). Patient chose to only correct the eyelid asymmetry. Day-1 following left Mullerectomy surgery (**b**) and 3 months postoperative appearance (**c**) with good eyelid symmetry

15.2.3 Surgeries of the Levator Muscle

Among various procedures performed for the correction of upper eyelid retraction, three primary levator muscle surgeries are commonly performed. These include levator *recession*, full-thickness *blepharotomy*, and levator *recession with eyelid spacers* (Fig. 15.9).

15.2.3.1 Levator Recession

While removal of Muller muscle suffices for mild retraction, for moderate cases, levator muscle recession has to be added to it or performed in isolation for adequate correction. It can be performed through either trans-conjunctival, or transcutaneous eyelid crease (Baylis) approach.

Levator recession is commonly used as an add-on second surgery beyond Mullerectomy for correction of moderate lid retraction. In 1965, Henderson described the combination of Mullerectomy and graded recession of the levator by a posterior approach [2].

Putterman refined Henderson's procedure by using local anesthesia for the graded approach [10]. He pointed out, that levator recession was required in a minority of cases after Muller muscle excision [8]. He also proposed that the focus of surgery should be in the temporal two-thirds, the aponeurosis is recessed in a graded manner, and a spacer is unnecessary [11].

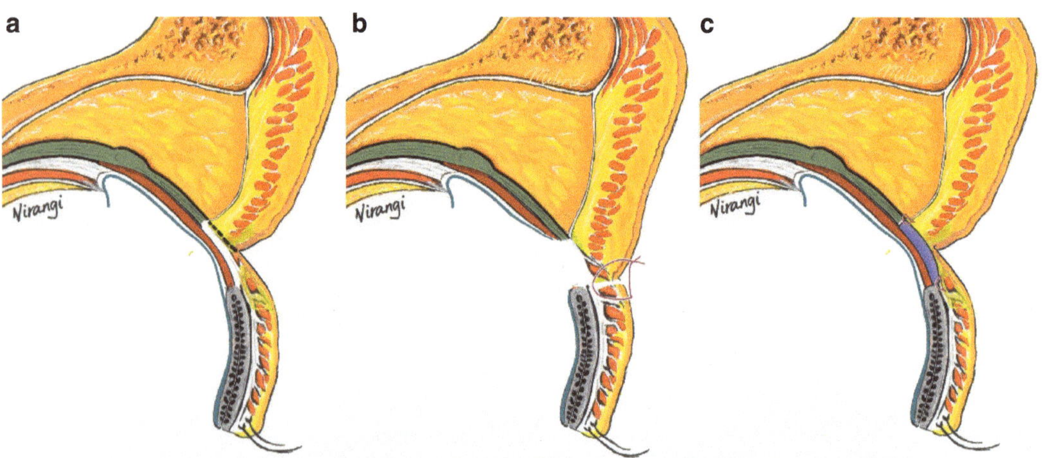

Fig. 15.9 Schematic diagram showing levator muscle surgeries in the management of moderate to severe upper eyelid retraction. Levator recession (**a**), Full-thickness blepharotomy (**b**), and levator recession with spacer graft (**c**)

Levator recession through the anterior approach is described here (Figs. 15.10, 15.11, and 15.12). Via an eyelid crease incision, the upper border of the tarsus is exposed, levator insertion is separated from the tarsus, to allow its recession until the desired eyelid drop is noted. In patients with significant lateral flare, the lateral horn of the levator has to be released to provide normal contour (Fig. 15.13). Anterior approach levator recession allows addressing the eyelid crease and symmetry of tarsal plate show (Fig. 15.14) and is therefore superior to posterior approach surgery.

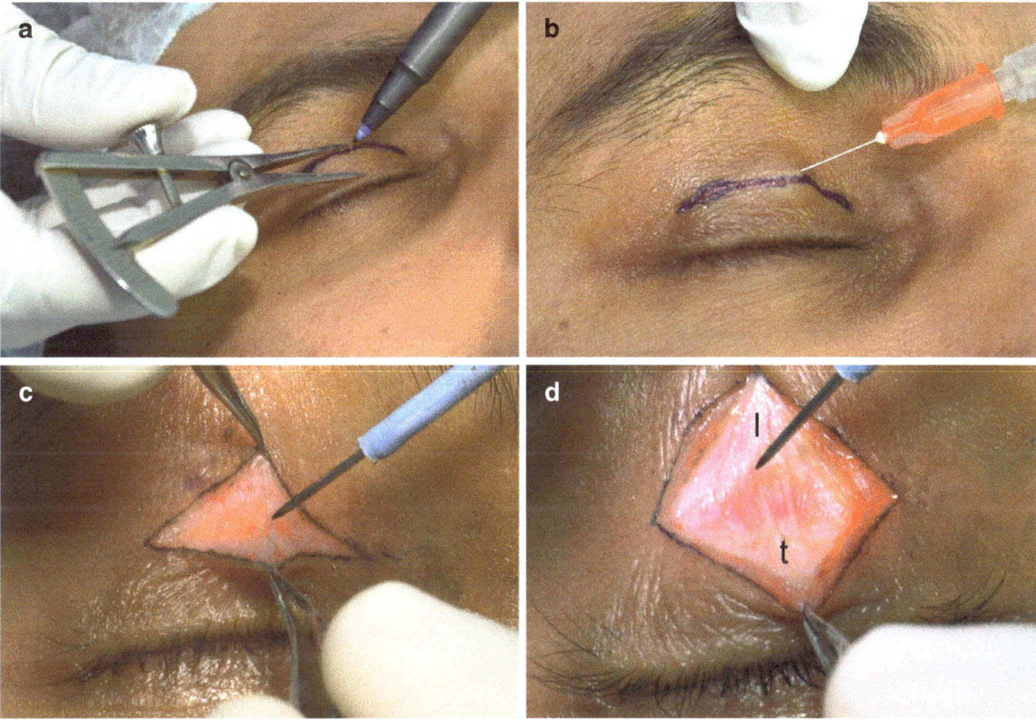

Fig. 15.10 Transcutaneous levator recession surgery (Baylis approach). The eyelid crease is marked at 7 mm from lashline (**a**), and local infiltration anesthesia (0.5 ml of 2% Xylocaine with 1:100,000 adrenaline) is given (**b**). Skin and orbicularis is incised with monopolar cautery (**c**) to expose the tarsus (t) and the levator (l) muscle (**d**)

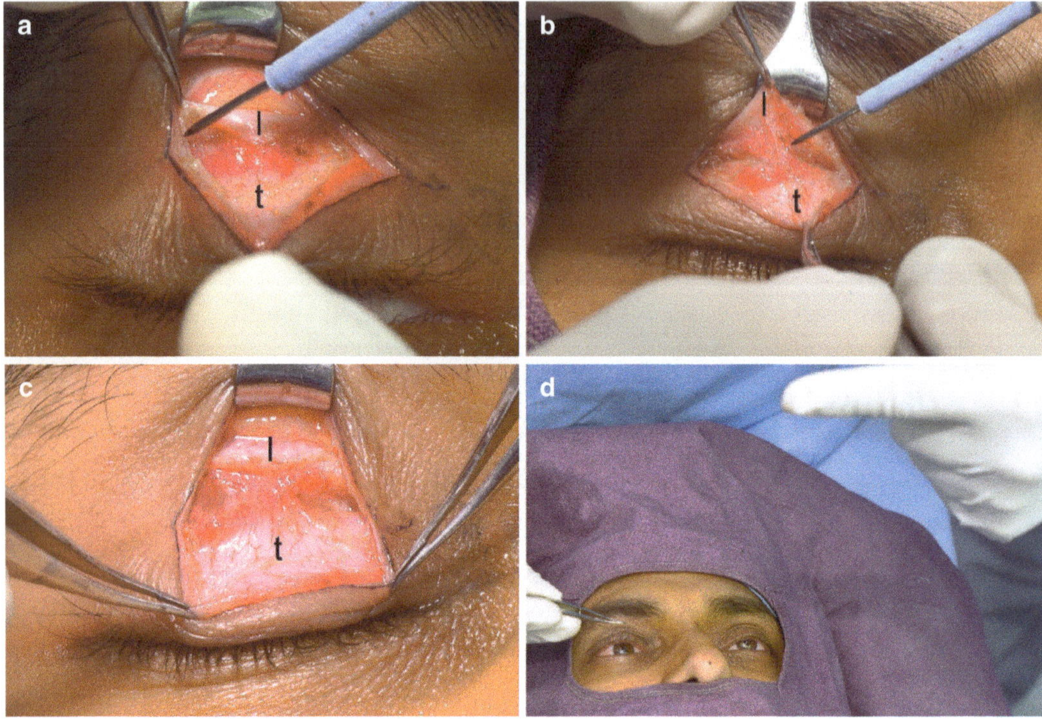

Fig. 15.11 Transcutaneous levator recession surgery (Baylis approach) *continued*. The levator is disinserted from the tarsus in a graded manner (**a**–**c**) while assessing the drop in eyelid position (**d**). Lateral horn is usually disinserted (**a**)

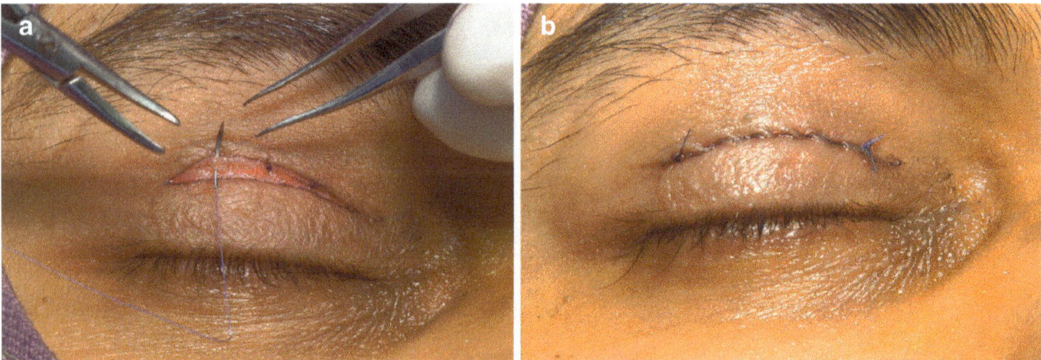

Fig. 15.12 Transcutaneous levator recession surgery (Baylis approach) *continued*. The wound is closed in layers: orbicularis (**a**) with Vicryl 6-0 suture, and skin (**b**) with Prolene 6-0 suture

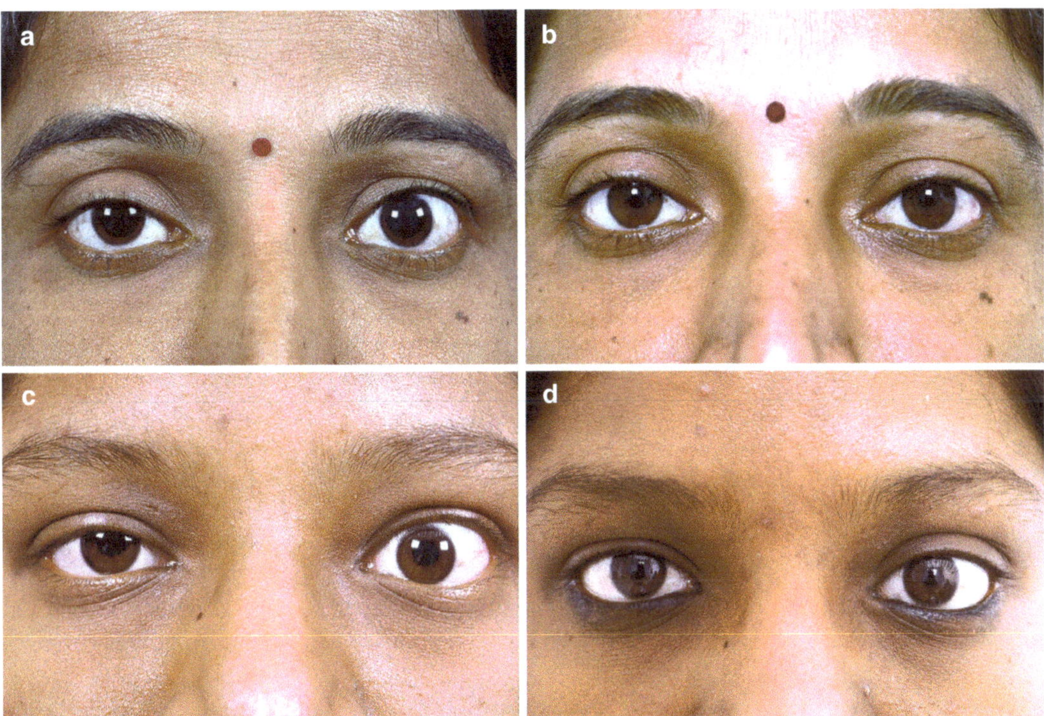

Fig. 15.13 Left upper eyelid retraction in a case of mild inactive TED (**a**, **c**). Good cosmetic correction following transcutaneous levator recession surgery with release of the lateral horn (**b**, **d**). Note the reduced tarsal plate show preoperatively (**a**, **c**). Note the equalization of tarsal plate show post-operatively (**b**, **d**)

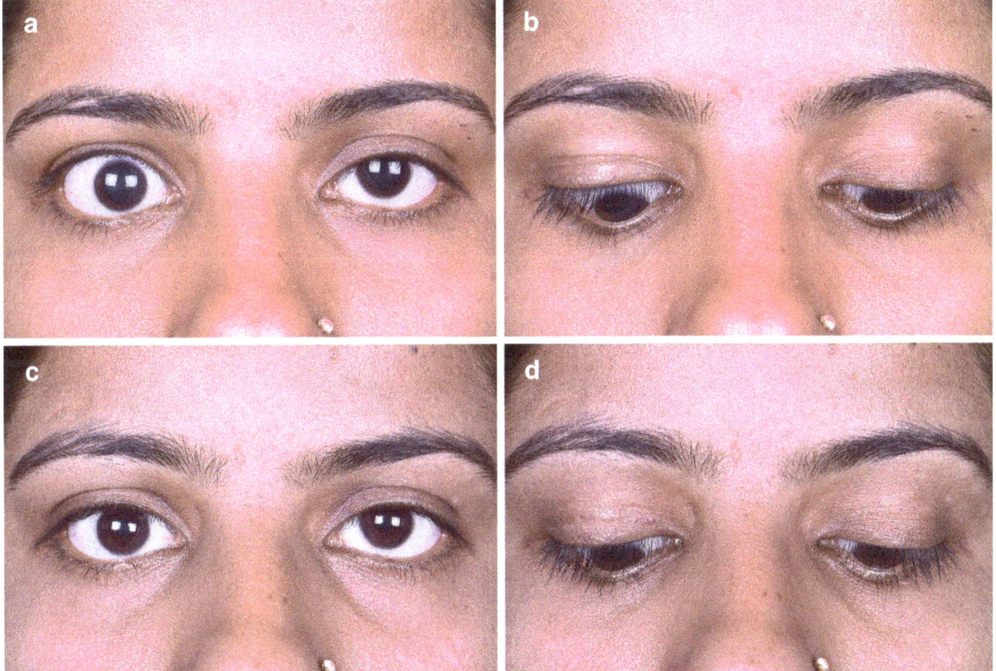

Fig. 15.14 A 23-year-old female with right moderate upper eyelid retraction (**a**) with downgaze lag (**b**). Three months following transcutaneous levator recession surgery (**c**), with eyelid scar hidden in the upper lid crease (**d**)

15.2.3.2 Full-Thickness Blepharotomy

This procedure is recommended for *moderate* upper eyelid retraction, and involves a full-thickness eyelid incision, from skin to conjunctiva, at the level of the eyelid crease (Fig. 15.9).

In 1999, Koornneef first communicated the graded full-thickness anterior blepharotomy procedure that was later published by Elner et al. in 2003 [12, 13]. In order to preserve the lid contour and prevent ptosis in the visual axis, Hintschich suggested preserving a central pedicle of conjunctiva to avoid a flat contour [14]. Once the desired lid height and contour have been achieved, only the skin and orbicularis is resutured. A review of surgical techniques in the correction of upper eyelid retraction in thyroid eye disease reported graded full-thickness anterior blepharotomy to be predictable, reproducible and a simple surgical procedure to master [15].

The surgical technique is described here (Figs. 15.15, 15.16, and 15.17). Via eyelid crease, dissection is carried out through the orbicularis to reach the upper edge of tarsus and the septum. The levator, Muller muscle, and conjunctiva are then incised just above the tarsal plate in a full-thickness fashion, until the desired lid height and contour is obtained. A central band of conjunctiva is left intact to avoid contour flattening. Only the anterior lamella (orbicularis and skin) is closed. This allows adequate and differential lengthening of the posterior lamella, thereby correcting the retraction in moderate cases (Fig. 15.18).

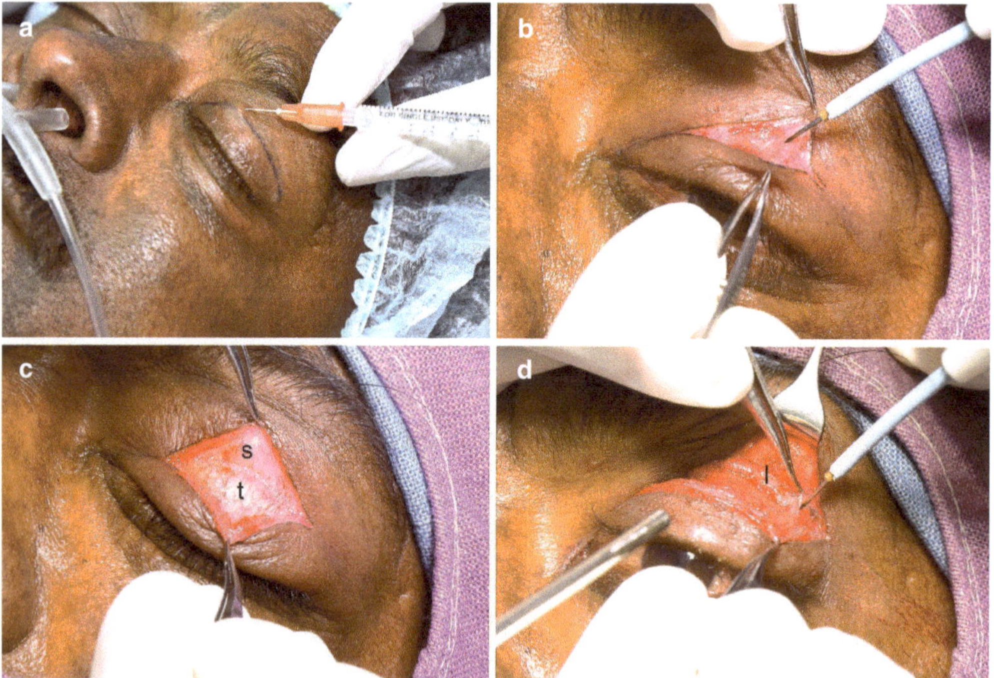

Fig. 15.15 Full-thickness Blepharotomy surgery (Koornneef): The eyelid crease is marked, and infiltrated with 0.5 ml of 2% Xylocaine with 1:100,000 adrenaline (**a**). The skin and orbicularis are incised with monopolar radiofrequency cautery (**b**). The tarsus (t) and septum (s) are exposed (**c**). The septum is opened to expose the levator (l) aponeurosis (**d**)

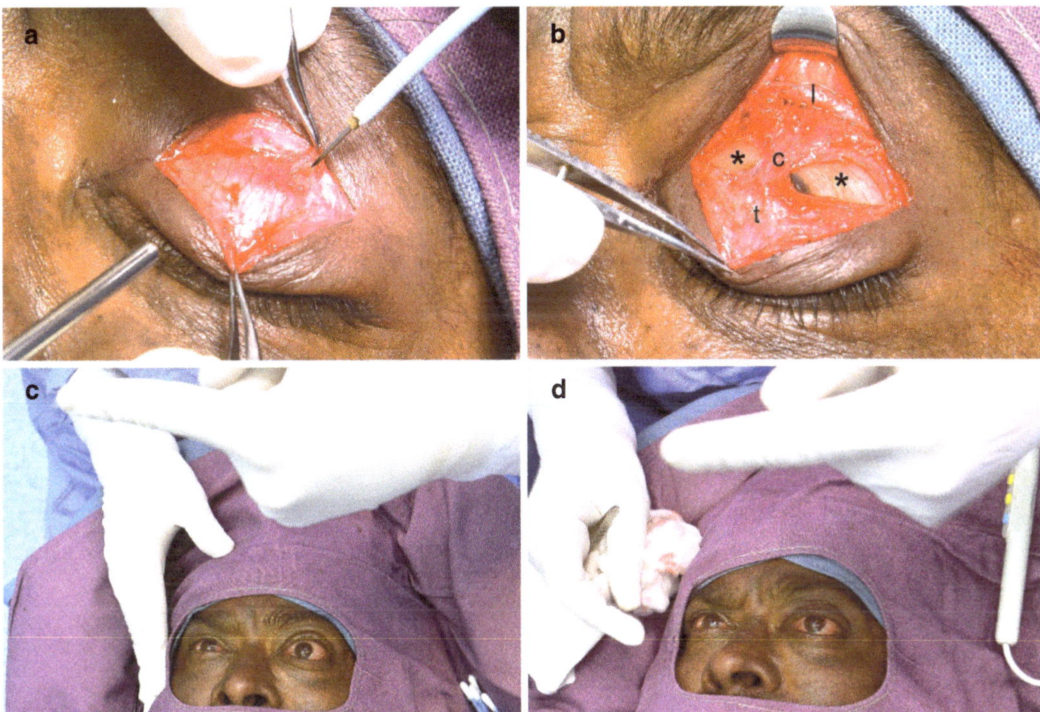

Fig. 15.16 Full-thickness Blepharotomy surgery (Koornneef) *continued*: The levator, Muller, and conjunctiva are then cut full thickness at the upper edge of the tarsus (**a**) to create a full-thickness blepharotomy (**b**). Note the recessed levator (l), the band of conjunctiva (**c**) attached to the tarsus (t), and the ocular surface visible through the full-thickness blepharotomy (asterisk). The central band of conjunctiva is left intact to avoid contour flattening. Note the intraoperative assessment of lid height, performed before (**c**) and after (**d**) blepharotomy by turning off the overhead lamp, and asking the patient to gaze in primary position

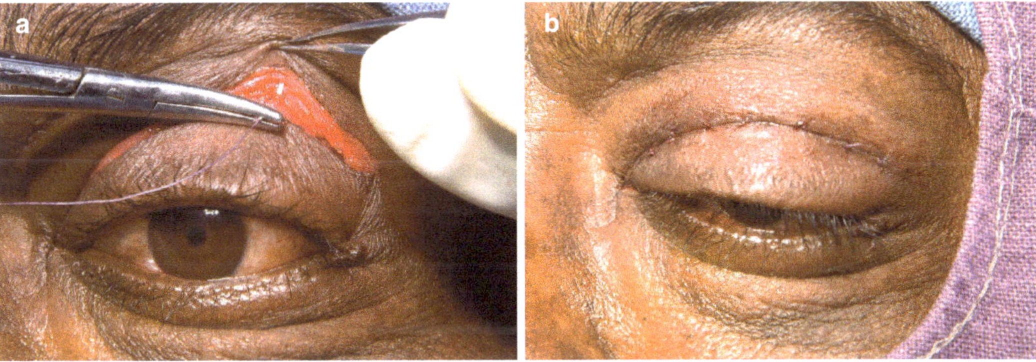

Fig. 15.17 Full-thickness Blepharotomy surgery (Koornneef) *continued.* The posterior lamella is left to epithelize, whereas the orbicularis (**a**) and skin (**b**) are closed in layers

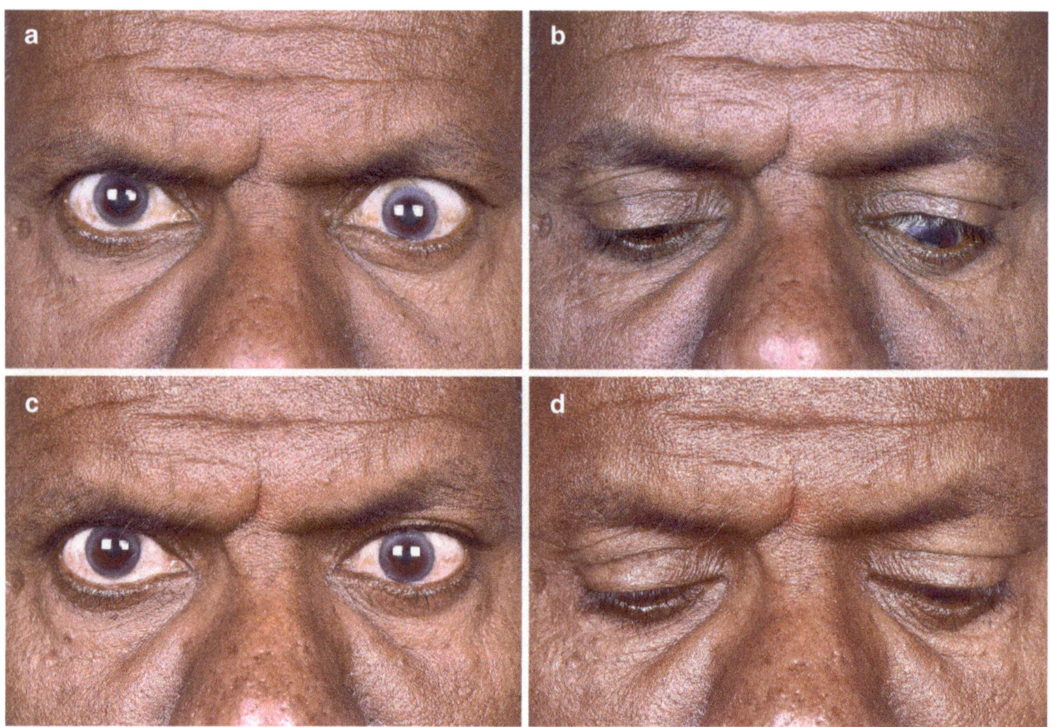

Fig. 15.18 Severe left upper eyelid retraction (**a**) with downgaze lag (**b**) in a 65-year-old male with inactive thyroid eye disease. Note the improvement in retraction following full-thickness blepharotomy (**c**), with resultant improvement in downgaze lag (**d**)

15.2.3.3 Levator Recession with Eyelid Spacers

Callahan first introduced the concept of using an absorbable spacer to lengthen the levator [16]. Later, various materials were reported as potential eyelid spacers such as donor sclera, autogenous tarsus, goretex, and mersilene mesh [17–22]. After 1980s, reports of spacer materials for this purpose are sparse [23]. Recently, Dermis fat graft and autologous tarsoconjunctival graft from upper eyelid to lower eyelid have been described for correction of eyelid retraction [24, 25]. Though not the author's personal choice, spacers can be used to further lengthen the upper or lower lid to augment lid recession (Figs. 15.9c and 15.20).

15.2.3.4 Adjustable Sutures in Eyelid Retraction Surgery

Small was the first to use an adjustable suture in order to control the lid margin position during surgery or in the early post-operative period [26]. This was further readdressed by Collin and Tucker [27, 28]. Adjustable sutures are not used by the majority of surgeons probably because the final results are seen only 4 or 6 weeks after surgery.

15.3 Lower Eyelid Retraction

Lower eyelid retraction is an often missed but significant sign of thyroid eye disease, and can be classified as mild (1 mm), moderate (2–3 mm), and severe (>3 mm) based on inferior scleral show in primary gaze (Fig. 15.19). Temporary nonsurgical correction for lower eyelid retraction can be achieved by hyaluronic acid gel injections [29] Chapter 5 Fig. 5.5. Surgically, two broad types of procedures have been described in the literature: *recession* of lower eyelid retractors, or *extirpation*, both being reported with and without an eyelid spacer graft (Fig. 15.20) [30]. Both can be performed either from the anterior transcutaneous or posterior trans-conjunctival route.

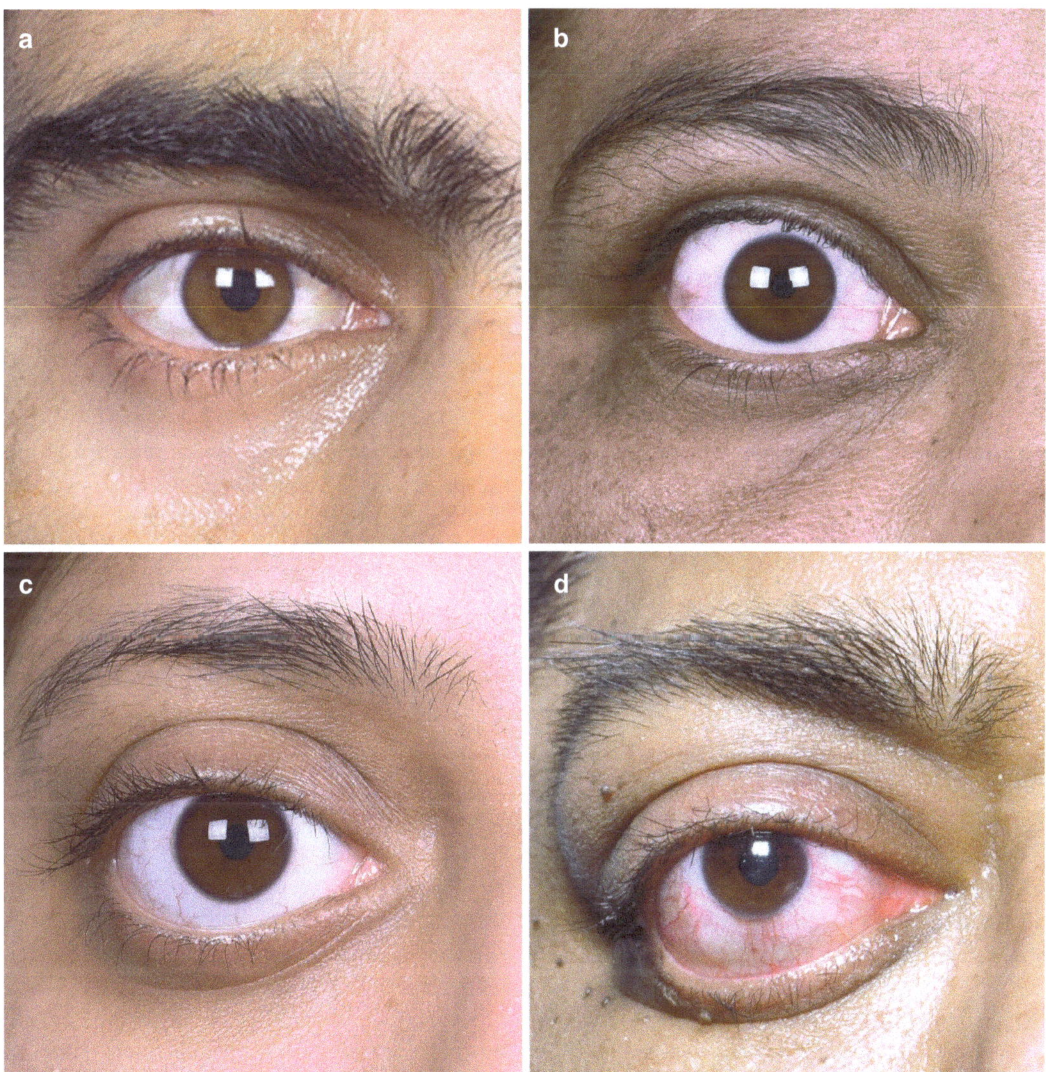

Fig. 15.19 Clinical grading of Lower Eyelid retraction. Normal position of the lower eyelid (**a**). Mild retraction with 1-mm scleral show (**b**), moderate retraction with 2–3 mm scleral show (**c**) and severe retraction with >3 mm scleral show (**d**)

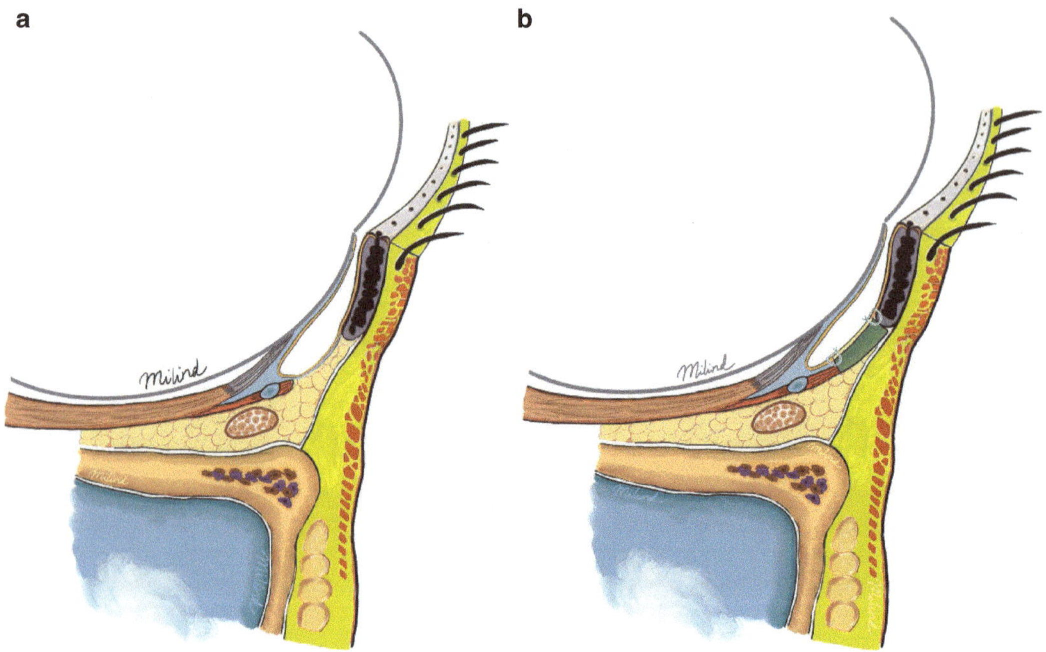

Fig. 15.20 Schematic diagram showing options for correction of lower eyelid retraction. Retractor release (**a**), and posterior lamellar spacer graft (**b**)

15.3.1 Recession of Lower Eyelid Retractors

The trans-conjunctival approach is preferred by most surgeons. The lower eyelid is everted on a Desmarre retractor and an infratarsal conjunctival incision is placed, starting from the lower pole of the caruncle, extending laterally just short of the lateral canthus (Fig. 15.21). The retractors are dissected from the orbicularis and septum anteriorly, and the conjunctiva posteriorly. This separation extends down to the fornix. The recessed retractors are either left alone in this recessed position or excised [18, 22, 31].

Variants of this procedure have been reported, namely composite recession of septum and retractors, use of adjuvants like 5 Fluorouracil or Mitomycin C, and simultaneous midface lift [30].

A good cosmetic correction can be obtained with trans-conjunctival recession of retractors, and can be augmented with an extreme lateral tarsorrhaphy (Fig. 15.22). The anterior approach is less popular, and is reported in the literature only when the eyelid surgery is associated with transcutaneous orbital decompression or when an alloplastic spacer is used to lift the eyelid [31, 32].

15.3.2 Recession of Retractors with Spacers

It is generally believed, that if the retraction is severe (>3 mm), a "spacer" interposed between the edge of recessed retractors and the lower border of the tarsus can improve the eyelid margin elevation. Homologous spacers include donor sclera or tarsus, and autologous spacers include tarso-conjunctival graft, auricular cartilage, hard palate mucosa, and dermis. Bioengineered dermal matrix such as Alloderm, or alloplastic materials such as polyester mesh (Mersilene), polytetrafluoroethylenes (Gortex), and high-density porous polyethylene (Medpor) have been reported.

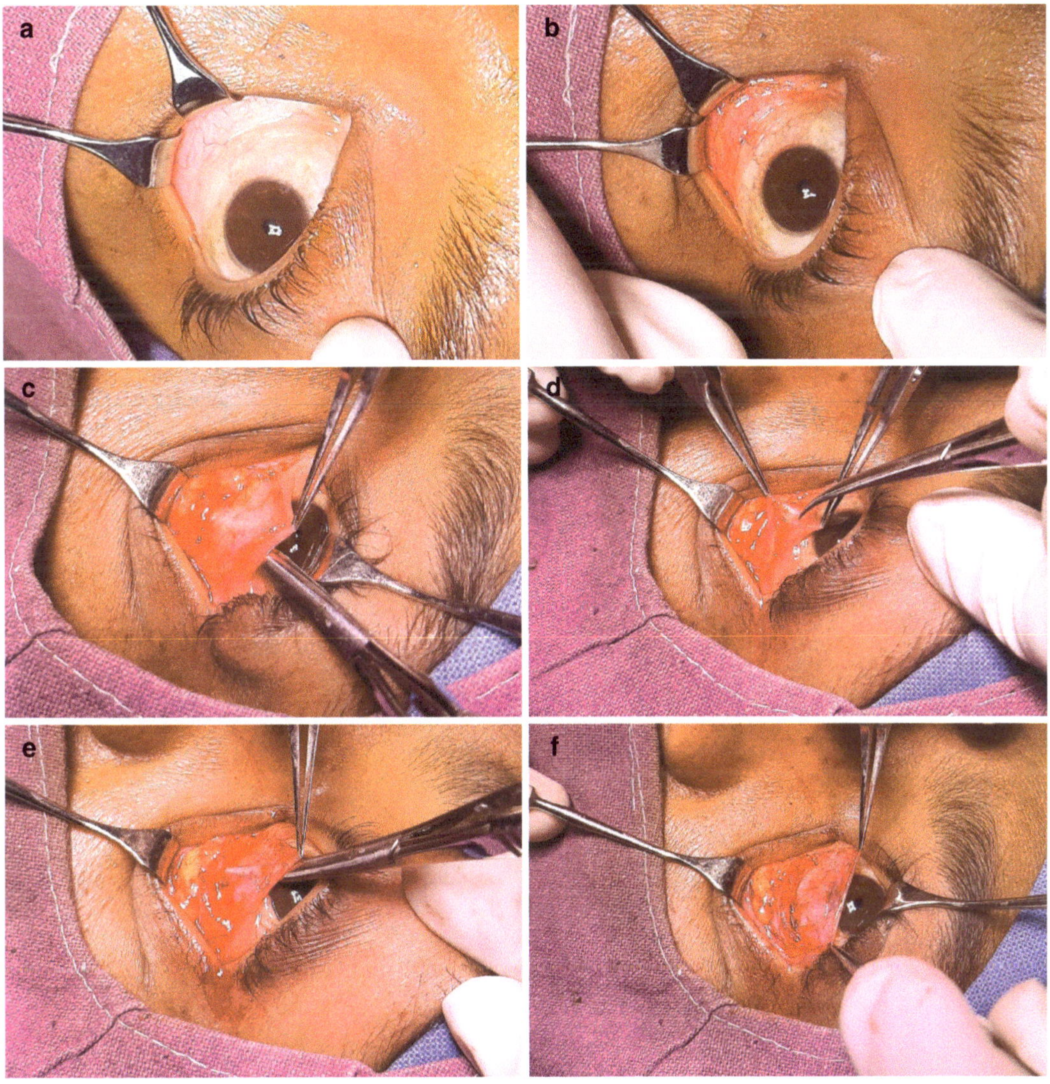

Fig. 15.21 Lower eyelid retractor release. Inferior forniceal exposure (**a**) and incision over palpebral conjunctiva (**b**). Fat/floor decompression if planned, can be performed first through the incision. The proximal end of conjunctival incision is picked up and pulled over the eyeball. The retractor is attached to it, thereby hiding the closed scissors held below this layer (**c**). The retractors and conjunctiva are separated from each other to allow recession of retractors (**d**). The scissor held below this plane is now easily visible trans-conjunctivally (**e**). Retractors are thus allowed to recess into the fornix (**f**)

An upward traction suture (Fig. 15.22b) is helpful in maintaining the upward pull during the healing phase so that the wound healing does not allow regression back to the retracted state. Often times, lower eyelid retractor lysis is performed along with orbital decompression surgery, and when preferentially combined with floor decompression, the downward shift of the eyeball aids in correcting the scleral show (Fig. 15.23).

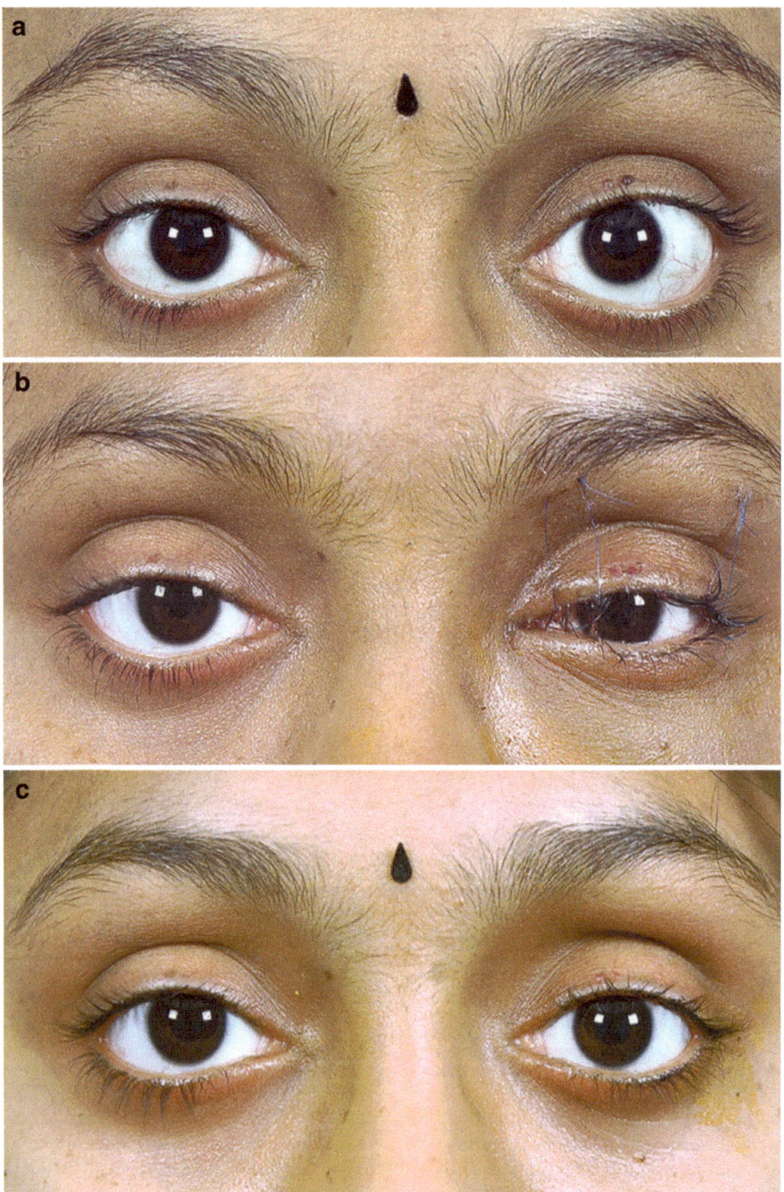

Fig. 15.22 Left inferior scleral show (**a**) with mild proptosis. Fat decompression, lower eyelid retractor release with fat-pearl grafting and post-operative lower eyelid traction suture (**b**) leads to a good cosmetic outcome (**c**)

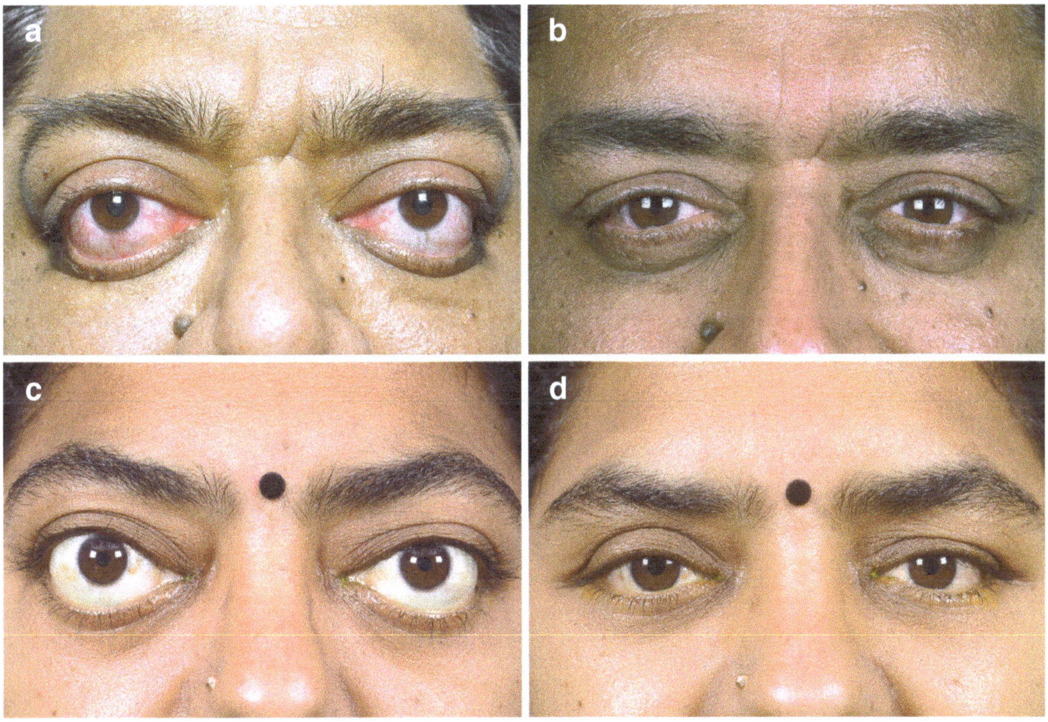

Fig. 15.23 Severe lower eyelid retraction (**a**, **c**) with moderate-to-severe proptosis. Along with orbital decompression, a lower eyelid retractor release was also performed to achieve good correction of proptosis as well as the eyelid retraction (**b**, **d**). Note that floor decompression was deliberately chosen as an option in both cases to allow downward displacement of the eyeball, thereby aiding in the correction of lower eyelid retraction

15.4 Summary

In summary, the spectrum of technical variations, and spacers described for the correction of eyelid retraction strongly suggests that the results are variable with any type of surgery, and there is no standardized approach. The upper lid retractors (levator and Muller muscle) can be weakened separately or in combination by an anterior or posterior approach. The muscles can be recessed, partially resected, or lengthened. Various materials have been tried as spacers between the recessed retractors and the tarsal border, but the results were not better than those obtained by just weakening the retractors. Residual lateral retraction is a well-known phenomenon, and most surgeons do more aggressive surgery laterally. Similar to ptosis surgery, patients undergoing correction of eyelid retraction should be made aware that it is not an exact science, and there is a possibility of revision or touch-up procedures in the post-operative period for better symmetry.

References

1. Goldstein I. Recession of the levator muscle for lagophthalmos in exophthalmic goiter. Arch Ophthalmol. 1934;11:389–93.
2. Henderson JW. Relief of eyelid retraction: a surgical procedure. Arch Ophthalmol. 1965;74:205–16.
3. Cruz AA, Ribeiro SF, Garcia DM, Akaishi PM, Pinto CT. Graves upper eyelid retraction. Surv Ophthalmol. 2013;58(1):63–76.
4. Shorr N, Seiff SR. The four stages of surgical rehabilitation of the patient with dysthyroid ophthalmopathy. Ophthalmology. 1986;93:476–83.
5. Naik MN, Vasanthapuram VH, Joseph J, Murthy SI. Microbial keratitis in thyroid eye disease: clinical features, microbiological profile, and treatment outcome. Ophthalmic Plast Reconstr Surg. 2019;35(6):543–8.
6. Waller RR. Eyelid malposition in Graves' ophthalmopathy. Trans Am Ophthalmol Soc. 1982;80:855–930.
7. Baylis HI, Cies WA, Kamin DF. Correction of upper eyelid retraction. Am J Ophthalmol. 1976;82:790–4.
8. Putterman AM, Urist M. Surgical treatment of upper eyelid retraction. Arch Ophthalmol. 1972;87:401–5.
9. Putterman AM, Fett DR. Miiller's muscle in the treatment of upper eyelid retraction: a 12-year study. Ophthal Surg. 1986;17:361–7.
10. Putterman AM. Surgical treatment of thyroid-related upper eyelid retraction. Graded Müller's muscle excision and levator recession. Ophthalmology. 1981;88(6):507–12.
11. Chalfin J, Putterman AM. Muller's muscle excision and levator recession in retracted upper lid. Treatment of thyroid-related retraction. Arch Ophthalmol. 1979;97:1487–91.
12. Elner VM, Hassan AS, Frueh BR. Graded full-thickness anterior blepharotomy for upper eyelid retraction. Trans Am Ophthalmol Soc. 2003;101:67–73.
13. Elner VM, Hassan AS, Frueh BR. Graded full-thickness anterior blepharotomy for upper eyelid retraction. Arch Ophthalmol. 2004;122:55–60.
14. Hintschich C, Haritoglou C. Full thickness eyelid transsection (blepharotomy) for upper eyelid lengthening in lid retraction associated with Graves' disease. Br J Ophthalmol. 2005;89:413–6.
15. Kazim M, Gold KG. A review of surgical techniques to correct upper eyelid retraction associated with thyroid eye disease. Curr Opin Ophthalmol. 2011;22(5):391–3.
16. Callahan A. Levator recession with reattachment to the tarsus with collagen film. Arch Ophthalmol. 1965;73:800–2.
17. Meltzer MA. Surgery for lid retraction. Ann Ophthalmol. 1978;10:102–6.
18. Flanagan JC. Retraction of the eyelids secondary to thyroid ophthalmopathy—its surgical correction with sclera and the fate of the graft. Trans Am Ophthalmol Soc. 1980;78:657–85.
19. Brown BZ. The use of homologous tarsus as a donor graft in lid surgery. Ophthalmic Plast Reconstr Surg. 1985;1:91–5.
20. Morax S, Hurbli T. Choice of surgical treatment for Graves' disease. J Craniomaxillofac Surg. 1987;15:174–81.
21. Downes RN, Jordan K. The surgical management of dysthyroid related eyelid retraction using Mersilene mesh. Eye (Lond). 1989;3(Pt 4):385–90.
22. Doxanas MT, Dryden RM. The use of sclera in the treatment of dysthyroid eyelid retraction. Ophthalmology. 1981;88:887–94.
23. Hedin A. Is scleral transplantation necessary in the treatment of upper eyelid retraction? Orbit. 1985;4:115–20.
24. Kuzmanović Elabjer B, Miletić D, Bušić M, Bišćan Tvrdi A, Bosnar D, Bjeloš M. Dermis-fat graft for correction of recurrent severe upper eyelid retraction in Graves' orbitopathy. Acta Clin Croat. 2018;57(1):173–6.
25. Lee NG, Habib L, Hall J, Freitag SK. Simultaneous ipsilateral transconjunctival repair of upper and lower eyelid retraction in thyroid-associated ophthalmopathy. Orbit. 2019;38(2):124–9.
26. Small RG. Upper eyelid retraction in Graves' ophthalmopathy: a new surgical technique and a study of the abnormal levator muscle. Trans Am Ophthalmol Soc. 1988;86:725–93.
27. Collin JR, O'Donnell BA. Adjustable sutures in eyelid surgery for ptosis and lid retraction. Br J Ophthalmol. 1994;78:167–74.
28. Tucker SM, Collin R. Repair of upper eyelid retraction: a comparison between adjustable and non-adjustable sutures. Br J Ophthalmol. 1995;79:658–60.
29. Goldberg RA, Lee S, Jayasundera T, et al. Treatment of lower eyelid retraction by expansion of the lower eyelid with hyaluronic acid gel. Ophthalmic Plast Reconstr Surg. 2007;23:343–8.
30. Ribeiro SF, Shekhovtsova M, Duarte AF, Velasco Cruz AA. Graves lower eyelid retraction. Ophthalmic Plast Reconstr Surg. 2016;32(3):161–9.
31. Harvey JT, Anderson RL. The aponeurotic approach to eyelid retraction. Ophthalmology. 1981;88:513–24.
32. Wong JF, Soparkar CN, Patrinely JR. Correction of lower eyelid retraction with high density porous polyethylene: the Medpor® lower eyelid spacer. Orbit. 2001;20:217–25.

Eyelid Conditions in Thyroid Eye Disease in East Asians

16

Gangadhara Sundar

16.1 Introduction

Thyroid Eye Disease (TED) (also called Thyroid Orbitopathy, Graves Orbitopathy, Thyroid-Related Inflammatory Orbitopathy) is a relatively common condition, yet poorly recognized and frequently mismanaged. Compared to the Western world, there exist several variations in the knowledge, attitude, and practice of Thyroid Orbitopathy in Asians with patient, general physician, and ophthalmologist-related factors. These factors have direct implications on the diagnosis, management, and clinical outcomes. Moreover, the clinical presentation may also be frequently different owing to inherent variation of orbital bony anatomy, soft tissue involvement (extraocular muscles, fat, fibrous connective tissue—intermuscular septum, orbital septum, retaining ligaments, etc.), and tissue response to medical and surgical intervention [1].

Eyelid changes are the most common and early presentation of thyroid eye disease. When typical eyelid signs are present (i.e., upper eyelid retraction, lid lag, temporal flare, etc.) along with a history of hyperthyroidism with or without underlying strabismus and proptosis, the diagnosis is often obvious. However, a definitive clinical diagnosis can be challenging in the early active inflammatory phase of the disease, especially for the general ophthalmologist, when there is no associated thyroid dysfunction or orbital or strabismus signs, commonly resulting in misdiagnosis and mismanagement [2].

G. Sundar (✉)
Diplomate, The American Board of Ophthalmology, Orbit and Oculofacial Surgery/Thyroid Eye Disease Service, Department of Ophthalmology, National University Hospital, National University of Singapore, Singapore
e-mail: Gangadhara_sundar@nuhs.edu.sg

S. Rath, M. N. Naik (eds.), *Surgery in Thyroid Eye Disease*,
https://doi.org/10.1007/978-981-32-9220-8_16

16.2 Challenges in the Diagnosis and Management of TED

Some factors related to patients, general physicians, and ophthalmologists that pose challenges in the diagnosis and management of thyroid eye disease are highlighted in Table 16.1.

Bottom line, it should be remembered that Thyroid Eye Disease is a clinical diagnosis, supported by laboratory tests (thyroid function tests, autoantibodies when positive) and/or imaging, but not ruled out in their absence.

Table 16.1 Patient, general physician, and ophthalmologist-related factors resulting in delay in diagnosis and improper management of TED patients

Patient-related factors	Physician/Endocrinologist-related factors	Ophthalmologist-related factors
Lack of awareness of disease entity	Limited awareness of disease entity	Unaware of the prevalence of condition, nonspecific early clinical signs
Higher threshold to seek attention	Absence of definitive confirmatory tests at initial presentation	Lack of access or failure to refer to a specialist who can make a definitive clinical diagnosis, especially in the absence of specific confirmatory test
Misled by initial misdiagnosis	Diagnosis ruled out even when considered clinically, because of normal Thyroid Function Tests (TFTs), absence of autoantibodies, "normal" imaging findings (early orbitopathy, fat predominant orbitopathy with normal extraocular muscles)	Unfamiliar with treatment modalities, outcomes of proactive management in early active phase of the disease and limited experience in managing the condition
Poor knowledge and attitude to medical and surgical advice—personal, family, and socioeconomic reasons	Failure to refer to experienced specialists during the onset and early phases of the disease	Expecting symptomatic treatment or observation to be effective for all patients with TED regardless of severity
Tissue considerations: Bony anatomy, variable soft tissue involvement (extraocular muscles, fat, intermuscular septum, and other fibro-connective tissues)	Assumption that management of thyroid dysfunction will resolve the signs and symptoms of TED	

16.3 Eyelid Signs in East Asians

Eyelid and ocular signs can be classified into those manifested in early and late TED. Upper eyelid, lower eyelid, and other ophthalmic signs—typical (easy to diagnosis) and atypical (often missed, misdiagnosed, and mismanaged) signs are shown in Table 16.2.

Acquired epiblepharon is a relatively unique yet frequently encountered condition in East Asians (Fig. 16.2). Pathophysiologic mechanisms include increased orbital pressure, from edema and/or infiltration with resultant extraocular muscle and/or fat volume enlargement, causing anterior migration of globe and orbital soft tissues. This in turn, in the presence of relatively

Table 16.2 Typical and atypical signs in early and late Thyroid Eye Disease

Typical signs	Atypical (nonspecific) signs
Early disease	Late disease
Upper and/or lower eyelid puffiness (edema and erythema) (Fig. 16.1a)	Conjunctival injection, chemosis, and conjunctivochalasis (nonspecific and hence missed)
Intermittent and variable eyelid retraction often masked by voluntary closure (from photic discomfort, dryness, and exposure)	Ptosis (myasthenia gravis) (Fig. 16.1b)
Maybe unmasked with dim lights, ocular surface anesthesia, candid clinical examination, etc.).	Upper eyelid crease: New onset when previously absent or superior migration of preexisting crease
Infrequent blink, lid lag (levator muscle inflammation and edema)	Unilateral presentation
	Symptoms preceding obvious clinical signs
	Active orbitopathy in the absence of obvious conjunctival injection, chemosis, caruncular edema, etc. "Silent Active Disease" (SAD)
Early disease	Late disease
Upper eyelid retraction, with temporal flare	Acquired epiblepharon
Lid lag (levator fibrosis)	Masked eyelid retraction from overlying brow fat expansion, brow ptosis, and/or dermatochalasis
Lagophthalmos	Ptosis (levator dehiscence, new-onset myasthenia, overcorrected eyelid retraction repair, severe dermatochalasis, etc.)
Lower eyelid retraction	Persistent unilateral disease (masked bilateral asymmetric disease)
Bilateral and symmetrical features	Masked eyelid retraction and underlying strabismus from ocular surface discomfort
	Superior limbic keratoconjunctivitis (rare in East Asians in TED)

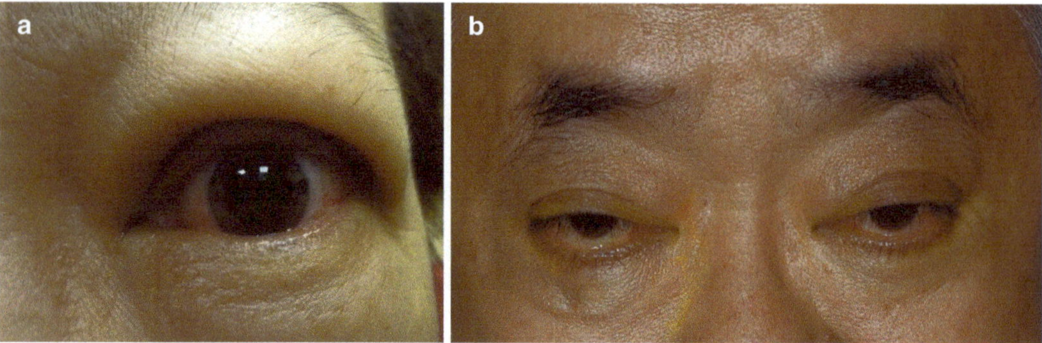

Fig. 16.1 (a) Eyelid puffiness and erythema in early active TED. (b) TED presenting as ptosis in a patient with coexistent myasthenia gravis

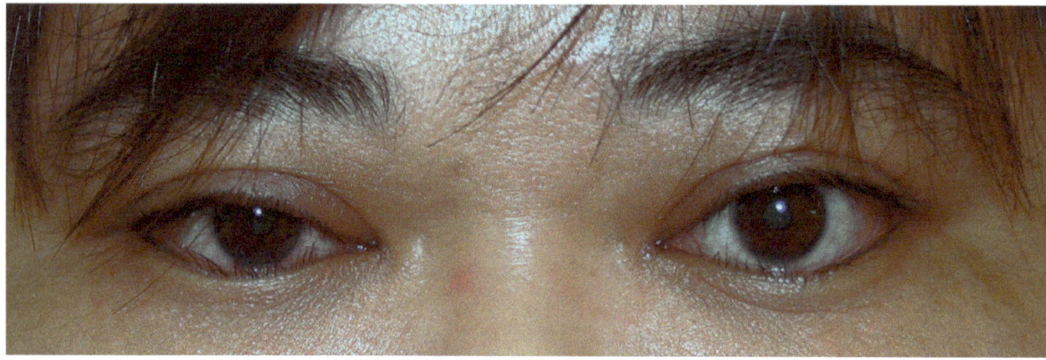

Fig. 16.2 Acquired epiblepharon in an East Asian patient with active TED

tight eyelids and frequent association of myopia with larger globes in this population, results in overriding of the anterior over the posterior lamella causing a lash-conjunctival and lash-corneal touch [3, 4].

"Silent Active Disease" (SAD) is yet another important feature observed in Asian and in East Asian patients (Fig. 16.3) [5]. This is a condition where there are progressive signs (proptosis, strabismus, and visual loss) and symptoms from underlying inflammatory and structural soft tissue changes in the absence of perceptible signs of inflammation of the ocular or adnexal surface, i.e., conjunctival erythema, chemosis, injection, or eyelid erythema. In fact, these are also frequently misdiagnosed and occasionally even

present with vision-threatening optic neuropathy. In such situations, unless the degree of suspicion is high, appropriate color vision testing, perimetry and imaging requested, they are often missed.

Much less frequently, obvious clinical features may be masked by ocular surface discomfort and either involuntary or voluntary closure of the eyes (Fig. 16.4).

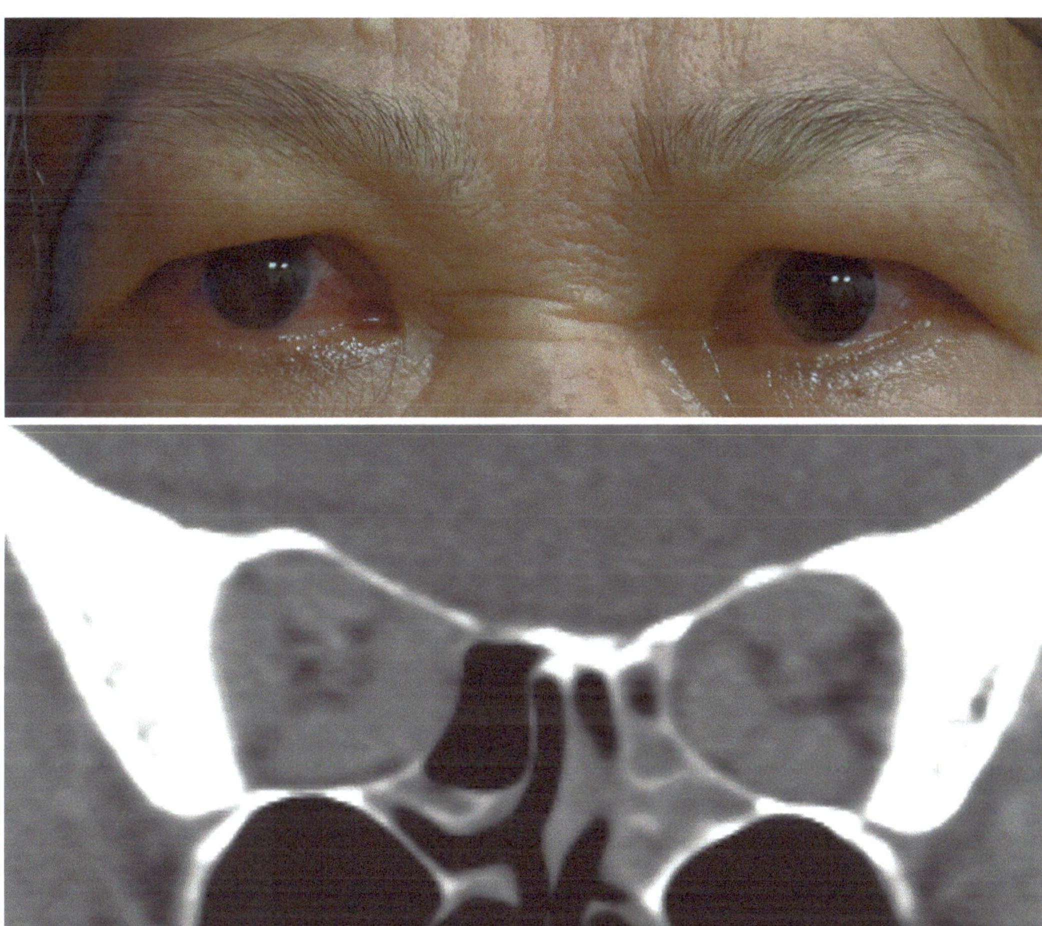

Fig. 16.3 "Silent Active Disease" in a 75-year-old patient (top). Note the absence of obvious clinical signs of inflammation. Coronal CT scan of the same lady showing apical crowding (bottom)

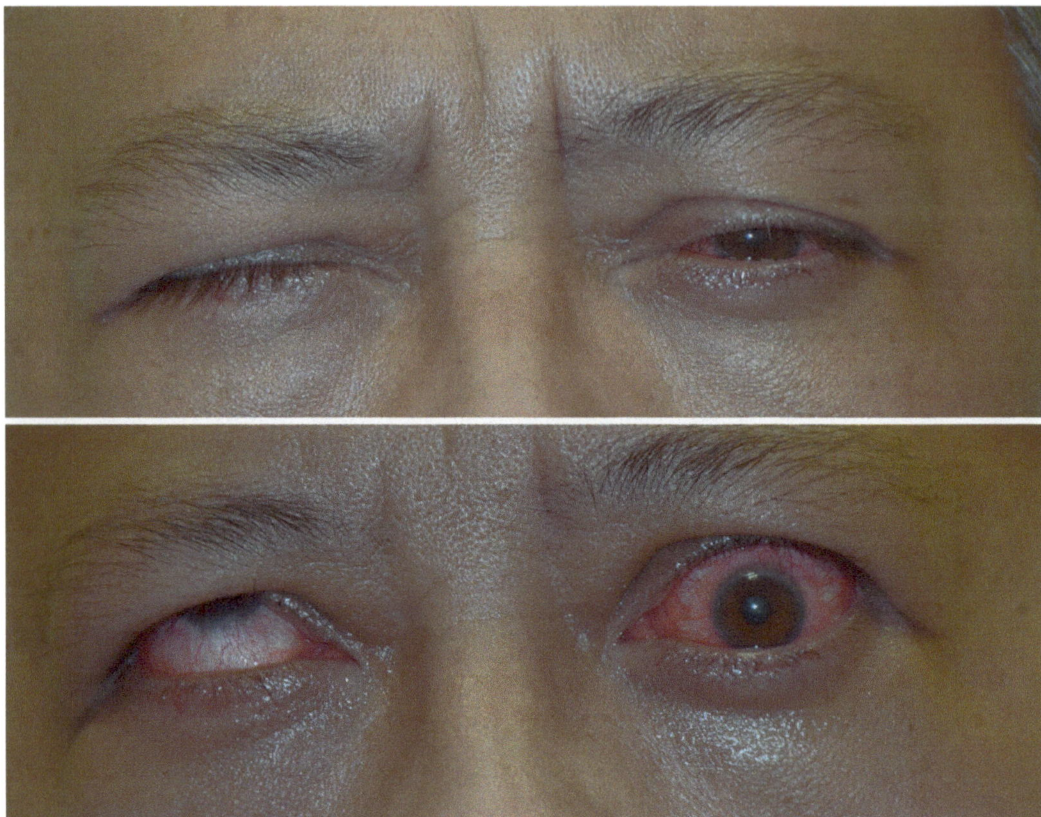

Fig. 16.4 Unmasking of underlying strabismus and upper eyelid retraction in a 60-year-old patient with active severe TED

16.4 Consequences of Eyelid Retraction and Epiblepharon

Upper and/or lower eyelid retraction, lid lag, acquired epiblepharon, and other clinical features may have either esthetic and/or functional consequences, which result in significant affliction of quality of life. Corneal complications include fine to coarse localized keratopathy limited to areas of exposure or lash-cornea touch. It thus warrants intervention, either by aggressive lubrication alone, by minimally invasive techniques (early active or mild inactive disease) or surgical intervention (moderate to severe disease during the burnt-out phase). Likewise, conventional surgical techniques of epiblepharon management may also not work in this situation. Severe exposure keratopathy with proptosis may result in corneal ulceration and even perforation resulting in blindness, warranting more aggressive procedures such as an urgent orbital decompression with blepharotomy and/or tarsorrhaphy.

16.5 Management Considerations

Most eyelid signs may be managed conservatively and expectantly. However, those with functional and esthetic compromise may be managed based on their symptoms, quality of life, and acceptance of procedures with realistic expectations. An overview of management of eyelid retraction with or without active inflammatory disease is shown in Table 16.3.

Table 16.3 Management of upper eyelid retraction in Early Active Disease

Degree of eyelid retraction	Management
Mild disease, minimal Quality of Life affliction	Observation, conservative measures (head elevation, eye protection, lubricants, moisture goggles at night, frequent conscious blinking of eyes)
Moderate disease, significant Quality of Life affliction	Management of primary orbital inflammatory disease—Pulsed high-dose intravenous methylprednisolone infusions (Fig. 16.5) (3)
Mild—moderate disease (primarily esthetic affliction)	Temporizing procedures • Neuromodulators (e.g., botulinum toxin 2.5–10 units) • Tissue fillers (e.g., hyaluronic acid) (Fig. 16.6) • Corticosteroid injections (triamcinolone): Upper eyelid (10 mg) and Orbital (30 mg)

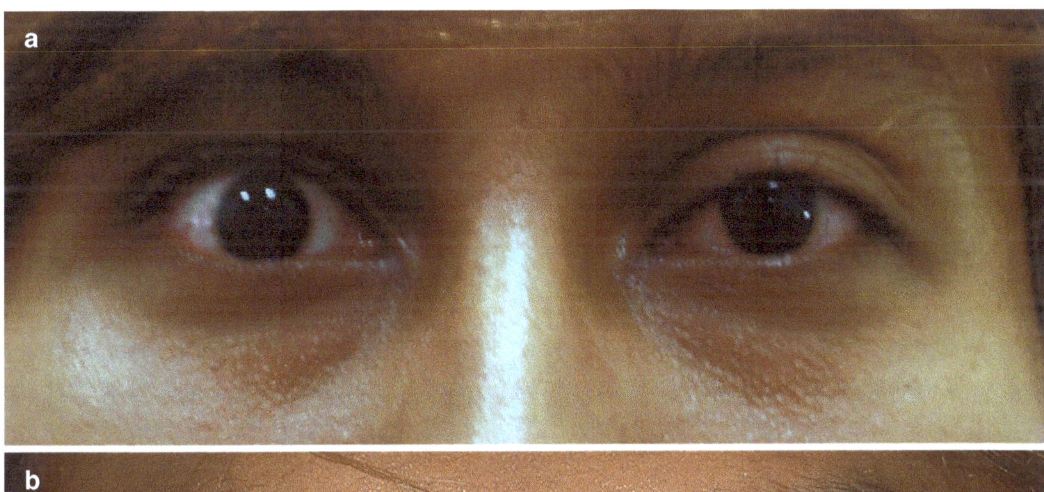

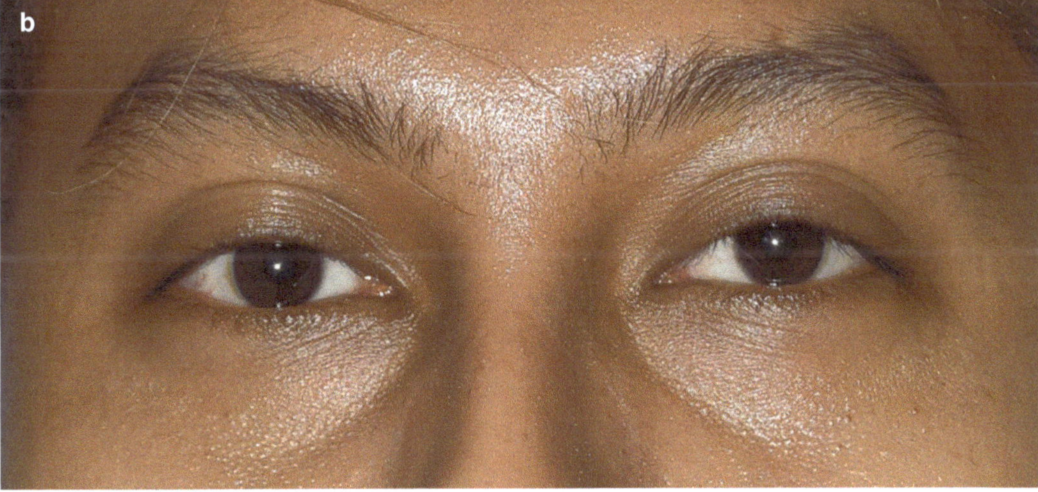

Fig. 16.5 Recent onset right upper eyelid retraction (Mild Active TED) (**a**) reversed with high dose (NUH) Intravenous Methylprednisolone protocol (**b**)

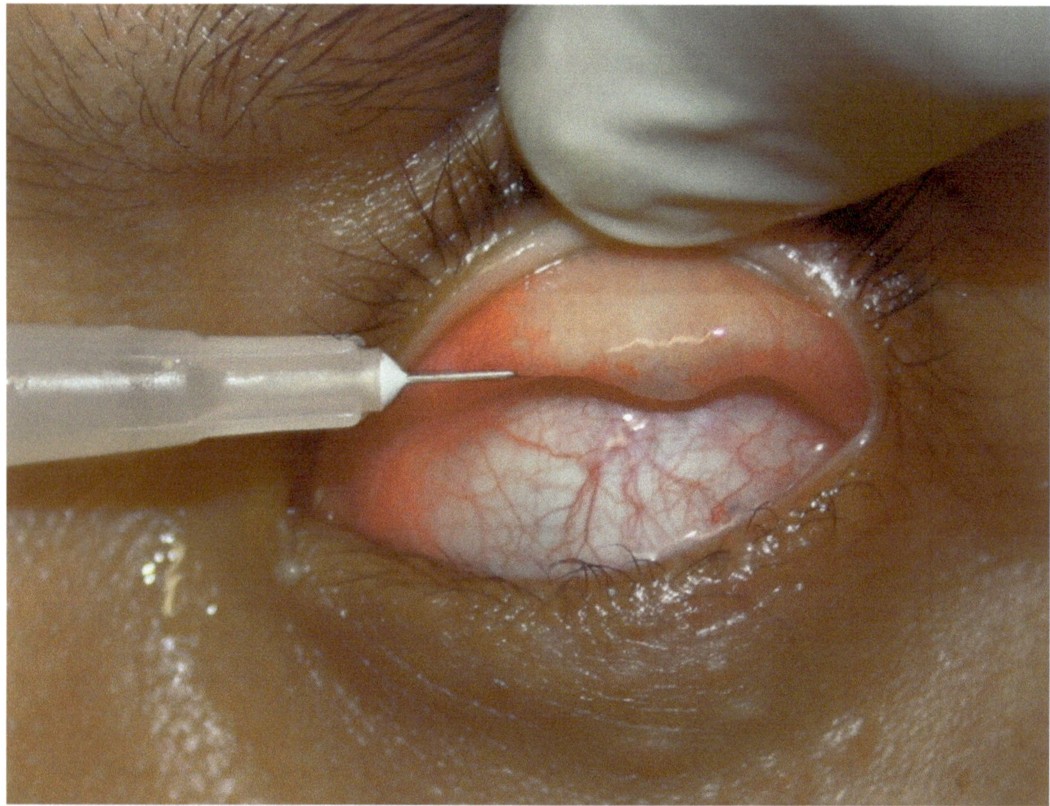

Fig. 16.6 Supratarsal tissue filler injection for left upper eyelid retraction

16.6 Management of Eyelid Retraction in Late "Inactive" Disease

Eyelid retraction may be surgically addressed based on the presence and severity of underlying orbitopathy (proptosis), exposure keratopathy, compressive optic neuropathy, strabismus, or just disfiguration. There is evidence and a trend toward addressing underlying orbital volumetric and pressure changes in addition to extraocular muscle length normalization prior to strabismus and eyelid retractor repair for optimal results. An overview of eyelid retraction and epiblepharon is shown in Table 16.4.

Table 16.4 Management of eyelid retraction and epiblepharon in late inactive disease

Degree of eyelid retraction	Management
Mild eyelid retraction, minimal Quality of Life affliction	Lubricants, eye protection, e.g., moisture goggles at night, sunglasses, etc. Tissue fillers (upper eyelid)
Upper eyelid	
1. Anterior (transcutaneous) approach	a. Levator stretching b. Levator disinsertion with/without spacers (9) c. Blepharotomy (Fig. 16.7) i. Full-thickness complete blepharotomy ii. Graded blepharotomy (10)
2. Posterior (transconjunctival) approach	2a. Muller's muscle resection b. Muller's muscle resection with levator stretching
3. Combined approaches (11)	3a. Retractor management posteriorly and crease management anteriorly b. Blepharotomy may occasionally be combined with an orbital decompression if severe and patient desirous of a single-stage rehabilitation
4. Others	4. On occasion, correction of underlying strabismus may address apparent upper eyelid retraction (Fig. 16.8)
Lower eyelid	
A. Eyelid retraction 1. Anterior approach	Transcutaneous approaches to the lower eyelid are generally avoided as they result in prominent and visible scars and the pathology is more of the middle and posterior lamellae
2. Posterior approach (12)	These are the most commonly performed procedures, after addressing underlying proptosis (either a fat alone or a fat and bony wall orbital decompression) a. If only middle lamellar scarring is present a middle lamellar release may be performed with the introduction of a spacer (Alloderm®, donor sclera) may be considered (Fig. 16.9) b. Alternatively, and more commonly, when both posterior lamella and middle lamella are shortened, a hard palate mucosal graft may be used to augment the posterior lamella of the eyelid with gratifying results. It is important to secure adequate release of the lower eyelid retractors and combine lower eyelid elevation to obtain good outcomes
3. Combined approaches (anterior and posterior)	Combined eyelid surgery with orbital surgery or strabismus surgery: Occasionally, orbital decompression may be combined with a lower eyelid retraction repair either by a near full-thickness blepharotomy sparing the eyelid skin or retractor release with middle lamella and/or posterior lamellar augmentation. In special cases with predominant orbital fat and lower eyelid retractor stretching performing a generous lateral orbital floor decompression alone may improve lower eyelid retraction.
B. Acquired epiblepharon	Epiblepharon with minimal proptosis: modified Hotz procedure Epiblepharon with significant proptosis: Orbital decompression alone or with modified Hotz procedure

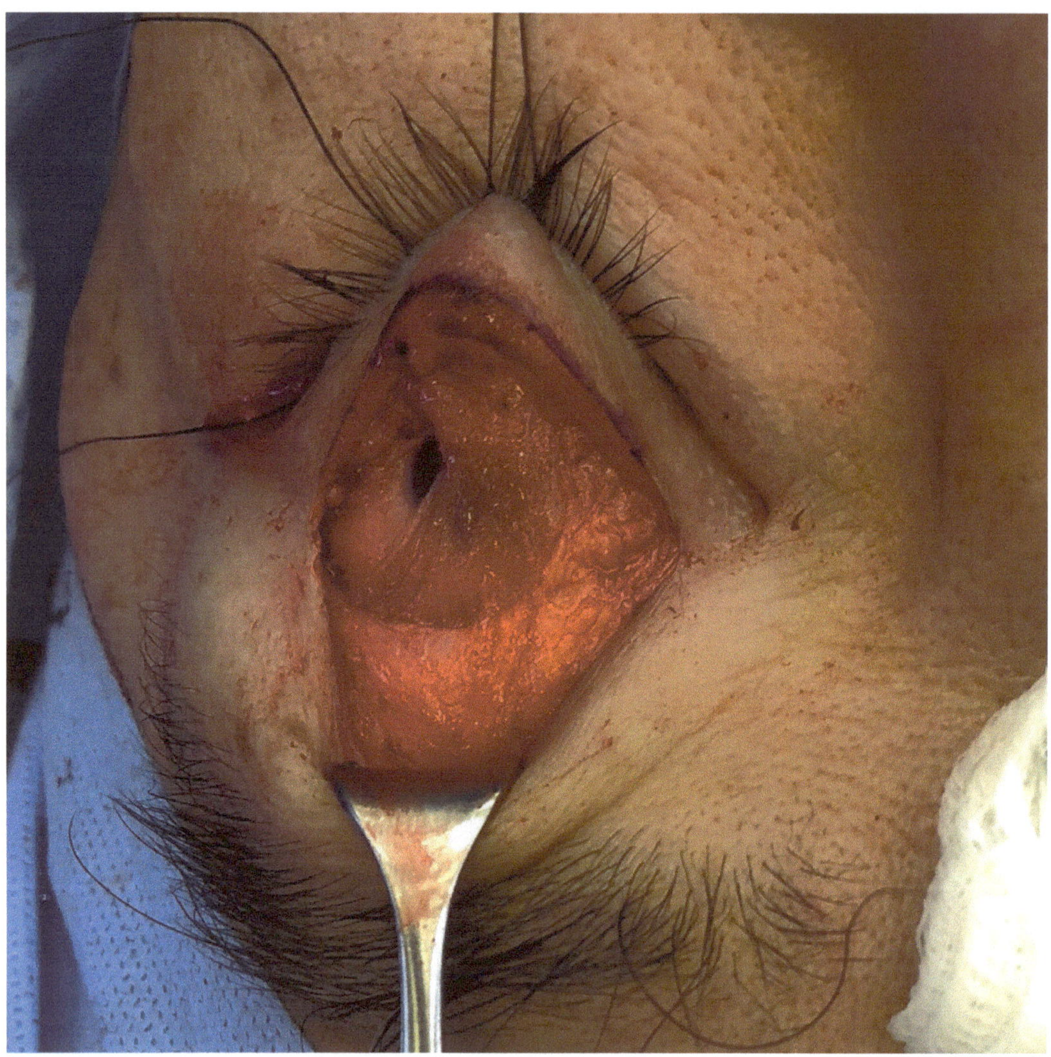

Fig. 16.7 Graded blepharotomy for upper eyelid retraction in inactive TED

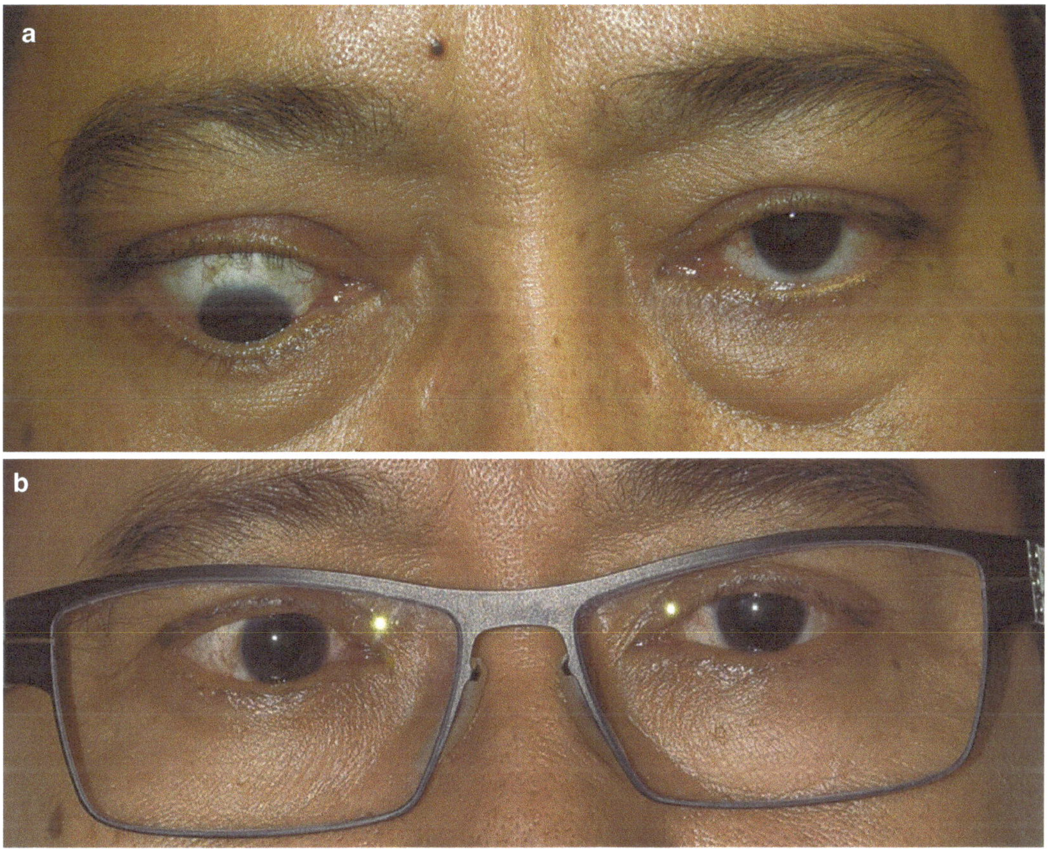

Fig. 16.8 Pseudoretraction of upper eyelid (**a**) corrected following strabismus correction for right hypotropia (**b**)

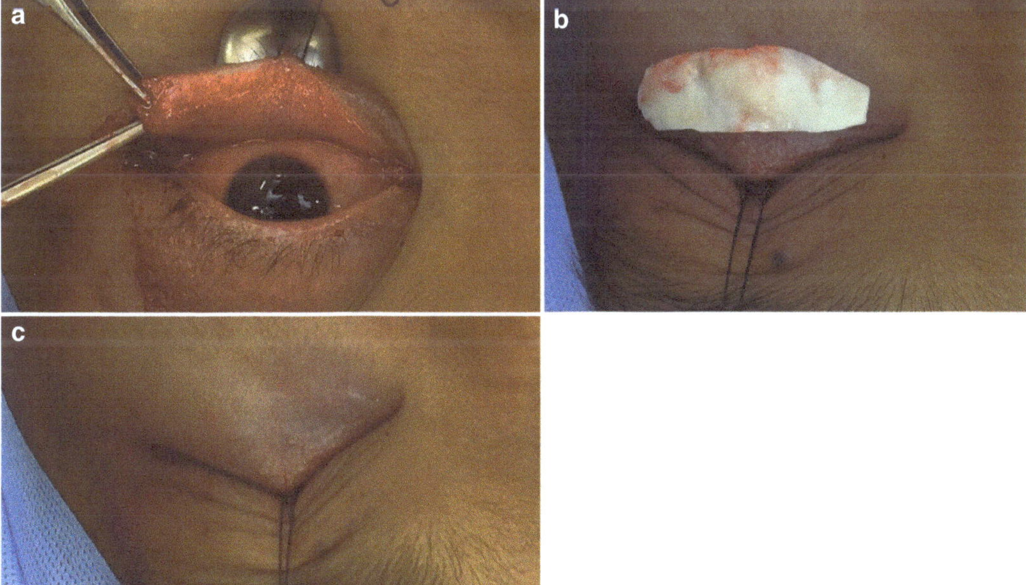

Fig. 16.9 Left lower eyelid retraction repair. Inferior middle lamellar release (**a**). Middle lamellar spacer (Alloderm®) graft (**b**), Frost traction suture of the lower eyelid post-operatively (**c**)

16.7 Postoperative Management

General measures include maintenance of euthyroid status, good general health, provide globe protection, avoid smoking, etc. Ophthalmic management post-operatively includes placing stretching reverse Frost sutures (upper eyelid retraction) or Frost sutures (lower eyelid retraction) to maintain eyelid traction during the early post-operative recovery phase. Occasionally, traction exercises may be of help in patients with mild early post-operative undercorrections. Revision surgery may be indicated to achieve better symmetry and contour. If underlying orbital disease has not been addressed, an orbital decompression may aid post-operative eyelid surgery results.

16.8 Outcomes and Complications

In general, most patients are positively benefited from eyelid surgery, performed either as a primary or secondary procedure (14). Patients should, however, be counselled regarding post-operative complications, both major (potentially blinding) and minor, e.g., undercorrections, overcorrections (Fig. 16.10), asymmetry of eyelid height and/or contour, possible need for repeat procedures) and have realistic expectations.

While some minor abnormalities may be conservatively managed, others may require a revision procedure.

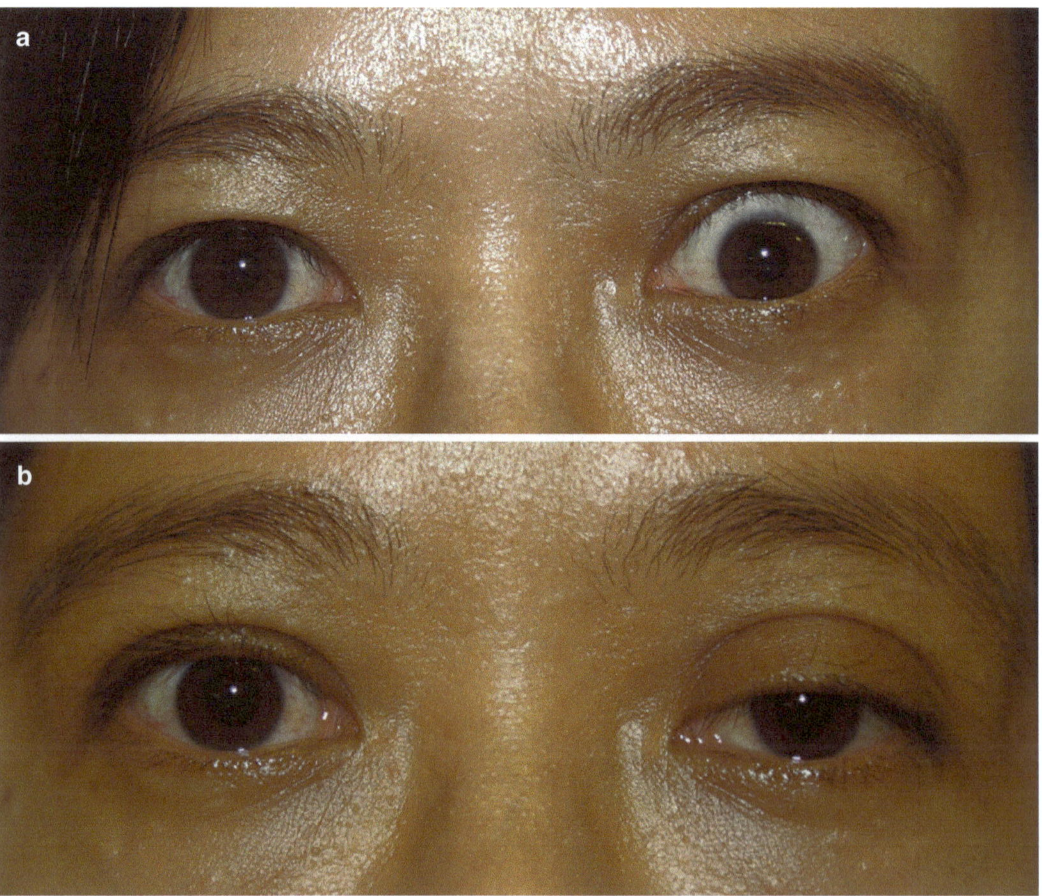

Fig. 16.10 Left upper eyelid ptosis (**b**) from over-correction of left upper eyelid retraction repair (**a**)

16.9 Conclusion

In summary, eyelid and orbital consequences in East Asians have both common and unique features with sociocultural perspectives, medical, and surgical considerations. A clearer understanding regarding both typical and atypical features, pathogenesis, and stages of disease, knowledge of medical and surgical interventions go a long way in managing patients affected by TED effectively.

References

1. Sundar G. Eyelid and eyebrow surgery in East Asians in expert techniques in ophthalmic surgery. New Delhi: Jaypee Publishers; 2016.
2. Lim NC, Sundar G, Amrith S, Lee KO. Thyroid eye disease: a Southeast Asian experience. Br J Ophthalmol. 2015;99(4):512–8.
3. Park SW, Khwarg SI, Kim N, Lee MJ, Choung HK. Acquired lower epiblepharon in thyroid associated ophthalmopathy of Koreans. Ophthalmology. 2012;119(2):390–5.
4. Sundar G. Congenital and acquired Epiblepharon. https://eyewiki.aao.org/Congenital_and_acquired_epiblepharon.
5. Hiromatsu Y, Eguchi H, Tani J, Kasaoka M, Teshima Y. Graves' ophthalmopathy: epidemiology and natural history. Intern Med. 2014;53(5):353–60.

Periorbital Aesthetic Considerations in Thyroid Eye Disease

17

Milind N. Naik

17.1 Introduction

Outcome measures of aesthetic rehabilitation for TED have been evaluated exclusively in relation to post-operative exophthalmometry and palpebral fissure height. However, there are several aesthetic concerns in the upper eyelid and brow region that are specific to TED, yet they have long been outside the purview of our traditional assessment of cosmetic rehabilitation of a TED patient. These include glabellar frown lines, brow fat expansion, and lacrimal gland enlargement.

Lower eyelid concerns not exclusive to TED, but often seen in these patients include eyelid bags, subconjunctival fat prolapse, and under-eye hollows. To address these concerns, patients are often treated with Botulinum toxin, Hyaluronic acid fillers, and Blepharoplasty. This chapter discusses the aesthetic concerns in TED patients, and their management.

17.2 Functional Anatomy

It is of paramount importance that the surgeon knows the dynamic and functional anatomy so as to give aesthetically and functionally pleasing results. The *eyebrow* is normally at the level of the superior orbital rim in men and slightly above it in women. The male eyebrow is rather flat, whereas the female eyebrow arches higher laterally (Fig. 17.1). The *upper eyelid crease* is a critical surgical landmark and is formed by the cutaneous expansion of the levator aponeurosis. It is generally 7–8 mm above the lid margin in females, and slightly lower in males [1]. The *Eyelid fold* is formed by the preseptal skin and orbicularis muscle, which is draped over the upper lid crease. The *Orbital septum* extends 360 degrees from the orbital rim, to fuse with the levator aponeurosis, outer tarsal borders, and

M. N. Naik (✉)
Ophthalmic Plastic Surgery Service, LV Prasad Eye Institute, Hyderabad, India
e-mail: milind@lvpei.org

S. Rath, M. N. Naik (eds.), *Surgery in Thyroid Eye Disease*,
https://doi.org/10.1007/978-981-32-9220-8_17

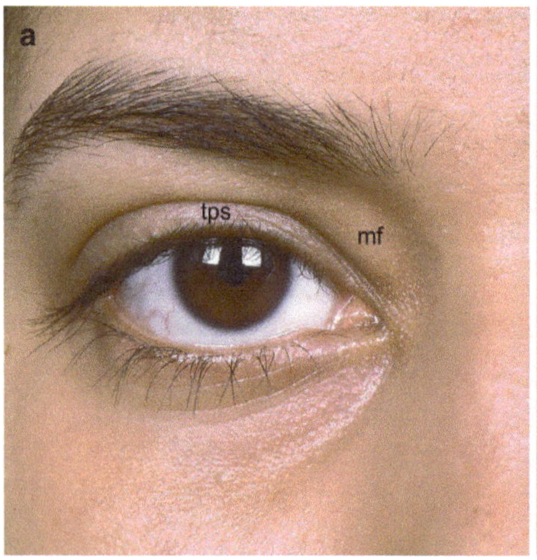

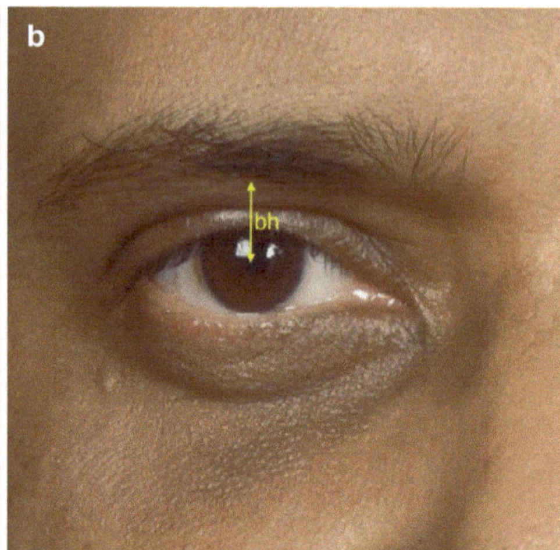

Fig. 17.1 Differences between a female (**a**) and a male (**b**) periorbital region. The female eyebrow arches upward and outward, whereas the male eyebrow is flat, leading to a shorter brow height (bh). In a female, the eyelid crease is higher, leading to a broader tarsal plate show (tps). Medial fat pad (mf) in the upper eyelid is usually a cosmetic concern for the female

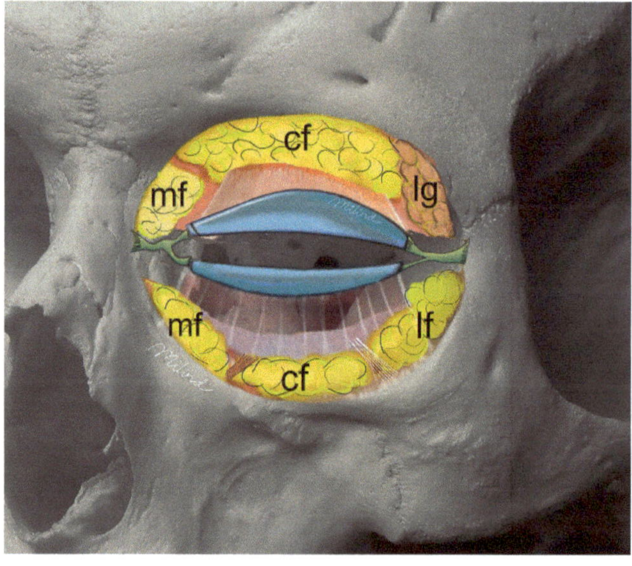

Fig. 17.2 Periorbital fat pads, left orbit. Upper eyelid has two fat pads, central (cf), and medial (mf). The superior oblique tendon separates the two fat pads. Laterally, upper lid has no fat pad since that space is occupied by the lacrimal gland (lg). Lower eyelid has 3 fat pads, medial (mf), central (cf), and lateral (lf). The central and medial fat pads are separated by the inferior oblique muscle. The central and lateral fat pad is separated by lateral raphe, a condensation within the capsulopalpebral fascia

canthal ligaments. The septum is inserted low in oriental eyelid anatomy, and has implications in cosmetic lid surgery [1]. The *Orbital* fat is contained within the orbit by the orbital septum [2]. The upper lid has 2 fat pads (medial and central), with the lacrimal gland occupying the lateral position (Fig. 17.2). The *lower lid crease* is usually 2–3 mm below the medial eyelid margin and 5–6 mm below the lateral eyelid margin [3]. The lower eyelid has three well-defined fat pads, medial, central, and lateral.

The periorbital anatomy in an aging eye and a patient of TED is quite different (Fig. 17.3). The retro-orbicularis oculi fat is increased, often exaggerating the lateral upward arching of the brow. The brow fat span is expanded in TED, and the corrugators are overacting, often leading to prominent dynamic or static glabellar lines (Fig. 17.3).

Negative vector: This concept plays an important role in lower lid treatments. The vector concept defines how far anteriorly the eyeball is placed in relation to the inferior orbital rim (Fig. 17.4). In most patients, a line dropped vertically from the cornea touches the inferior orbital rim. In patients with a negative vector, the inferior orbital rim falls posterior to this line [4]. These patients may be at risk for lower lid retraction or hollowed out appearance post blepharoplasty.

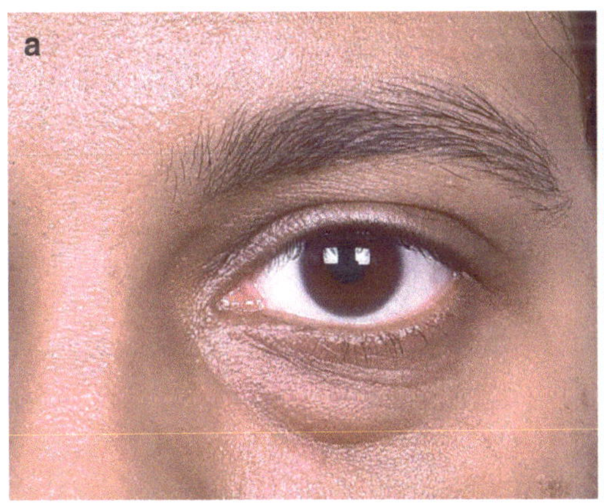

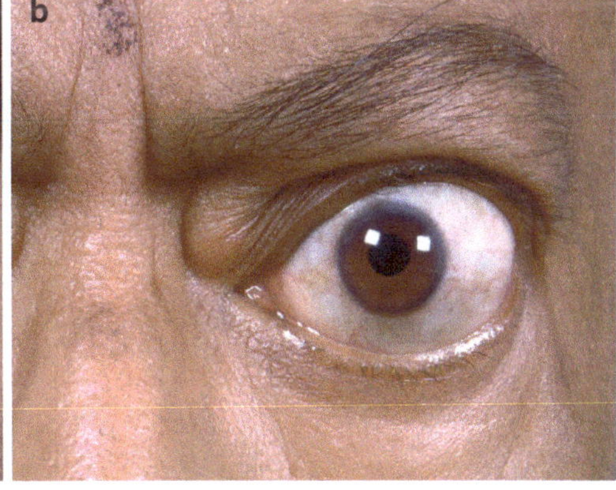

Fig. 17.3 Comparison of periorbital soft tissue changes in aging (**a**) and thyroid eye disease (**b**). Note the normal glabellar region, brow volume loss, and lower eyelid fat bags as seen in aging (**a**). In contrast, note the findings in TED (**b**). Apart from proptosis and eyelid retraction, note the prominent glabellar lines (static and dynamic), brow fat expansion with lateral arching, and prominent medial fat pad in the upper eyelid

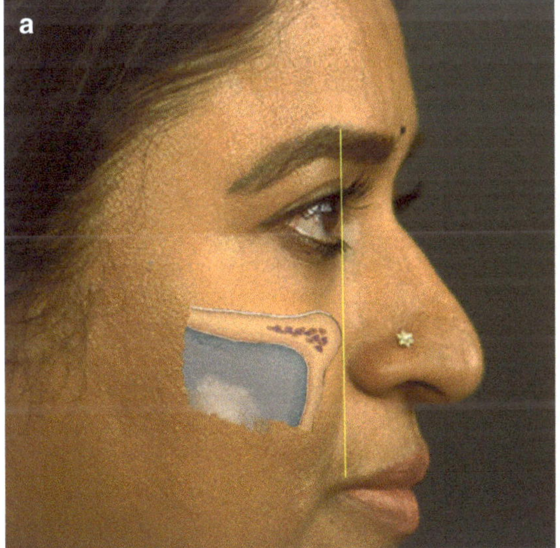

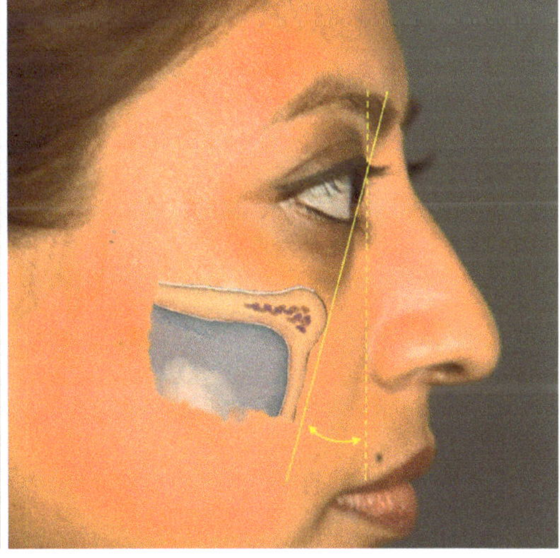

Fig. 17.4 The negative vector. In a normal person, the plane of cornea lies behind or is in line with the plane of the inferior orbital rim (**a**). In patients with a prominent eye (**b**), the corneal plane is placed ahead of the orbital rim (negative vector). The negative vector provides less bony support to the lower eyelid soft tissues, thereby increasing the tendency to scar downward

17.3 Periorbital Changes Specific to TED

Traditionally, the four stages for aesthetic surgical rehabilitation of thyroid eye disease have chronologically focused on proptosis, strabismus, eyelid retraction and lastly excess eyelid fat/skin [5]. Orbital decompression has minimal effect on the anterior periorbital or extraorbital soft tissues (Fig. 17.5). These need special attention for complete cosmetic rehabilitation of a patient affected by TED.

17.3.1 Glabellar Frown Lines

The glabellar muscles corrugator supercilii and procerus are protractors of the upper lid, and they aid the orbicularis oculi in eye closure. They protect the eyes in bright sunlight by medial and downward movement of the eyebrow. They represent muscles of facial expression that are active in anger or perplexity. In TED, the upper eyelid retraction, photophobia, and ocular discomfort act as a stimulus for the contraction of these protractors, thereby inducing an excessive frown response in these patients [6].

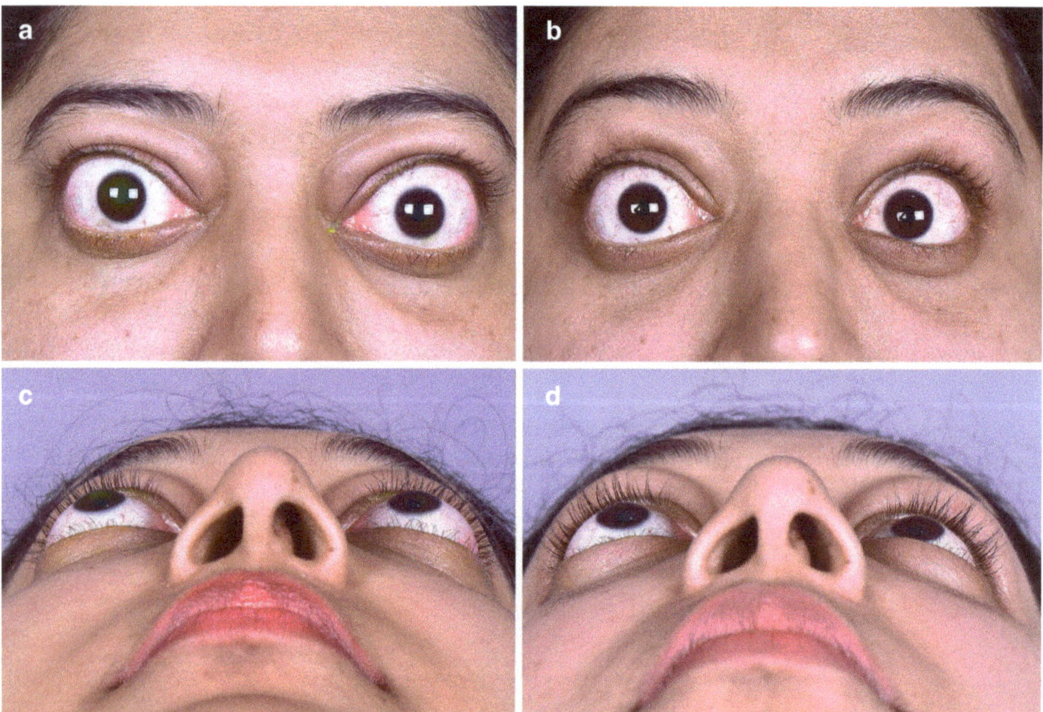

Fig. 17.5 A 26-year-old female with bilateral proptosis, and eyelid retraction (**a**, **c**). Same patient after two-wall balanced orbital decompression showing improvement in exophthalmometry, but no change in pre-septal soft tissue expansion (**b**, **d**)

Relaxing these muscles by injecting appropriate amount of Botulinum toxin can reduce the frown expression, or the angry look in patients with TED [6]. In the glabella, there are typically five injection sites: one at each medial end of the corrugator, one at each lateral end of the corrugator (1 cm above the orbital rim at the mid-pupillary line), and a single injection into the procerus (Fig. 17.6). A dose of 20–30 units for women, and 30–40 units for men is recommended for glabellar frown lines (Fig. 17.7) [7]. The dose can be considerably reduced if the patient wants only a reduction in action rather than complete akinesia. Side effects include brow ptosis and blepharoptosis.

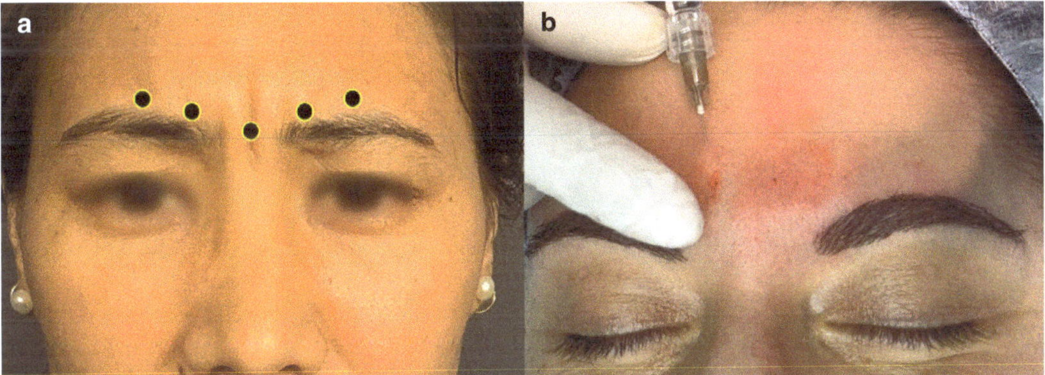

Fig. 17.6 Botulinum toxin type A (Xeomin) 25 units injected at 5 sites for the treatment of glabellar frown lines (**a**). Central point between the eyebrows is for procerus muscle, injected superficially. One point each on either side for lateral part of corrugator, in the mid-pupillary line. One point each on either side, mid-way between the central point and lateral point. Corrugator injections are placed deep, staying above, and beyond the orbital rim. Subdermal hyaluronic acid injection being performed for static glabellar lines (**b**)

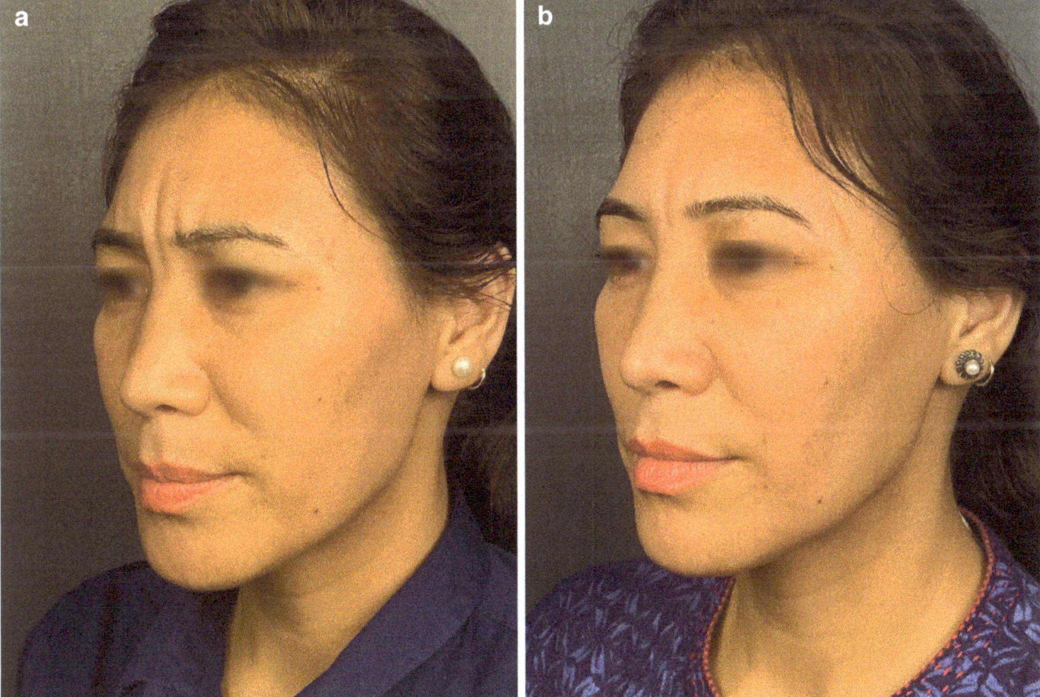

Fig. 17.7 Vertical glabellar frown lines formed by the contraction of the corrugator supercilii muscle (**a**). Significant reduction in the lines following Botulinum toxin injection (**b**)

17.3.2 Brow Fat Expansion

TED affects the upper eyelid/brow complex quite differently as compared to aging changes. It has been shown that the brow fat pads enlarge in TED (Fig. 17.3) [8]. The retro-orbicularis oculi fat and supraorbital contour expands in thyroid eye disease due to enhanced adipogenic potential of eyebrow fibroblasts [9, 10]. It is also reported that aesthetic disfigurement of brow volumetrics can persist even after orbital decompression or correction of eyelid retraction (Fig. 17.5) [11, 12].

17.3.3 Lacrimal Gland Enlargement/ Prolapse

Enlargement of the lacrimal gland is noted in Graves' patients, which can lead to a visible bulge at the lateral third of the upper eyelid that can become prominent in downgaze, or can become more visible after upper blepharoplasty (Fig. 17.8) [13].

Repositioning of the prolapsed lacrimal gland is an added component of upper blepharoplasty in select cases and contributes to improved aesthetics. After skin or skin–muscle excision in an upper blepharoplasty, the septum is opened, and the prolapsed lacrimal gland is identified (Fig. 17.9). The superolateral orbital rim periosteum is exposed, and the gland is fixed to the periosteum with one or two fixation sutures (Fig. 17.10). Following successful fixation, the gland would stay behind the orbital rim, and would not prolapse out with gentle pressure over the eyeball. Lacrimal keyhole, when performed as a part of lateral wall decompression (Chapter 10), provides additional space for the gland to stay within the orbital boundaries.

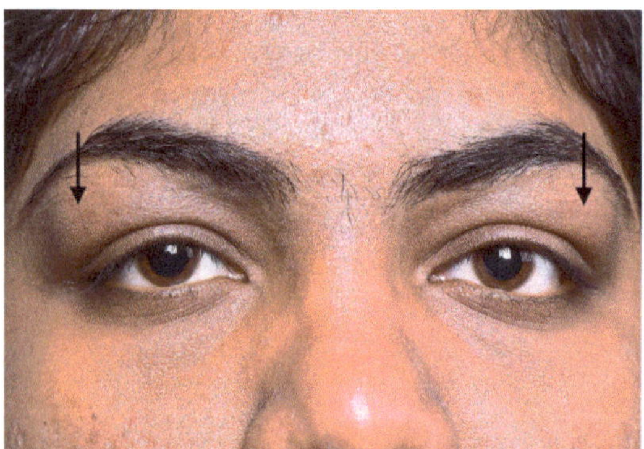

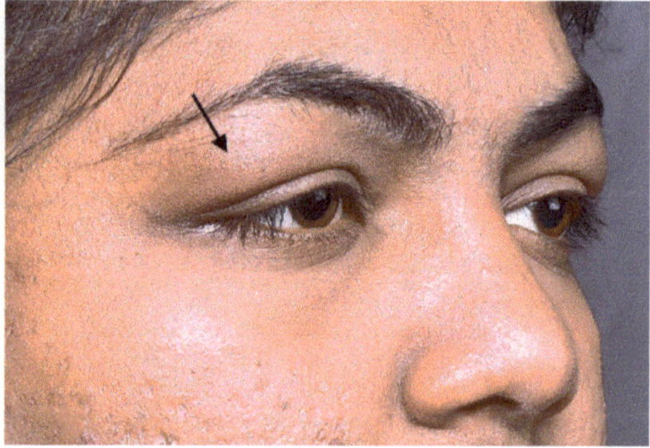

Fig. 17.8 Prominent lacrimal gland (arrow) in a patient with hypothyroidism and mild thyroid eye disease

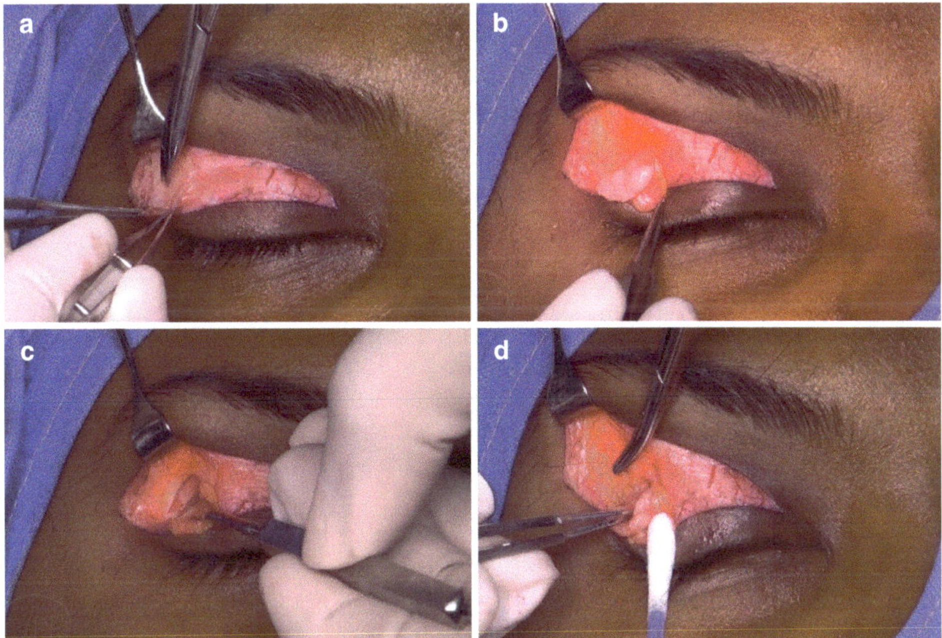

Fig. 17.9 Fixation of a prolapsed lacrimal gland as a part of upper eyelid blepharoplasty. Orbital septum is opened close to the superolateral orbital rim (**a**). Prolapsed lacrimal gland is identified as fibrous pale structure (**b**). Superior orbital rim is exposed (**c**). Vicryl 6-0 suture is passed through the periosteum of the superolateral orbital rim (**d**)

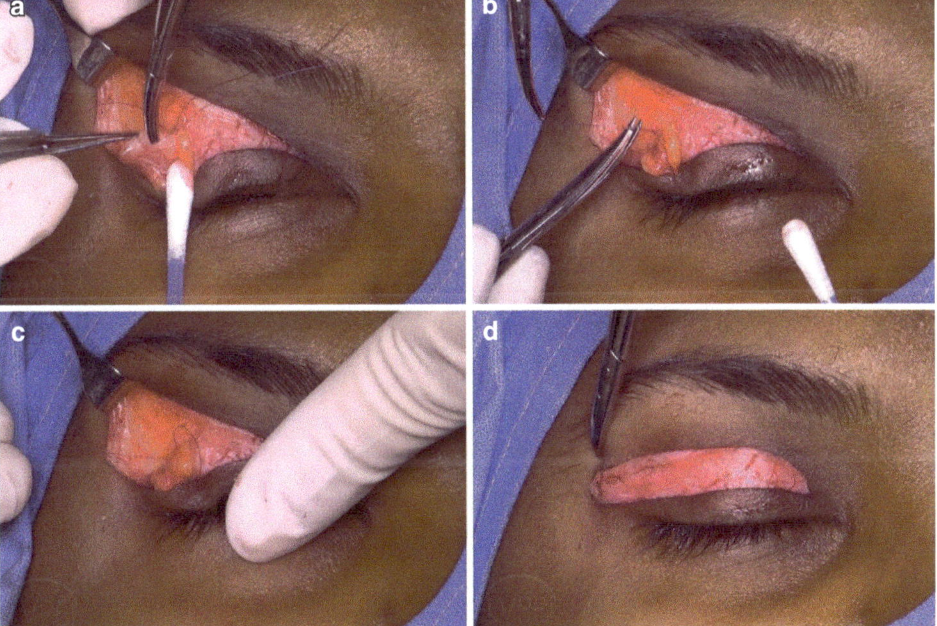

Fig. 17.10 The fascia or outer edge of the prolapsed lacrimal gland is included in the suture bite (**a**), and sutured back to the periosteum (**b**). More than one suture can be placed, to ensure that the gland does not prolapse out even on applying pressure over the globe (**c**). Orbital septum is closed (**d**)

17.3.4 Subconjunctival Fat Prolapse

Orbital fat is located within the intraconal and extraconal space and is contained by Tenon capsule, periorbita, and orbital septum. Tenon capsule envelops the eyeball, from the limbus to the optic nerve. It is pierced by the tendons of the extraocular muscles [14].

Just as the extraconal fat can prolapse causing the well-known eyelid bags, subconjunctival fat herniation is rare but possible spontaneously [15]. Age-related attenuation of Tenon capsule can spontaneously allow intraconal fat to prolapse as a subconjunctival mass [16]. It is possible that raised intraorbital pressure in patients with TED may augment the anterior prolapse of orbital fat [17].

It typically occurs in the lateral canthal area beneath the temporal or superotemporal bulbar conjunctiva as a soft yellowish mass with a convex anterior margin and faint superficial blood vessels (Fig. 17.11). It is usually bilateral, but may also be unilateral.

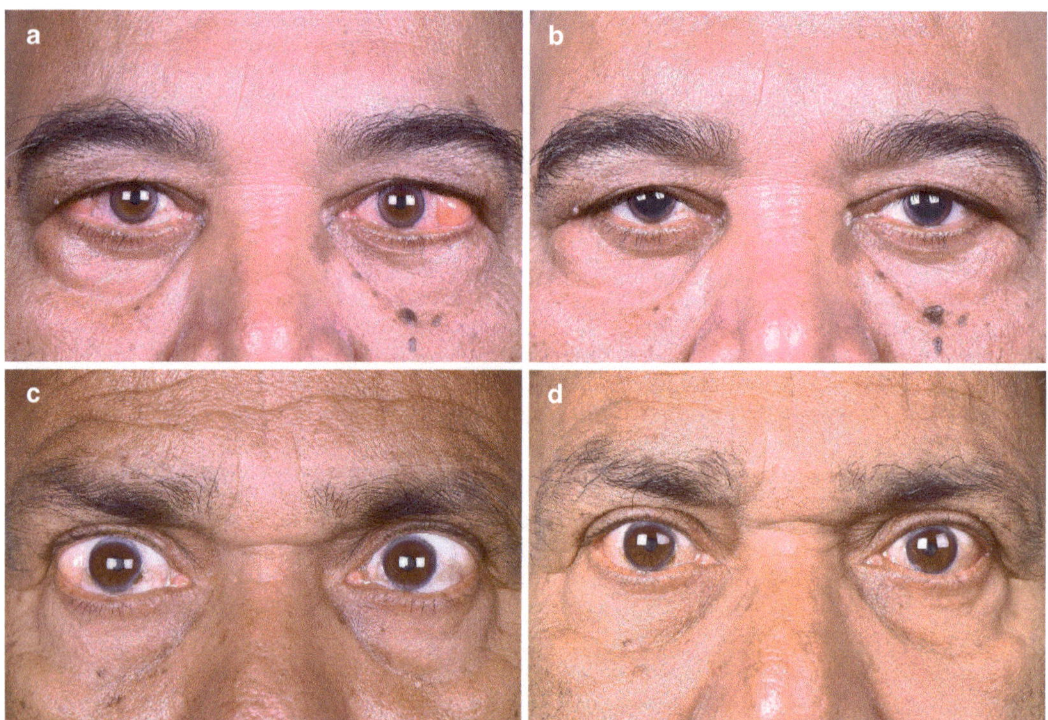

Fig. 17.11 Subconjunctival fat prolapse in patients with thyroid eye disease. Preoperative (**a**, **c**) and post-operative (**b**, **d**) photos following trans-conjunctival fat excision

17.4 Lower Eyelid Hills and Valleys

The soft tissue contour changes around the eye (hollows and elevations) require Fillers or fat where there is a loss of volume, and surgical excision where there is an apparent excess. These can be best understood as either valleys or hills and are applicable to the lower lid aging changes [18]. The valleys in the lower eyelid region that are pertinent in TED are *tear trough* and the *zygomatic hollow*.

17.4.1 Tear Trough (Orbital Rim) Hollow

The tear trough depression is an important feature of eyelid and midface aging. It is defined as the depression of the medial lower eyelid just lateral to the anterior lacrimal crest and limited in its inferior aspect by the inferior orbital rim [18]. This region corresponds anatomically with the location of the lacrimal sac, hence the term "tear trough" (Fig. 17.12).

The Orbital rim hollow corresponds with the location of the orbital rim or orbitomalar ligament. Medially, it is synonymous with the "tear trough." Laterally, it follows the circular contour of the inferior orbital rim (Fig. 17.13). In the mid-pupillary line, overlying the infra-orbital foramen, the orbital rim hollow widens into a triangular pit.

Amongst all the valleys, the *tear trough* (orbital rim hollow) receives the maximum attention with respect to treatment modalities. Hyaluronic acid fillers, and autologous fat transfer are the two commonly employed techniques to fill this valley (Fig. 17.14). Several commercial preparations of Hyaluronic acid fillers are available, along with recommendations for use [19]. In the majority of cases, filling is required in the medial half (medial to the mid-pupillary line). One of the widely discussed and grave complication of filler injection is "blindness" caused by retrograde migration of the filler particles, thereby causing central retinal artery occlusion [20]. It is important for ophthalmologists to be aware of this complication.

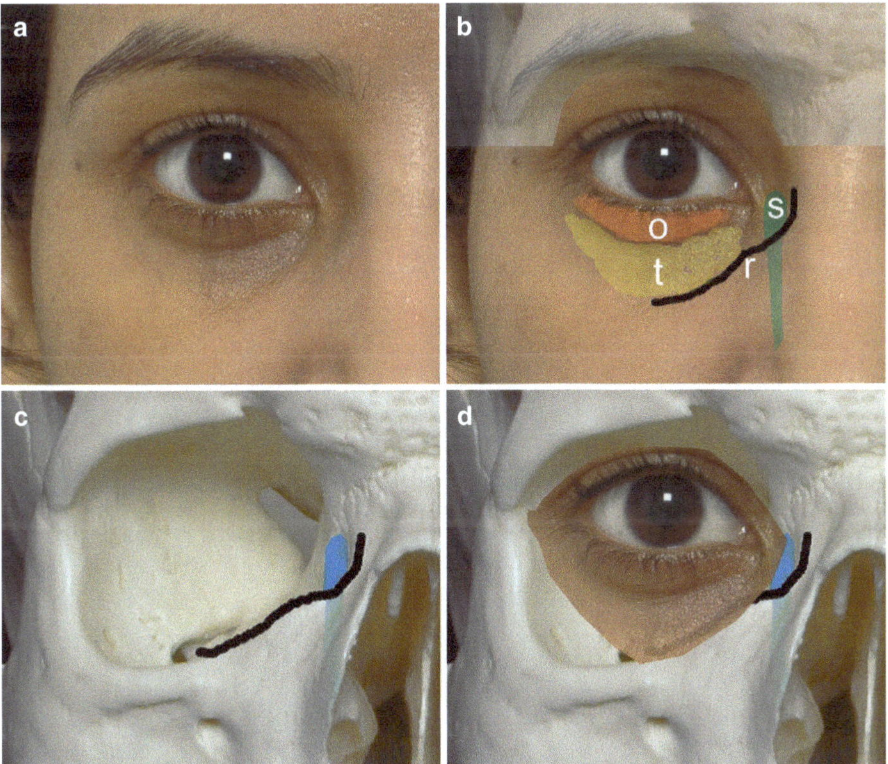

Fig. 17.12 The right eye demonstrating the Hills and Valleys around the eye (**a**). Note the orbicularis roll (o) and the tear trough (t) in relation to the inferomedial orbital rim (r) in image (**b**). The lacrimal sac (s) lies medially (**c, d**), continuing below the orbital rim as the nasolacrimal duct. The "tear trough" therefore does not lie over the orbital rim (**c**), but often lateral and superior to it (**d**)

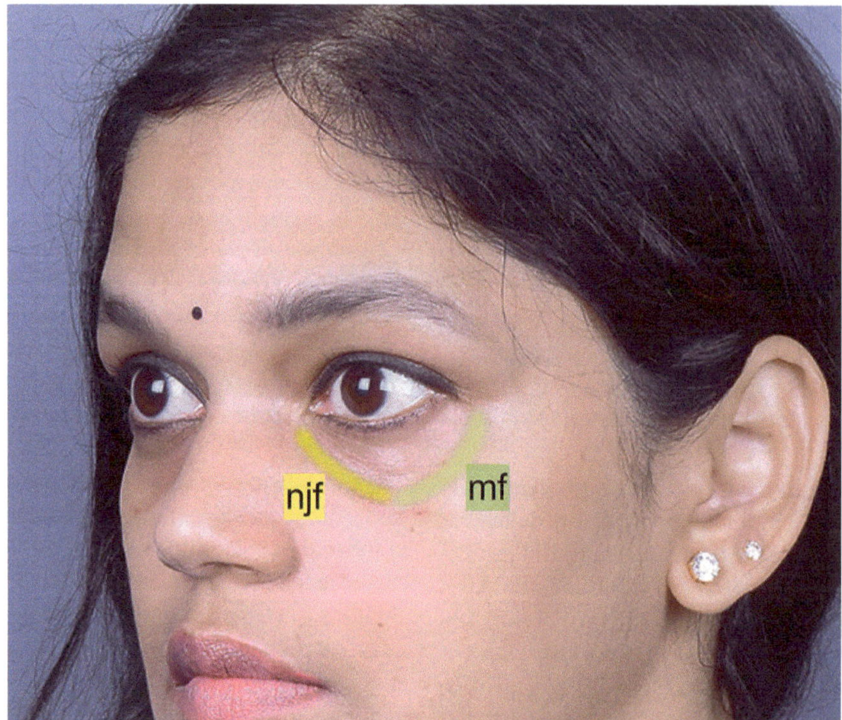

Fig. 17.13 The lower eyelid merges with the skin of the cheek, with no specific demarcation in youth. The nasojugal fold (njf) runs from the medial canthus along the orbital rim, and the malar fold (mf) runs from lateral canthus along the orbital rim. These two valleys deepen with age, giving a tired or hollowed look

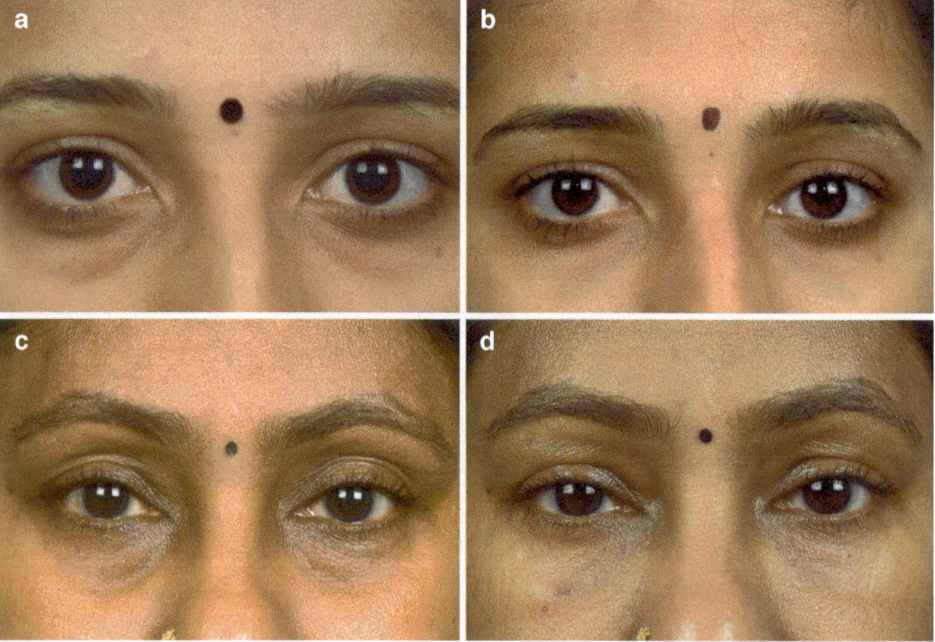

Fig. 17.14 Tear troughs are under-eye hollows that can make a person look old or tired (**a**, **c**). Hyaluronic acid filler (Belotero Balance) was used in these cases, to fill the hollow (**b**, **d**). Note the improvement in the apparent pigmentation caused by shadowing effect

17.4.2 The Zygomatic Hollow

It corresponds to the location of the orbitozygomatic ligament (Fig. 17.15). It lies along the origin of the levator labii superioris and zygomatic muscles. The zygomatic hollow is bound by the triangular malar fullness above and by the lateral cheek fat below [18].

The *Zygomatic hollow* receives attention with respect to the filling of the malar volume loss. Filling the zygomatic hollow along with the tear trough restores the malar volume and thereby the malar prominence.

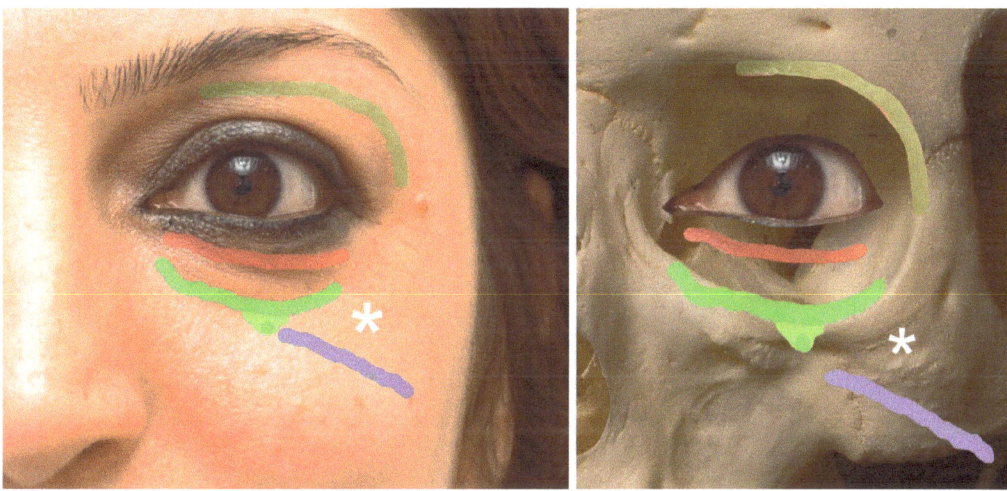

Fig. 17.15 The left eye demonstrating the three periorbital hollows. The red line marks the eyelid crease hollow that divides the orbicularis roll (above) and fat bag (below). The green line marks the orbital rim hollow. Medially it represents the tear trough. Note the widened triangular pit along the mid-pupillary line. The orbital rim hollow marks the lower limit of fat bag. Orbital rim hollow can sometimes be visible along the superior orbital rim. The violet line represents the zygomatic hollow, which extends inferolaterally from the mid-point of orbital rim hollow. The triangular area between the lateral half of the orbital rim hollow and the zygomatic hollow is termed as the triangular malar mound (asterisk)

17.5 The Hills

17.5.1 Orbital Fat Prolapse

This could be considered as the commonest lower lid "hill" that presents to the ophthalmologist or cosmetician. Orbital fat prolapse is bound superiorly by the septal confluence hollow, and inferiorly by the orbital rim hollow [18]. The fat mound is often compartmentalized by the inferior oblique and the arcuate expansion into a central, medial, and lateral fat pad (Fig. 17.16). The fat actually lies in a deeper plane, behind the orbital septum. This orbital fat is the same anterior extraconal fat that is encountered during orbital decompression surgery. In moderate to severe cases of TED, orbital decompression alone makes this fat less prominent anteriorly. In milder cases of TED, this orbital fat requires conservative fat removal or repositioning [21].

17.5.2 Fluid Bags

Several configurations of fluid retention can happen in the periorbital region in a patient with TED. These include pre-malar swelling, fluid festoons, and triangular malar mound (Fig. 17.17). *Pre-malar* or *cheek swelling* has been reported as a subtle under-diagnosed entity in patients with TED [22]. *Fluid festoons* within the lower eyelid can very much mimic fat bags, as they often occupy the same anatomic location, and are often bound by the inferior orbital rim. The swelling, however, is in the plane of the subcutaneous tissue, and has distinct differences from a fat bag (Fig. 17.16). The *triangular malar mound* or malar festoon is a fluid bag located inferolateral to the orbital rim [18]. It is bound above by the orbital rim hollow, and below by the zygomatic hollow (Fig. 17.17d). Prominent triangular malar mounds often run in families and can be variable, but are also found in patients with thyroid disorder due to the increased fluid retention in this region.

While pre-malar fluid is associated with hyperthyroidism and higher chances of dysthyroid optic neuropathy [22], the others simply represent areas of fluid retention, and are difficult to treat. A blepharoplasty is ineffective in a fluid bag, and in fact can worsen it due to disruption of the lymphatics. When using hyaluronic acid fillers for the orbital rim hollow, patients with triangular malar mounds should be preferably avoided, since the gel can imbibe more fluid, and look unnatural.

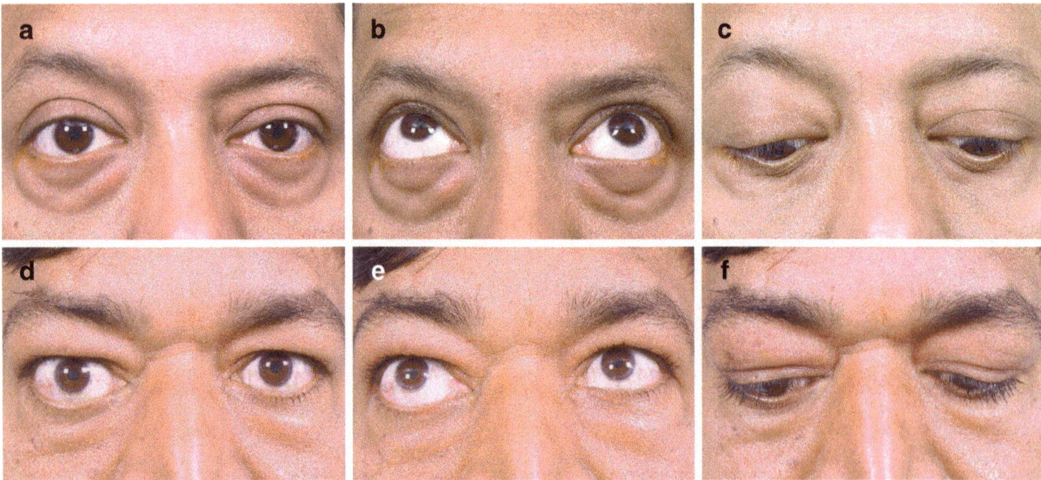

Fig. 17.16 Differentiating lower eyelid fat bags (**a–c**) from fluid bags (**d-f**). Note the compartmentalization of the fat bags (**a**), increase in upgaze (**b**), and decrease in downgaze (**c**). Fat bags are bound inferiorly by orbital rim hollow. In comparison, fluid bags are not compartmentalized, and do not change much with gaze. Its borders are indistinct and may not always be restricted by orbital rim hollow

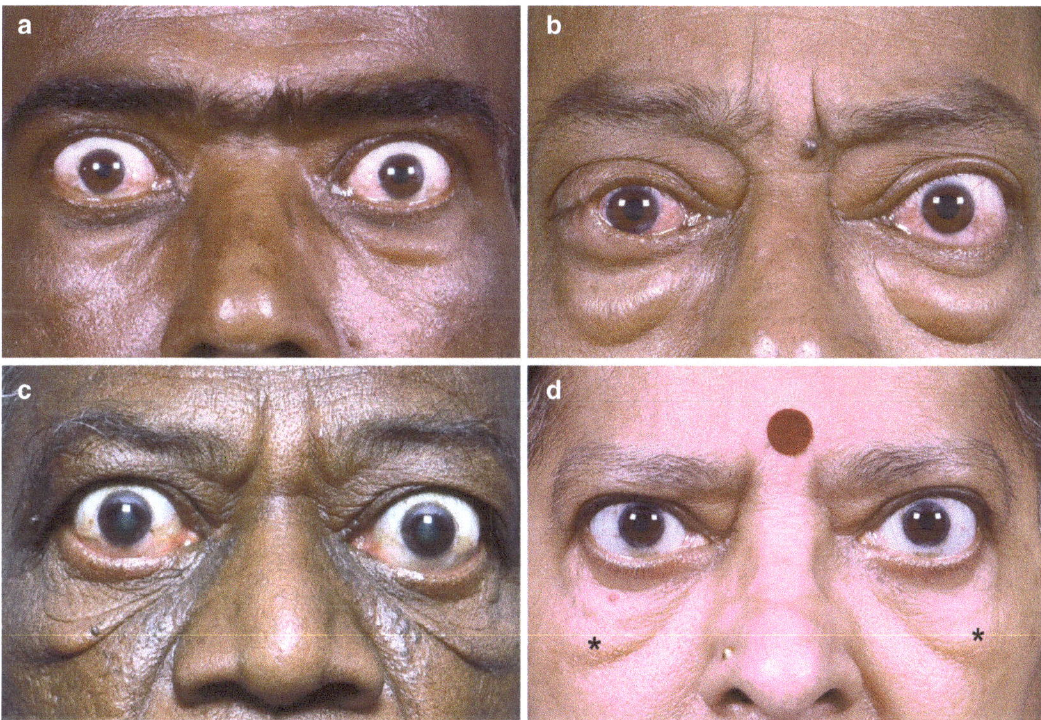

Fig. 17.17 Right pre-malar edema (**a**), active fluid festoon (**b**), chronic partially collapsed fluid festoon (**c**) and triangular malar mound shown with asterisk (**d**) in patients with thyroid eye disease

17.5.3 Upper Eyelid Blepharoplasty

In the setting of TED, upper eyelid blepharoplasty primarily involves the removal of excess overhanging skin, pre-aponeurotic fat, and/or retro orbicularis oculi fat (ROOF). Although this has been traditionally described to be the last step in the surgical paradigm [5], recent literature suggests simultaneous corrections considering the aesthetic impact of surgery on patients with TED [23, 24].

Assessment of photographs prior to the occurrence of TED is important to restore the appearance. Blepharoplasty may be performed under local or general anesthesia depending upon the surgical plan, patient and surgeon preference and need for concomitant operations like correction of lid retraction, or orbital decompression. The eyelid step can often be performed under local anesthesia in the same sitting, before the patient is induced for orbital decompression. The author believes that TED patients often have a low pain threshold, and hence IV sedation or general anesthesia is preferable.

Although it is recommended that a minimum 20 mm of vertical upper lid skin should be preserved in a blepharoplasty surgery for normal eye closure, in patients with TED with residual prominence of the eye, more skin can be left to avoid lagophthalmos and resultant exposure.

The excess skin is removed, via a classic blepharoplasty incision. Other *modifications* during an upper blepharoplasty in a patient with TED include fat sculpting, recession of levator, lateral canthal resuspension, and fixation of prolapsed lacrimal gland (Figs. 17.18 and 17.19). Excess of retro-septal fat and retro-orbicularis oculi fat (ROOF) may be safely excised through the incision. Gentle pressure on the patient's globe can make the orbital fat more prominent while the patient is in a recumbent position. Overall, under-correction is preferred to prevent hollowing.

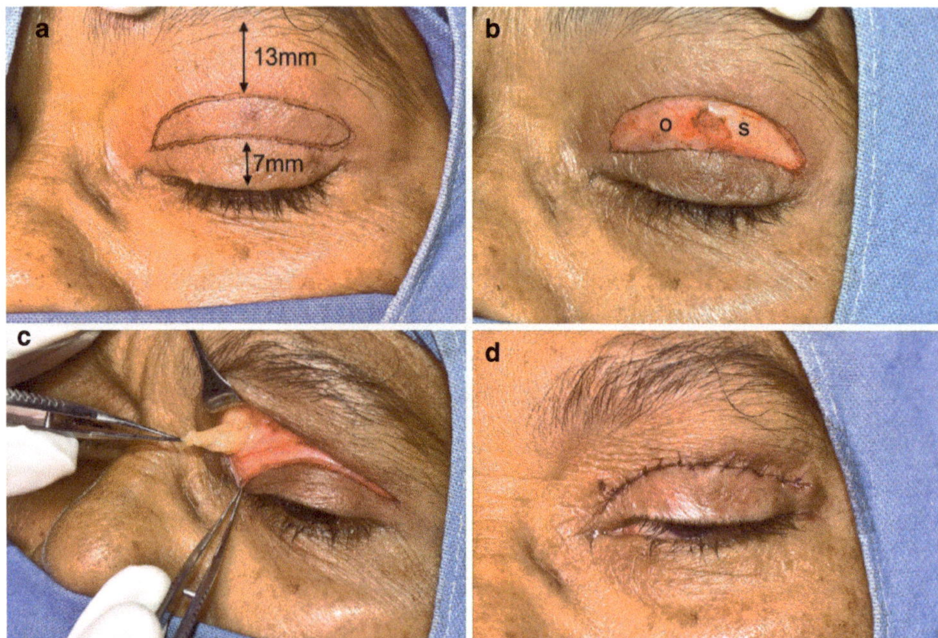

Fig. 17.18 Upper eyelid blepharoplasty. The eyelid crease is marked 7–8 mm from the lashline, and another incision 13 mm from the brow (**a**). The incision is made with Radiofrequency monopolar cautery (**a**). Medially, it converges towards the medial canthus, whereas laterally it stays parallel to the eyelid margin. Medial half, the orbicularis (o) is preserved, whereas in the lateral half, it is removed to expose the septum (s) (**b**). Medial fat can be excised if excess (**c**). Wound is closed with interrupted 6-0 vicryl sutures (**d**)

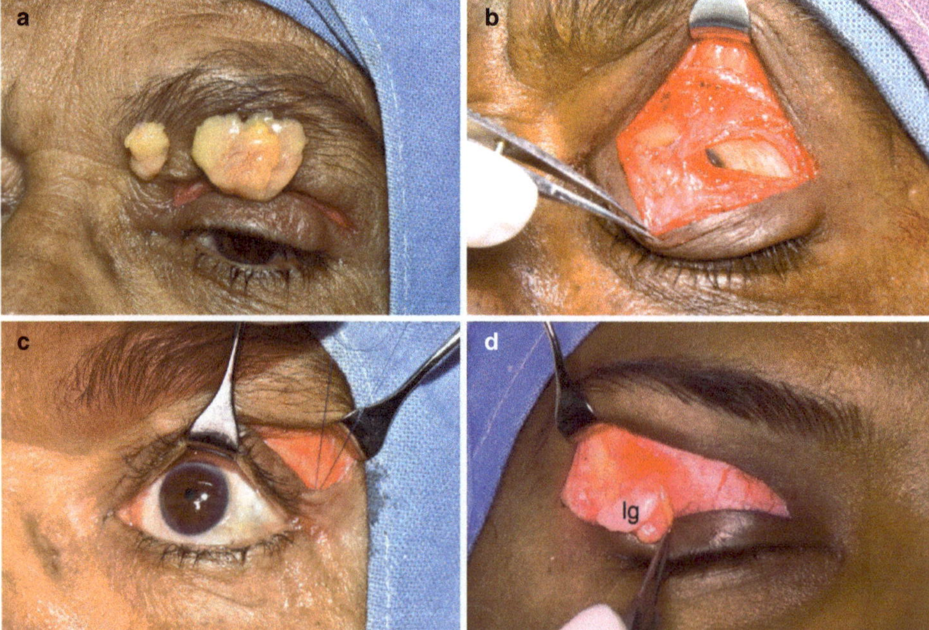

Fig. 17.19 Modifications that may be done during upper lid blepharoplasty. Excess fat can be removed, even from central fat pad (**a**). Levator muscle recession for eyelid retraction (**b**). A minimally invasive lateral canthal resuspension can be done to raise the lateral canthus by fixing it to the periosteum of the lateral orbital rim (**c**). In cases of lacrimal gland prolapse, the gland (lg) is identified and fixed within the bony orbital rim (**d**)

17.5.4 Lower Eyelid Blepharoplasty

A number of aesthetic changes in the lower eyelid can be apparent, such as skin laxity, orbital fat prolapse (eyelid bags), canthal laxity, and fluid bags or malar festoons.

Fat bags should be differentiated from fluid festoons, since the management is entirely different (Fig. 17.16). Mild cases of TED with predominantly fat space expansion may be concerned about their lower lid bags (Fig. 17.20). Such cases can be treated with a Blepharoplasty, rather than a decompression. Most orbital surgeons who deal with TED today have developed a customized aesthetic approach to surgery in which the specific anatomic problems are identified and the operation is individualized to address these problems [24].

There are two principal surgical approaches to a lower lid blepharoplasty: transcutaneous and transconjunctival. The transconjunctival approach is preferred in young patients. It leaves no external scar and reduces the chance of eyelid retraction, scleral show, and post-operative ectropion than other methods [25, 26]. The transcutaneous approach is preferred if there is excess skin that requires excision [27]. Aesthetic refinements in a prominent eye have several intricacies, and it is important to understand these as most patients with TED seek cosmetic rehabilitation to restore their looks [28].

For transconjunctival lower lid blepharoplasty, the inferior fornix, eyelid skin, and lateral canthus are anesthetized with 1% lidocaine containing 1:100,000 epinephrine (Figs. 17.21 and 17.22). Surgery is performed through an infratarsal palpebral conjunctival incision with a radiofrequency monopolar cautery or CO_2 laser. Gentle pressure on the eyeball prolapses the fat compartments and aids in the identification of the medial, central, and lateral fat pads. Conservative

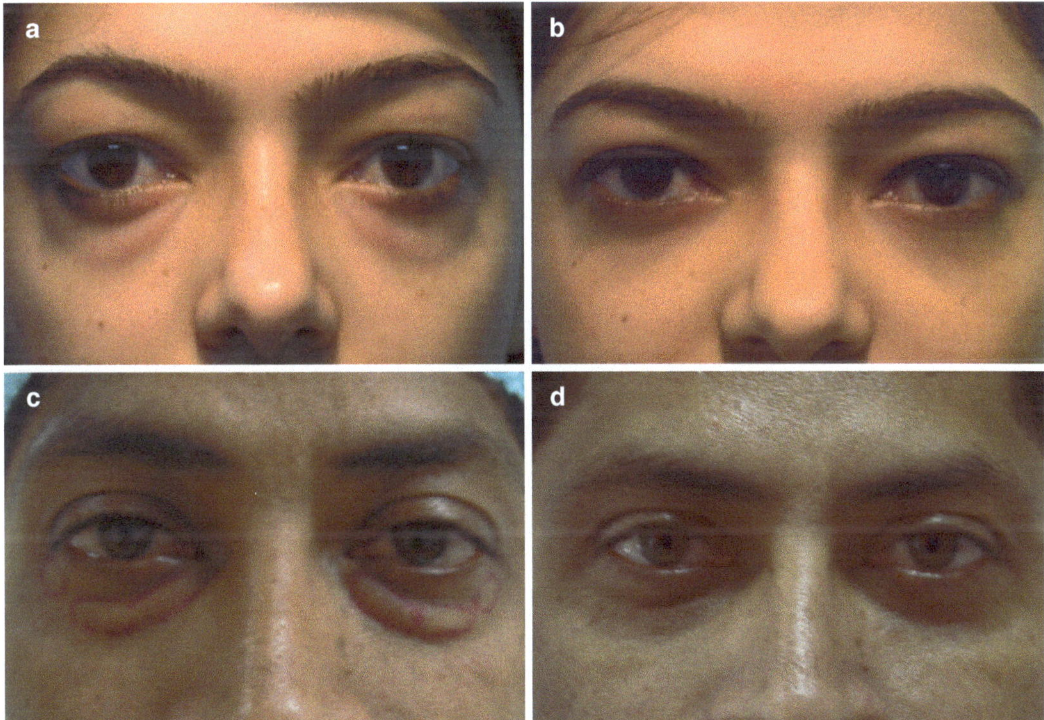

Fig. 17.20 Preoperative (**a**, **c**) and post-operative (**b**, **d**) photographs following transconjunctival lower eyelid blepharoplasty with conservative fat excision. No external scar, no conjunctival sutures, and no scarring of the orbital septum are the advantages of the transconjunctival approach

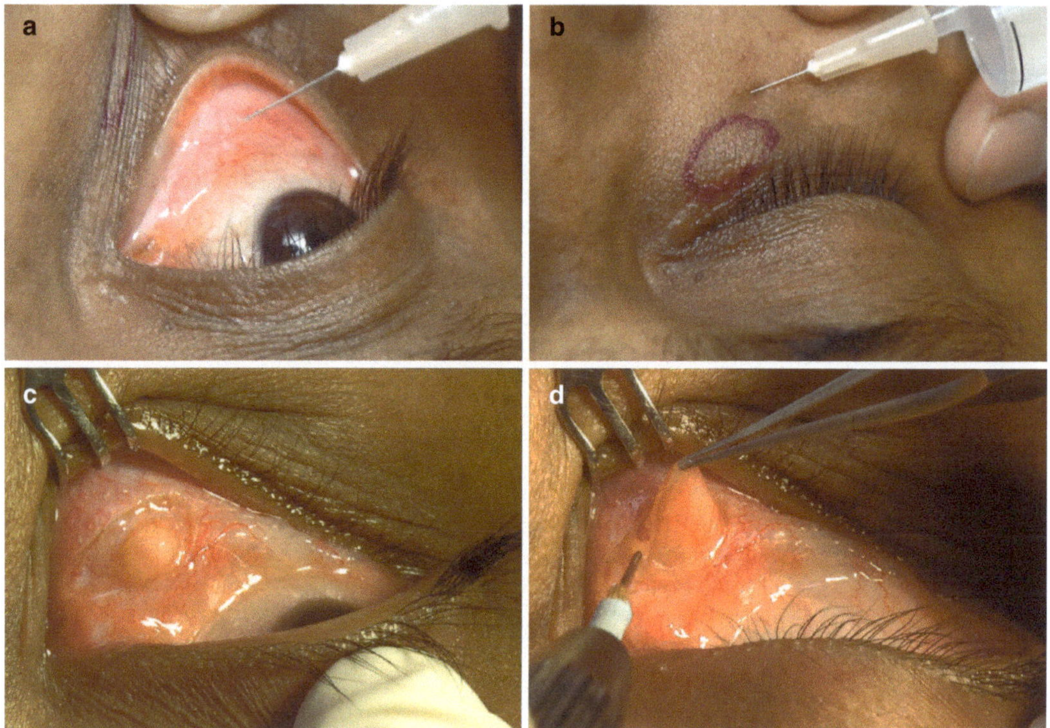

Fig. 17.21 Transconjunctival blepharoplasty (Surgeon's view). Injection of local anesthetic into the inferior conjunctival fornix (**a**) and infraorbital nerve block (**b**). Stab incision over palpebral conjunctiva to expose orbital fat (**c**). The fat is covered in layers of septae that need to be incised to release the fat (**d**)

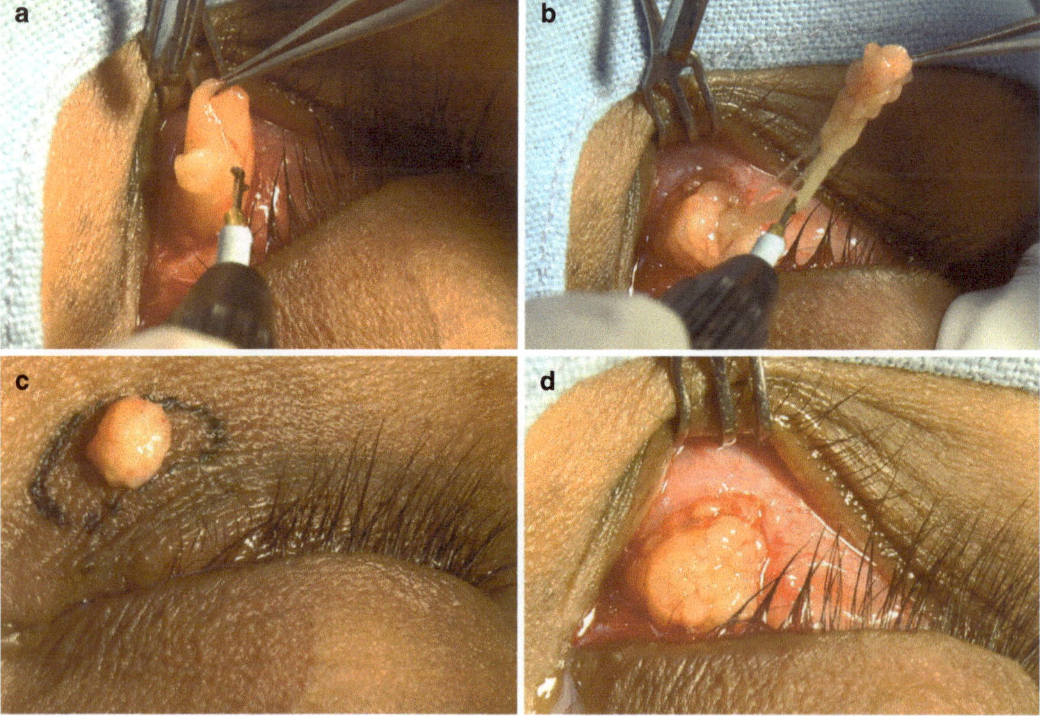

Fig. 17.22 Transconjunctival blepharoplasty *continued*. Once the fat prolapses, it is excised piecemeal (**a**, **b**) while checking the amount of fat removed and the changes in the contour (**c**). Fat prolapsing beyond the orbital rim can be excised (**d**)

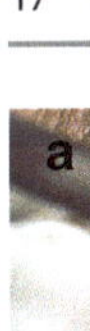
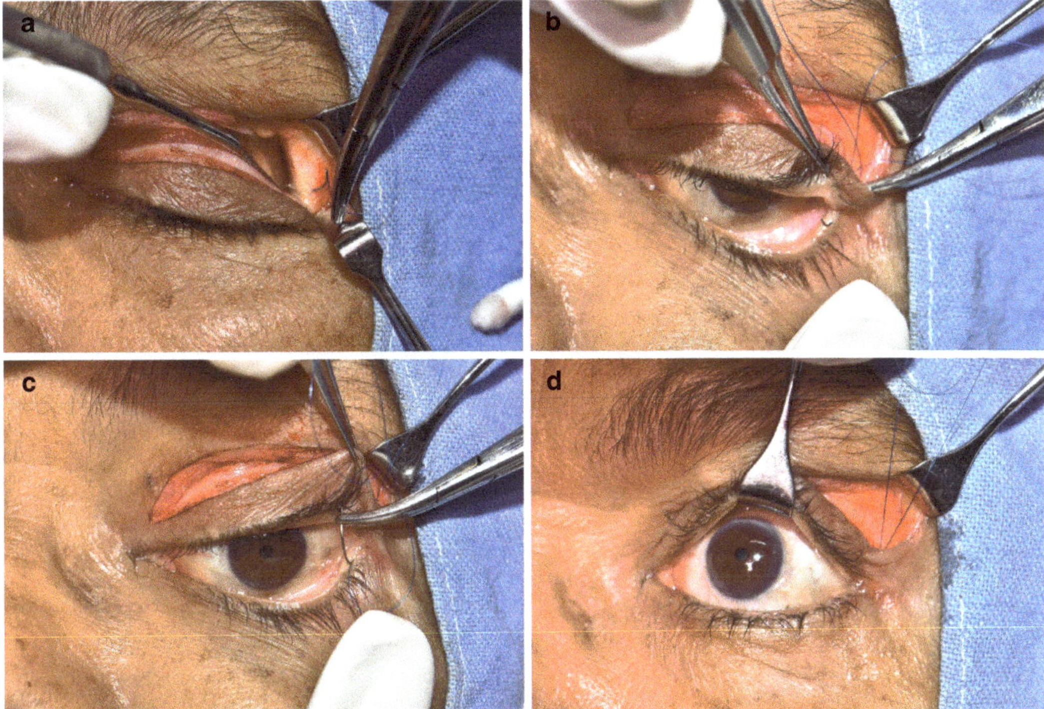

Fig. 17.23 Minimally invasive lateral canthal resuspension that can be performed through a Blepharoplasty or a superolateral eyelid crease stab incision. Superolateral orbital rim is exposed and 6-0 Prolene suture is passed through the periosteum just above the lateral canthal position (**a**). Same needle is passed in the sub-orbicularis plane to bring it out through the lateral-most meibomian gland orifice of the lower lid (**b**). The needle is entered back through the same opening, taking a slightly different route to hitch a part of lateral tarsus (**c**). The suture is again passed through the superolateral periosteum, and tied to achieve horizontal eyelid tightening (**d**). The same effect as that of a lateral tarsal strip is achieved, with minimal dissection

fat removal is achieved. The trans-conjunctival incision is left to heal by epithelization without any sutures. Excellent aesthetic outcome is achieved in most cases (Fig. 17.20). Lateral canthoplasty if performed along with lower eyelid blepharoplasty, should be done with caution in patients with a negative vector as it could increase the inferior scleral show (Fig. 17.23) [28].

Transcutaneous lower lid blepharoplasty is chosen when excess skin or orbicularis needs to be excised along with the prolapsed fat.

The more aggressive "skin-muscle flap" method is also approached through a subciliary incision, undermining the skin, and orbicularis. Dissection can be continued along the orbital septum to the level of the orbital rim. Periorbital fat is approached through small incisions in the septum. Orbicularis muscle fibers and skin can be excised at closure however, damage to the orbicularis may lead to lower lid malposition and orbicularis denervation.

17.6 Conclusion

Aesthetic rehabilitation of thyroid orbitopathy is extremely relevant to the affected patients, especially because the disease is common in young and middle-aged females. Despite adequate focus on orbital decompression and eyelid retraction surgery in the past, the attention to other soft tissue aesthetic concerns has only gained importance in recent times.

Awareness of facial aesthetic changes other than proptosis and eyelid retraction is the need of the hour. Established treatments for these concerns can be combined with orbital decompression whenever possible. Although these can be looked at in a sequential manner as the classic surgical paradigm in TED, patients would be surely pleased if we take them into consideration and address them along with the classic surgeries like decompression and eyelid retraction surgery.

References

1. Bosniak SL, Zilkha MC. Cosmetic blepharoplasty and facial rejuvenation. Philadelphia: Lippincott-Raven; 1999.
2. Castanares S. Blepharoplasty for herniated intraorbital fat; anatomical basis for a new approach. Plast Reconstr Surg. 1946;8(1):46.
3. Codner MA, Kikkawa DO, Korn BS, Pacella SJ. Blepharoplasty and brow lift. Plast Reconstr Surg. 2010;126(1):1e–7e.
4. Jelks GW, Jelks EB. The influence of orbital and eyelid anatomy on the palpebral aperture. Clin Plast Surg. 1991;18(1):183–95.
5. Shorr N, Seiff SR. The four stages of surgical rehabilitation of the patient with dysthyroid ophthalmopathy. Ophthalmology. 1986;93:476–83.
6. Olver JM. Botulinum toxin A treatment of overactive corrugator supercilii in thyroid eye disease. Br J Ophthalmol. 1998;82(5):528–33.
7. Carruthers J, Fagien S, Matarasso SL. Botox consensus group. Consensus recommendations on the use of botulinum toxin type a in facial aesthetics. Plast Reconstr Surg. 2004;114(6 Suppl):1S–22S.
8. Goldberger S, Sarraf D, Bernstein JM, Hurwitz JJ. Involvement of the eyebrow fat pad in Graves' orbitopathy. Ophthalmic Plast Reconstr Surg. 1994;10(2):80–6.
9. Hwang CJ, Khadavi NM, Papageorgiou K, et al. Histopathology of brow fat in thyroid-associated orbitopathy. Ophthalmic Plast Reconstr Surg. 2012;28(1):27–9.
10. Thornton IL, Clark J, Sokol JA, Hite M, Nunery WR. Radiographic evidence of prominent retro and suborbicularis oculi fat in thyroid-associated orbitopathy. Orbit. 2016;35(1):35–8.
11. Papageorgiou KI, Ang M, Chang SH, Kohn J, Martinez S, Goldberg RA. Aesthetic considerations in upper eyelid retraction surgery. Ophthalmic Plast Reconstr Surg. 2012;28(6):419–23.
12. Papageorgiou KI, Hwang CJ, Chang SH, Jarullazada I, Chokron Garneau H, Ang MJ, King AJ, Mancini R, Douglas RS, Goldberg RA. Thyroid-associated periorbitopathy: eyebrow fat and soft tissue expansion in patients with thyroid-associated orbitopathy. Arch Ophthalmol. 2012;130(3):319–28.
13. Harris MA, Realini T, Hogg JP, Sivak-Callcott JA. CT dimensions of the lacrimal gland in graves orbitopathy. Ophthalmic Plast Reconstr Surg. 2012;28(1):69–72.
14. Koorneef L. New insights in the human orbital connective tissue. Result of a new anatomic approach. Arch Ophthalmol. 1977;95(7):1269–73.
15. Jordan DR, Tse DT. Herniated orbital fat. Can J Ophthalmol. 1987;22(3):173–7.
16. Stangos AN, Hamédani M. Spontaneous subconjunctival orbital fat prolapse: presentation of four cases. Klin Monatsbl Augenheilkd. 2006;223(5):415–7.
17. Chang E, Wilson MW, Smith ME. Orbital imaging in thyroid eye disease. In: Dutton JJ, Haik BG, editors. Thyroid eye disease. New York: Marcel Dekker; 2002. p. 303.
18. Naik MN. Hills and valleys: understanding the undereye. J Cutan Aesthet Surg. 2016;9:61–4.
19. Matarasso S, Carruthers J, Jewell ML, Restylane Consensus Group. Consensus recommendations for soft-tissue augmentation with nonanimal stabilized hyaluronic acid (Restylane). Plast Reconstr Surg. 2006;117(3 Suppl):3S–34S. discussion 35S–43S
20. Beleznay K, Carruthers JDA, Humphrey S, Carruthers A, Jones D. Update on avoiding and treating blindness from fillers: a recent review of the world literature. Aesthet Surg J. 2019;39(6):662–74.
21. Naik M. Blepharoplasty and periorbital surgical rejuvenation. Indian J Dermatol Venereol Leprol. 2013;79:41–51.
22. Kim BJ, Kazim M. Prominent premalar and cheek swelling: a sign of thyroid-associated orbitopathy. Ophthalmic Plast Reconstr Surg. 2006;22(6):457–60.
23. Bernardini FP, Skippen B, Zambelli A, Riesco B, Devoto MH. Simultaneous aesthetic eyelid surgery and orbital decompression for rehabilitation of thyroid eye disease: the one-stage approach. Aesthet Surg J. 2018;38(10):1052–61.

24. Douglas RS. Commentary on: simultaneous aesthetic eyelid surgery and orbital decompression for rehabilitation of thyroid eye disease: the one-stage approach. Aesthet Surg J. 2018;38(10):1062–4.
25. Rizk SS, Matarasso A. Lower eyelid blepharoplasty: analysis of indications and the treatment of 100 patients. Plast Reconstr Surg. 2003;111:1299–306. discussion 1307–8
26. Zarem HA, Resnick JI. Minimizing deformity in lower blepharoplasty. The transconjunctival approach. Clin Plast Surg. 1993;20:317–21.
27. Adamson PA, Strecker HD. Transcutaneous lower blepharoplasty. Facial Plast Surg. 1996;12:171–83.
28. Richter DF, Schwaiger N, Wiedner M. Aesthetic refinements in patients with prominent eyes. Facial Plast Surg. 2015;31(6):633–44.

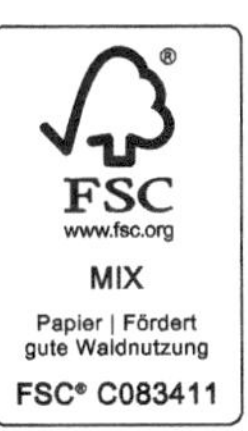

Zeitfracht Medien GmbH
Ferdinand-Jühlke-Straße 7
99095 Erfurt, Deutschland
produktsicherheit@kolibri360.de